W9-BUO-990

HAMILTON HALL, M.D., F.R.C.S. (C), is an internationally respected orthopaedic surgeon, best known for his specialty in back ailments. He is on staff of Women's College Hospital and the Orthopaedic and Arthritic Hospital in Toronto. In 1974, he founded the Canadian Back Institute and is currently director of this growing organization. He is a popular lecturer around the world, so popular, in fact, that when he delivered a public lecture at the Ontario Science Centre, the crowds caused a traffic jam in the streets.

Dr. Hall's first book, *The Back Doctor*, was published in hardcover in 1980 in Canada, the U.S., the U.K., and Australia. It went into ten editions in six countries, in four languages, and was a Canadian bestseller in paperback. His second book, *More Advice from the Back Doctor*, was also a number-one national bestseller.

Dr. Hall currently lives and works in Toronto.

HAMILTON HALL M.D.

More Advice From The Back Doctor

M&S

An M&S Paperback from
McClelland & Stewart Inc.
The Canadian Publishers

An M&S Paperback from McClelland & Stewart Inc.

First printing January 1989
Trade paperback edition 1988
Cloth edition 1987

Reprinted 1992, 1994

Canadian Cataloguing in Publication Data

Hall, Hamilton, 1938 –
More advice from the back doctor

(M&S paperbacks)
Includes index.
ISBN 0-7710-3769-4

1. Back – Care and hygiene.   2. Backache.
I. Title.
RD768.H36   1989   617′.56   C88-094737-3

Cover photo by Peter Paterson
Anatomical illustrations © Margot Mackay, ANSCAD, BSc, AAM
Other illustrations © Peter Honor

Printed and bound in Canada

This book is not intended to replace the services of a physician. Any
application of the recommendations set forth in the following pages is
at the reader's discretion and sole risk.

McClelland & Stewart Inc.
The Canadian Publishers
481 University Avenue
Toronto, Ontario
M5G 2E9

Contents

INTRODUCTION

Eight years ago, I set out to write my first book, *The Back Doctor*, realizing there were countless numbers of people out there who needed information to help them overcome back pain. I expected to reach a lot of them, but I never dreamed my message would travel virtually around the world.

I got the first inkling of the book's wide acceptance when publishers in Britain and Australia joined with those in Canada and the United States to produce the initial editions. Next, other publishers translated my words into French, Hebrew, and Dutch (in The Netherlands I am now proud to be known as De Rugdokter).

But the most delightful evidence of a world-girdling interest in my message came to me in a personal letter. The writer was Dr. Jay Keystone, an acquaintance of mine during our days as resident physicians in Toronto. Since my field was orthopedic surgery and Jay's was tropical medicine, our differing schedules set us on diverging paths. Over the years I lost touch with him and had no idea that he'd developed a bad back. All that changed in 1983, when I received his one-page letter from Hyderabad, India. Jay explained he was on a sabbatical studying leprosy and was writing in haste to describe an experience he felt was just too good to keep to himself. His letter went on:

Yesterday I was invited to meet an octogenarian Anglo-Indian retired school principal who lives not far from my hotel. She was the friend of a missionary and also of the British physician under whom I am studying in Hyderabad.

I was taken to the back of a rather run-down school where several small hotel-like rooms were located. Here, we found a little old Indian lady whose mental faculties were very well preserved. She sat in a darkened room, surrounded by her belongings, which were rather meager.

After a round of tea and biscuits the conversation turned to my painful back, which has worsened as a consequence of riding along bumpy roads in three-wheeled "auto-rickshaws." I could hardly believe my eyes when from under a pile of dust-covered books she pulled out a copy of *The Back Doctor*. I am now reading your book, which I was unable to find at several Toronto book stores because they ran out of stock!

By the time I sat down to begin this sequel, I was convinced not only that I had found a huge audience for my message but also that there was no shortage of fresh material of potentially wide interest. It's true that when friends and patients heard I was working on a second book, many wanted to know, "What could you possibly write that isn't already in your first book?" But for every reader who evidently regarded *The Back Doctor* as *the* complete book of its kind, there was another who told me, "The things you wrote were helpful, but I wish you'd said more about such-and-such."

And so, as well as introducing new topics, I have responded to many requests for information on subjects I dealt with only fleetingly in *The Back Doctor*.

Patients faced with the prospect of back surgery wanted more information on the nature of their operations and additional tips on the art of post-operative recovery. I have obliged. Other readers wanted me to elaborate on neck pain, a common complaint that deserves the full discussion found here. A number of people were concerned about the effects of back pain on sexual relations and pregnancy, and many were hesitant to broach the subject with their doctors. I have tried to address their concerns. Our knowledge of the chronic pain syndrome – a sadly misunderstood behavioral disease that too often afflicts back patients – has advanced so remarkably that I felt it would be useful to describe the condition in detail. And so, in thinking through the scope of the new book, I assigned each of these subjects a chapter of its own.

I also felt an obligation to respond to increasing concern over two widely discussed conditions that create back pain: osteoporosis, a sometimes troublesome aspect of the aging process; and spinal stenosis, about which surgeons have learned much since publication of *The Back Doctor*. (In fact, spinal stenosis has emerged as such a significant problem in my practice that I have revised my classification of the causes of common backache to include it as Type Four.)

The very nature of this demand for information suggested a format for the new book: why not assemble all the questions patients kept asking me, add a few questions I sometimes wish they *would* ask, and then provide my answers? Although I did not foresee what a comfortable choice it would prove to be, the more I worked with this question-and-answer approach, the better I liked it. It lends itself readily to the informal, conversational style that I favor when working with my patients. And I hope readers will feel, as I do, that it has enabled me to put across much useful information, including some fairly technical concepts, in a clear and meaningful way.

One additional point of style: like many other writers these days, I wish there were a singular pronoun in English, equivalent to "he" or "she," to refer to a person of either sex. I got around the problem in most cases by using such neutral words as "you" and "the patient." In a few instances, I resorted, reluctantly, to the clumsy he-or-she construction. But where those alternatives weren't workable, I simply said "he" – trusting my readers to realize that, where the context allowed, the one pronoun was intended to mean either a male or a female.

I must confess that the prospect of writing a second book presented several opportunities I found attractive for personal reasons. It would provide a chance to convey my enthusiasm for technological advances that represent good news for patients and doctors alike. (I am as enthusiastic about an emerging diagnostic tool called magnetic resonance imaging as I was about the invaluable CT scan when I wrote *The Back Doctor*.) A second book would enable me, as well, to bring readers up to date on my evolving concepts of back care, such as my increased appreciation for the therapeutic value of extension exercises. And it could serve as a platform from which to express my growing concern over the way personal injury lawsuits are discouraging some back patients from getting well.

In a new book I could also report the latest findings and developments at the Canadian Back Institute. This last possibility proved to be even more timely than I anticipated. While this book was going through the writing process, the Institute went through an exciting new stage in its evolution. The CBI had a modest beginning in 1974, as a series of informal lectures intended to help small groups of my own patients with their back problems. In its first metamorphosis, it developed into the Canadian Back Education Units, with branches in several Canadian provinces and U.S. states and an outpost in Perth, Australia.

Even after it adopted its present name and embarked on several research projects, the institute for several years remained essentially an educational organization. Then, less than two years ago, to fill the gap between the treatment it recommended and the treatment most patients received, the CBI broadened its scope significantly to become a comprehensive center for education, assessment, treatment, and training, employing modern techniques of non-invasive therapy while conducting research into the value of specific exercises for the various types of back pain. In the course of its research, the CBI, at last count, had studied and analyzed the problems and progress of more than 15,000 victims of common backache.

Now, encouraged by the favorable response of patients within reach of its charter headquarters, the new-style CBI is expanding to other locations, with every expectation of becoming a continent-wide operation by the early 1990s.

From the moment I first considered writing a second book, I realized that its fundamental message would have to be identical to that of *The Back Doctor*. After all, although my approach to back problems continues to evolve, my basic beliefs remain unchanged. In fact, CBI studies have now confirmed opinions I adopted years ago as simple, self-evident truths: that the more you know about your back, the better able you are to care for it, and that taking the responsibility for your own recovery helps guarantee a good result. I make no apology for restating these and other essential principles, but I have tried to present my ideas in a fresh and timely fashion, to reinforce what readers of *The Back Doctor* already know, while providing the essential information to others.

With the publication of my first book, some people formed the erroneous opinion that in prescribing exercises for the relief of back pain, I favored quite a different approach than that of my good friend Robin McKenzie. A physical therapist from New Zealand, Robin has worked with unfailing energy to demonstrate the value of a therapy program tailored to the patient's specific requirements. And more than any other person I am aware of, Robin has been instrumental in re-establishing the importance of extension exercising – an achievement I am happy to acknowledge. After reading this sequel, anyone familiar with Robin McKenzie's work should realize that there never has been any professional conflict between us.

Only time and my readers' responses will tell whether I have succeeded in creating the book I intended. If I have, some of the credit must certainly go to several individuals.

I am indebted to Tony Melles, senior physiotherapist and director of the Canadian Back Institute, and to the rest of its staff, whose contributions to the development of the CBI exercise program are reflected extensively in this book.

My discussion of the chronic pain syndrome owes much to the special expertise of Allan Walton, Dr. Rickey Miller, and Dr. David Corey, whose diligent work in this previously neglected area of human psychology continues to shed welcome light on a difficult problem.

The section on osteoporosis was prepared with the generous help of Dr. William Sturtridge, whose knowledge and experience as a specialist in metabolic bone disease and whose ability to speak intelligibly to a surgical confrere form a rare and invaluable combination.

Without the perseverance and gentle pressure of Hal Tennant, this book would never have been written. I welcome this opportunity to declare publicly how much I have learned from our long association about the vicissitudes of the English language and the subtleties of the writer's art. Hal has become more than a genial collaborator; he is a valued friend.

I am delighted that Peter Honor agreed to illustrate this text. I have used his pictures in my talks for years, to rave reviews. I always remember hearing from a doctor in California who wrote asking not for a copy of a speech I had delivered there but for copies of the cartoons I'd used!

A word of thanks to the Colberts, Nancy, Stanley, and David, whose expert guidance and sound advice have done so much to enlighten me on the ways of the publishing world.

Finally, I acknowledge the help and support of Ellen Seligman. As my current editor and my former back patient, she holds a unique perspective. Her professional insight and personal empathy have touched every chapter of this book.

Hamilton Hall, M.D., F.R.C.S. (C)
Toronto
November 1986

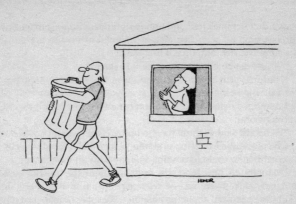

1. HAVE YOU HUGGED YOUR GARBAGE CAN TODAY?

No matter how many doctors or therapists you may see, or how many treatments or operations you may have, the basic responsibility for your back and its care rests with you.

You have a choice. You can allow your back to rule your life by influencing your every decision, however big or small. Or you can devise a strategy for taking charge, so that *you*, not your back pain, will determine how you live and what you do with your life.

Once you have resolved to take control, the trick is to pursue your strategy with single-minded determination – yet not allow it to become an obsession. The distinction between the two is not that hard to make if your intentions are clear and honest and your strategy is sound.

I can think of two patients whose attitudes readily illustrate the difference. One patient was a woman in her late forties who had been coming to me with a back problem for years. Originally an active person, she had developed the unfortunate habit of dwelling constantly on her back pain. As an ardent traveler, for instance, she would dramatize her suffering by hiring ambulances to take her to and from airports.

On one of her visits to me, I conducted my routine tests and found that her back had undergone significant improvement since the last time I'd seen her. But, as inclined as ever to accentuate the negative, she didn't see it that way.

"What are you doing these days?" I asked.

"Nothing," she said. "I've even given up grocery shopping. I can't lift the heavy bags."

I asked why she didn't have someone else carry her groceries out to her car.

"Well," she said, "I'd still have to unload them when I got home."

Of course she could have gotten help from a family member or neighbor or could have unpacked the bags an item at a time.

I'd forgotten how fond this woman was of the Yes-But game, and how skilled she was at rejecting any positive thought that might be expressed about her condition. Despite my many attempts to provide her with reassurance and constructive advice, she had remained determined to dwell on her problem and defy anyone to help her get better. I realized there was no point in making more suggestions; there is little a doctor can do or say when a person refuses to be helped.

Apart from back pain, her determination was about the only thing that woman had in common with another patient whose experience was related to me by a colleague. At the age of twenty-three, in a careless plunge into the shallow end of a swimming pool, Richard crushed three vertebrae in the thoracic, or middle, section of his spine. Fortunately there was no damage to the spinal cord.

After a short stay in the hospital, he visited several doctors, each of whom told him the same thing: although the fractures had created an obvious and painful bump on his back, there was nothing anyone could do for him. He simply had to get on with his life as best he could.

Unemployed, Richard went looking for work – *any* kind of work. But prospective employers turned him down, time and again, because of his back. Fed up with rejection, he got into an exercise program and began strengthening the uninjured parts of his back, so that they could take the load and ease the strain on those deformed vertebrae. After several months he got to the point where he could control the discomfort – but he still couldn't land a job.

Finally, he went into yet another job interview – with a new tactic: when he was asked whether he had any medical problems, he lied. He declared that his health was perfect. He never mentioned his back. The company hired him and sent him for a routine physical check-up. Since the slight deformity from the old fractures was still visible, he feared the jig was up. But in the examining room, Richard struck up a conversation about fitness and exercise and got the doctor so engrossed that the man never did get around to looking at Richard's back. Richard passed the medical, started work, and is now considered a valuable employee.

While I can't condone his lie, Richard's attitude offers a refreshing contrast to the Yes-But responses I heard from the other patient, and clearly illustrates the important part that positive thinking can play in overcoming even the most serious back problem.

You have often said publicly that roughly four out of five people in this part of the world will suffer from common backache at some time in their lives. Does that mean back pain is inevitable for most people?

Not at all. A great many people could avoid some or all of that pain if they practiced certain exercises regularly and adopted better habits in the course of their daily living.

Are you saying that most people abuse their backs without realizing it?

They do, in the sense that they place unnecessary strain on their spines, either without realizing it or at least without knowing how to avoid it. In their everyday activities, most people constantly subject their backs to many minor loads. These strains, combined with the natural wear and tear of aging, lead to back pain.

When the spine ages, the small joints connecting the vertebrae lose their smooth lining, and the roughened surfaces rub together. The discs become less resilient and bulge out between the bones, sometimes pressing on a nerve. Any of these conditions can produce severe, even excruciating, pain. In its early stages, however, this wear and tear is so gradual that most people are unaware of it. Then, one day, a person may unwittingly place a little more stress on the back than those worn parts of the spine can handle –

an unaccustomed twist of the trunk, for instance, or an attempt at an unusually heavy lift – and the result is a sort of "last straw" effect. That's when your spine will send you a clear message – in the form of a sudden attack of pain.

And I suppose the worse the wear has been up to that moment, the more painful the attack will be.

Oddly enough, that's not so. The amount of pain often has little relationship to the seriousness of the problem. You can suffer a lot of pain from a back condition that is in fact just a minor sprain on a vertebral joint, just as you can feel a great deal of pain from whacking your funnybone without actually damaging your arm.

At the other end of the scale, I've seen serious conditions, such as sustained pressure on a nerve, causing muscle weakness, that produced very little pain.

But you say people could avoid many of those painful attacks by adopting better living habits.

Certainly. The ways you stand, walk, sit, lie down, sleep, work, play, and go about all the other routine things you do every day, control how much load your spine must endure and whether a worn joint or disc will suddenly produce new pain.

And that's what you're referring to when you talk about having a strategy against backache. Can you suggest a standard set of rules?

I don't believe in uniform rules for everyone, because something that works well for one person may not work for another. It's better to develop an individual strategy based on a few general principles.

What are the general principles of good back care?

Apart from proper exercise and ordinary common sense about the things you expect your back to do, the one basic principle I like to cite is summed up in a phrase that was popular in the 1960s: "If it feels good, do it." If some position you use in standing or sitting or working makes your back feel good, it's the right position for you. It certainly won't cause trouble, and it probably reduces the load on your back.

Is the opposite true? If some activity hurts your back, is it harming your spine?

Probably not harming, in the sense of causing damage. It may hurt a little, or even a lot, because it's aggravating a sore spot, but it's unlikely to be causing physical injury. When you feel pain, your back isn't necessarily saying, "This is damaging me." More likely, it's saying, "Look out! You're making me do something I don't want to do." Even if you were in perfect condition, you'd get a similar message from various parts of your body if you ran the Boston Marathon or swam the English Channel. Tender though it may be, your back is far too tough to be harmed – that is, damaged – by a little extra exertion.

There may be times when you will consider it worthwhile to ignore that message from your spine and put up with a little extra pain to get on with your daily work or to carry on with some activity you particularly enjoy, like golfing. Or making love.

Of course there will be a great many more occasions when you will want to avoid pain because there is nothing to be gained by putting up with it and there's a lot to be gained by adopting the habits that make your back feel good.

That brings me to a more specific question: my back hurts when I wake up in the morning. Do you think I need a better mattress?

Possibly but not necessarily. The most important consideration is your sleeping position. I'd suggest sleeping on your back with a fat pillow under your knees, or on your side with your legs tucked up and a large pillow between your thighs. Experiment. Any position that makes you comfortable and prevents your back from aching in the morning is a good position for you.

What about sleeping on my stomach?

Generally speaking, you are better off not sleeping on your stomach. When you do, your back arches, squeezing the spinal joints together and often causing pain. However, if you've always found that position comfortable and it's the only way you can get a decent night's sleep, then it would be foolish to change. I'd suggest, though, that you try putting a thin pillow under your pelvis. This will modify the arch in your back and reduce the pressure on the small joints.

But don't a lot of people fall asleep in one position and wake up in another? And maybe sleep in a lot of other positions between times? I know I do.

Of course. And it can be one of those situations where you're damned if you do and damned if you don't. It's true that during sleep you may assume certain positions that will aggravate a bad back. On the other hand, a certain amount of shifting around is good for you. Sleeping in the same position for hours at a time may lead to temporary but painful stiffness of the joints in the morning.

If you make a point of it, you can train yourself to assume or avoid almost any position – just as we all train ourselves, from early childhood, not to fall out of bed while we're sleeping.

What if I sleep in my most comfortable position and still wake up with back pain?

In that case, your mattress could be to blame. If it sags, or is resting on a sagging base, it's probably not providing the support you need.

How much support does my back need? Should I consider putting a board under the mattress?

The right amount of firmness is a matter of personal preference. If a mattress feels right when you lie on it and lets you turn over without difficulty or discomfort, it's right for you. If you have a sleeping partner who is much heavier than you are, you might be more comfortable with an extra-firm mattress or one constructed with individual-acting coils to prevent a "trough" that keeps you sliding downhill.

As for the old board-under-the-mattress idea, that's passé – a relic of the time before the modern box-spring was in common use, when mattresses were generally supported on a sagging link-spring base. A board on a good box-spring won't make much difference, and if you put a board on top of the mattress, why bother with a mattress at all? You might as well just sleep on the board – or on the bare floor.

Would it be a good idea to switch to a waterbed?

A waterbed, particularly a heated one, is designed to help you relax and avoid the restlessness you were talking about a minute ago. Many people find a waterbed helpful since it provides full, contour support for the spine and reduces movement during sleep. Others say it makes their backs feel worse. I suspect that's because they change position so infrequently that their back joints become stiff. And so, again, it's a matter of individual choice. Rather than make the purchase and risk disappointment, why not try one out for a few nights? You may find a waterbed store that offers a money-back trial, or if you're planning a trip, you could look for a hotel or motel that has waterbeds. Or maybe you can stay with a friend who owns one.

What about lying in a hammock?

If you have back pain, I'd suggest limiting your time in a hammock to a couple of hours. Otherwise, you're likely to have trouble, for two reasons. First, it's impossible to lie in a hammock and maintain the normal curvature in your low back; there is no uniform support. And second, a hammock doesn't allow you to move around to avoid continuous pressure on the same part of your spine. If you try to roll over, the hammock rolls with you. That's the great appeal: the swaying action offers a sort of return-to-the-womb feeling. But it's hard on your back.

Sometimes in the morning my neck, especially, seems stiff. Would a special pillow help?

It's certainly worth a try. Your neck has a particular problem whenever you sleep on your side: with your head on the pillow and your shoulder on the mattress, your neck is often tilted to one side. Worse still, it is suspended, unsupported, like a clothesline between its two end poles. Naturally, it sags, and that increases the pressure on one side of the cervical spine. Attempts to avoid that sag have given rise to the design of special cervical pillows to ease the pressure on the neck. One popular type is known as the butterfly pillow because of its shape. You lie with your neck over the "body" of the butterfly, and as long as you remain that way, the "wings" on each side provide the stability you need to keep your head in the right position.

Other pillows, more elegant, are designed in shapes based on biomechanical studies, but their purpose is the same as that of the butterfly. Some of these give you support for the head as well as for the neck. Others are designed so that you can roll over.

Like everything else, these pillows have their enthusiasts and their detractors. In some cases, even the designers admit their pillows will seem uncomfortable at first. And this raises another point: some of these items are expensive, as pillows go, and only you can decide whether they're worth the money.

If waterbeds and special pillows are sometimes helpful at night, what about using various supports and aids during the day?

Back supports, foot-rests, and various other devices can provide temporary relief from back pain – and I'm all for that. But it's important to realize these aids are *passive* ways of achieving temporary relief, not substitutes for an active program of regular back care and exercise.

I saw someone with a portable folding foot-rest. What do you think of carrying something like that?

The principle is fine, although personally I wouldn't bother with one of those gadgets. They're like many safety devices that sound great in theory but seldom get used. However, if you like the idea of a portable foot-rest, and you're willing to spend the money on it, there's no reason why you shouldn't own one. But I've always been willing to take my chances on finding a low rail or step – whatever's handy.

What about posture? Are there certain habits you should adopt?

Yes, there are. You should begin by recognizing that your spine has a natural, moderate curvature that doesn't take kindly to extremes. Your back isn't comfortable when it's ramrod straight or when that natural contour is exaggerated.

Then how *would* you describe the best posture for standing?

Try to position your body directly under your head and neck. In an easy and relaxed manner settle your head in line with your shoulders, then gently tuck in your buttocks to tilt the top of your pelvis backward and reduce any excess curve in your lower spine. The effect should be one of standing up straight without strain. To further avoid discomfort while standing, change your position frequently to vary the pressure on all parts of your back.

From gym class I remember a posture called the "monkey slump," which relaxed our backs. Would that achieve the same thing?

No, the posture I am suggesting will leave you in no danger of being mistaken for an ape in the zoo. By all means do yourself a favor once in a while by standing in a slump for a few minutes, with your head and shoulders well forward and your arms dangling down. You'll find that stance relaxing because it stretches out the muscles in the upper back and reduces any excess curve in the lower spine. But it's not good as a regular form of posture. Besides looking silly, it creates a whole new pattern of increased load on the spine.

With proper posture, you're relaxing without actually slumping. You'll know, from the feeling of comfort, when you've got it right – especially if you have Type One back pain, which originates from pressure on worn joints. If you are overweight, you probably have a tendency to arch your back too much, and the strain-free posture will help relieve your pain.

Another elementary technique to reduce an excessive curve in your low back is to avoid standing for any length of time with both feet flat on the floor. Whenever possible, get one foot up onto a step or a stool. Of course, you will find yourself in situations where this kind of relief is not to be found, such as at a cocktail party where all the chairs have been moved out, and everybody has to stand around, flatfooted.

Department-store shopping can be painful, too. Most stores provide little seating and no foot rails. But there is usually some solution if you look hard enough. For example, if you take the escalators, not the elevator, you can stand on one step and rest one foot on the step above.

I was going to suggest supermarkets as a bad place, too, but at least you can rest one foot on the lower shelf of your shopping cart.

That's right. And while you're pushing the cart, you can lean over and take some of your upper body weight on your arms. As I mentioned earlier, varying your posture usually gives your back some relief.

Art galleries are difficult places for back sufferers. Typically they offer no place to sit down and nothing but miles of level floor, except for a staircase here and there. Most other indoor exhibitions and fairs can be just as difficult.

Now that you mention it, I realize that's probably why my back hurts whenever I have to stand around a long time waiting for a bus. Maybe I should try using the curb as a foot-rest.

That's not a bad idea if there's no danger from the traffic. Standing with one foot on your lunch box or briefcase is one good strategy. Even leaning against a building or a lamp-post will often help a little.

Yes. I've already discovered that, especially if I'm carrying a heavy package I don't want to put down. Are there any rules about carrying heavy objects?

Yes. I often tell my patients, "Never take out the garbage in your Sunday suit."

You've got to be kidding. If I have to carry out the garbage, what difference does it make whether I'm wearing good clothes or old ones?

I'm serious. If you're wearing your good clean clothes, you will instinctively hold the garbage bag away from your body. When you reach out and hold a load at arm's length, there's a leverage effect. The distance between your spine and the load magnifies the strain on your back. If that garbage is heavy, you can easily bring on a bout of back pain.

The most basic principle of all, when it comes to lifting any object, is to bring it in close to your body – hug it if you can – and save your back that way. This one fact is more important than all the other instructions you've heard about lifting with your back straight or bending your knees. If I thought people would take the idea seriously, I'd distribute a bumper-sticker asking, HAVE YOU HUGGED YOUR GARBAGE CAN TODAY?

Do you find more back problems among people who have to do a lot of standing, compared to people who are seated during much of a normal day?

It may not seem logical but sitting down is harder on the back than standing up. Sitting places a greater load on the discs in your spine. And that prolonged compression may cause changes in a disc, flattening it out somewhat and squeezing the material inside towards the outer shell. That sort of pressure can be painful.

Then I suppose it is a big help to sit in a comfortable chair.

The kind of seat you use can make a tremendous difference, but I would be careful with the word "comfortable." One of the great horrors in the world of chairdom is the so-called "comfy" chair – that overstuffed monster that looks inviting but feels almost as if it were designed to produce backache. Its arms are so high that you can't rest your own arms on them. The seat is so deep from front to back that you can't rest your feet comfortably on the floor. And the back of the chair is so soft that it provides no support. Your spine sags so much as you slump into it that you are forced into a flexed position. And the more "give" there is to the back of the chair, the more you have to bend forward to compensate.

A "comfy" chair looks comfortable because it is soft. Nobody likes the idea of sitting on a hard chair. But you have to sit in a "comfy" chair for only a short time to realize it is actually a back-trap.

Then am I better off with the other extreme – say, a hard bench?

Not necessarily. The hard, backless bench – the kind you see in many shopping-malls – can be almost as bad. But at least it allows you a choice of posture. If you find yourself having to use a bench like that, try sitting the way football players often do: hunched forward, with your hands or elbows on your knees. Taking the weight through your arms unloads your spine. In fact it's a great position for a three-minute rest, but if you stay that way too long you'll find that when you straighten up your back feels sore. Maybe that's what shopping-mall designers intend – making sure you won't sit too long without getting up and going into a store to buy something.

A bench, unlike the "comfy" chair, allows you to choose your own position and lets you change that position as often as you choose. I can think of eight or ten ways I might sit on an ordinary backless bench, and each one would provide some relief by varying the otherwise constant load on my spine. Even so, without a firm back support and suitable arm-rests, the bench is far from ideal.

Another difficult form of a seat is the Cape Cod chair, a wooden outdoor lounging chair with a seat quite close to the ground. The Cape Code has wide, flat arms and a back that tilts twenty degrees or so away from the vertical. The seat has wooden slats that slope sharply downward from front to back. It looks comfortably inviting, but, as you discover once you're seated, it's very awkward to get up again.

Most backache sufferers have had bad experiences as well with director's chairs, which have curved canvas backs that provide no support for the spine, and narrow seats that make position changes difficult.

Sometimes I wonder if there isn't a world-wide chair conspiracy against people with back problems, especially when I see modern chairs made of chrome or stainless steel that are so uncomfortable for the spine. Even the bean-bag chair, which has the merit of adapting itself comfortably to your body shape, can be as hard to get out of as the Cape Cod.

Is there such a thing as the perfect chair?

No, there isn't. We are not all the same shape and size, and the chair that suits one person may not suit another. A colleague of mine, a plastic surgeon, now retired, didn't like performing surgery while sitting on a standard stool. Instead he had his own seat designed. It looked for all the world like a big, old-fashioned tractor seat. To him, it was the ultimate in working comfort. And he wasn't alone. Whenever he was out of the operating room, several other surgeons used to compete for the privilege of sitting in that seat. But not everybody found it comfortable.

Of course you stand a better chance of achieving near perfection if you know exactly what you want and can afford to have it custom made.

I once visited the shop of a craftsman who specializes in custom-making chairs for maximum comfort. He had a simple system using a heavy mesh screen and movable wooden rods to shape a chair exactly to the contours of your back – and your backside. I was quite taken with his approach; he didn't try to impress me with a lot of scientific theory about the biomechanics of my spine. He just worked hard to make absolutely sure the end result would suit me perfectly. His whole approach was: "Let's build whatever feels comfortable to you."

What guidelines can you offer to a person who is looking for a good chair for an office job?

Find a chair that supports the small of your back with its normal forward curve, without rigidity or too much "give." The back of the chair should tilt backwards ten to twenty degrees, to suit your comfort and needs, and it should have a means of being locked into place at the angle you prefer. Make sure the seat is deep enough to support the length of your thighs and wide enough to allow easy position change. If you're going to be seated for long periods, you want to be able to shift from one side to another, to cross and uncross your legs, lean forward, lean back, and so on, to ease the stress.

The chair you're looking for should have arm-rests that allow you to transfer some weight from the upper body and temporarily reduce the load on your lower spine.

Check the height of the chair seat against your desk or work table to ensure that they combine to place your work surface at the level of your elbows when you are seated with your arms at your sides and your forearms held parallel to the floor. The chair should also let you rest your feet easily on the floor, to reduce the amount of weight taken by the backs of your thighs.

And even with the best possible chair, you might do well to place a stool or even a thick book on the floor in front of you, so you can prop one foot up now and then. Or do what I do: pull out a low desk drawer and rest your foot on that.

Is it a good idea to have a seat that can be easily raised and lowered?

With an adjustable chair, a person can obtain the seating height that seems exactly right, although this can also be achieved by trying out various chairs of fixed height. It seems like a good idea to vary the height of your seating from time to time while you work, but in my experience few people use adjustable chairs this way.

What about that new "kneeling chair," which has a seat with an extreme forward slope and a knee-rest that places nearly all your body weight on your knees. Does it employ some useful scientific principle?

The kneeling position automatically puts the forward curve of the low back into a neutral position, and that's good. But the design also puts a substantial load on your knees, and some older people may not like that for long. I wouldn't buy this chair just on the basis of how it feels during a tryout in the store; I'd want to test it personally during several days of actual use. Over time, you might find it very comfortable or you might discover that the kneeling chair is too confining since it deprives you of the chance to change position easily. Like many devices built to help the back, it's great for some and not so good for others.

Is there such a thing as the perfect way to sit?

The best position, for your back's sake, is probably a compromise between sitting rigidly upright, in the old schoolroom tradition, and slumping way down, as teenagers often do when watching TV or talking on the phone.

A couple of guidelines, based on biomechanics, are worth keeping in mind. First, forward bending increases disc load. So don't bend forward for long periods. Second, try to find some support for your lower back, from the chair itself, from a small cushion, or from a specially designed support.

Aren't specially designed supports just commercial gimmicks?

No, I consider them legitimate because they induce a posture that is physiologically normal – a forward curve at the neck, a backward curve of the thoracic spine, in the area of the shoulders, and a forward curve in the lumbar region, or lower spine. If you can maintain those curves in their correct proportions, you will go far in relieving your back pain. Of course, the advantages of an expensive contour support must be weighed against the benefits of a simple, inexpensive cushion. The choice depends on comfort, convenience, and cost.

So proper sitting posture means avoiding extreme positions?

Most of the time, yes. But even the extremes – slumping down and sitting bolt upright – can be used as brief variations to provide helpful relief. We all know that if we stay in any one position for long, such as in a movie theater or on a long car ride, our bodies and legs become cramped and sore. Sometimes a change is as good as a rest.

But what if you have to work at a desk with a knee hole so narrow and low that there's no room to use a foot-rest or cross your legs or move around much?

Try shifting occasionally from side to side, riding "side saddle," so to speak. Also, stand up and walk around two or three times an hour, to loosen up your muscles and joints.

So, that's another regular strategy to use – loosening up by moving around now and then.

That's right, and if you're on the lookout for chances to limber up, you'll sometimes find them in surprising places. For example, at Toronto's Pearson Airport, Terminal One contains several staircases that seem quite inconvenient to arriving passengers.

As you make your way to the luggage carousel, you have to walk
down narrow flights of stairs and then cope with a door that
will not stay open by itself. It's awkward, especially for anyone
toting carry-on baggage, but it has one big advantage: it provides
useful exercise for passengers who may have been sitting in a
plane for several hours with their backs and legs fairly immobile.
Getting down that staircase and opening that door involve walking,
flexing, twisting, and pushing with the arms. All these motions
help you stretch, and they may be especially welcome if you have
common backache.

This short interlude of exercise can be helpful even if you have
used all my standard tricks to protect your spine during the flight –
sitting with one foot up on a small case, keeping the seat belt
tightly fastened, supporting the hollow in the low back with a
small pillow, and choosing an aisle seat so you can get up easily
and move about.

**How would you rate the average airplane seat compared to the
typical automobile seat?**

For most people the airplane seat is a little better, but it's always
a matter of personal preference. Some new car seat designs are
very good but even the best of them will give some people backaches. One good step in car design would be to do away with
the bench seat. Among the horror tales of bad seating, the familiar
bench ranks right up there with the "comfy" chair.

Several years ago, I had a car I couldn't drive without a seat
cushion. I got a nasty backache whenever I sat in the driver's
seat without a pillow wedged behind the small of my back. If
my children didn't want me going out, they'd hide my pillow. When
I bought another car, I assumed I'd need the pillow, as always.
But in the new car I found the pillow quite uncomfortable, and
I discarded it. I've found it's wrong to make any absolute rule
about your back and its needs, since they will vary from one situation
to another.

Later I got a car with a steering wheel that tilts and a power
seat that's adjustable every which way. Now I'd hate to be without
those extras. Driving on a long trip you can assume many different
positions. You can ride for a while like a bus driver, with the
seat high and the steering wheel up close and almost horizontal,
like a sundial. Or you can place the steering wheel almost vertical,

like a clock on a wall, and then sit back as though driving a sports car. And between those two extremes there are a dozen possible variations.

What about other types of vehicles – bicycles, for instance? Are they hard on the back?

The biggest drawback to the bicycle is the small size of the seat. With a racing bike, especially, a large proportion of your body weight bears down on a relatively small surface, and so the concentration of load is high. This effect is somewhat offset by the fact that you are carrying much of your upper body weight on your arms. But that forward-bent position creates more load on the discs, so some of that advantage is nullified. If you have back problems, choose a conventional bicycle, not a racer.

I suppose motorcycle seats are pretty bad for backs.

Not necessarily. The motorcycle seat has evolved from a bicycle-style seat into a small bench, usually with a big pommel, and that's an improvement. Some motorcycles also have arm- and back-rests, which of course take some of the load off the spine.

What about horseback riding – is that bad for your back?

Not really. A good rider adopts a posture that is upright without being stiffly military, and that's good.

But what about the jarring effect when a horse trots or canters?

For beginners, that's a hazard, but once people learn to ride properly, they reduce that impact with their legs, minimizing the shock to their spines. Of course, most of us will have some backache after a long day in the saddle.

Earlier, you mentioned a colleague who liked to work on a tractor-type seat. Isn't it ironical that your back is better off when you drive a tractor than when you sit behind the wheel of a luxury automobile?

It's better off only because of the wide, contour seat that used to be standard on every tractor. Unfortunately, modern tractors have cabs with bench seats, which are hard on the back. The driver's back is subjected to a lot of jarring as he drives over rough terrain, but the worst punishment for his spine may come from vibration. Studies have shown that certain rates of vibration produce a corresponding resonance in the spine. If a machine vibrates at a certain frequency, and if that frequency happens to match the natural resonance of the spine, it will create waves of movement that can seriously aggravate back trouble.

This phenomenon explains why many people who do certain kinds of work – operating earth-movers, for instance – suffer from backache. It applies also to some truck drivers and, in fact, to almost any job where the person's body is subjected to constant vibration.

Is backache inevitable, then, for people in jobs like those?

I wouldn't say it's inevitable, but it's much more likely. Some people can go through a lot of physical aggravation without developing chronic backache. But even the people who are vulnerable can take steps to ward off trouble. Much of the vibration can be reduced, if not eliminated, by the use of spring-mounted seats or padding, or by better design of the machinery itself. There is a lot of research going on now to find out what vibrations are harmful and how they can be reduced, changed, or eliminated.

Does vibration cause a particular condition that you can diagnose?

No, vibration just accentuates the same kind of wear in the discs and back joints that you'd find in any patient with common backache.

You said earlier that sitting is harder on the back than standing. Are you better off, then, with a job where you sit for maybe an hour or two and then get up and do some other form of work?

It depends. That kind of job is great if you get up to move around, stretch, or do light work. It's not so good if you have to go from being sedentary to suddenly doing heavy lifting. This happens, for instance, with a truck driver who does his own loading and unloading. He works hard loading his truck for an hour or two, then drives for several hours while his back and legs stiffen up, and then jumps out of his cab and begins hoisting heavy objects again. It's hardly surprising when pain results from that abuse of a spine already affected by the normal wear and tear of aging.

But if that's his job, he can hardly avoid the problem.

Maybe not entirely, but he would be smart to take a tip from professional athletes, who know the importance of warming up before any strenuous activity. Before he tackles a loading job, the driver should walk briskly around his rig and do a little bending and stretching, maybe on the pretext of checking his tires or examining the freight. Anything to prepare the back muscles for the exertion ahead.

What other occupations are particularly difficult for people with back problems?

It's hard to think of a job that doesn't have some potential for causing backache, although some jobs, of course, are worse than others. Construction workers and dock hands often get backaches because they do a lot of bending, lifting, and twisting of the upper body. Nurses are vulnerable, too, often having to lift bedridden patients. The trouble usually starts with the unexpected lift or twist. The person has just started to lift when his partner drops the other end of a heavy box, or he accidentally slips on a wet floor and twists hard to avoid falling down. In such cases, the sudden load catches the muscles by surprise and the spine has to take most of the weight.

One of the toughest jobs on the back is hard-rock mining. To drill holes where dynamite sticks will be inserted into the rock face, a man has to lift a hundred-pound power hammer and hold it at shoulder height while it vibrates like mad. If any job can be described as back-breaking work, that's it. There are machines that can help do the job, but much of hard-rock mining is still done with human muscle – and backs. Hard-rock miners are a strong breed, and they need all that strength to protect their spines. For instance, if they have weak belly muscles, the load on their backs may just be too much.

A jack-hammer operator working on a paved street is a little better off, not having to bear the whole weight of the equipment while using it. But he must lift that heavy hammer continually, often twisting his upper body as he does so. His back would be a lot better off if he used his feet to turn his whole body at once.

Some other occupations belong on this "high risk" list, such as repetitious assembly-line jobs requiring lifting and turning from fixed positions. To increase my understanding of these causes of backache, I've toured many factories, including one where fire hoses are manufactured. There, workers use long metal poles to handle masses of rubbery goo, which they lift at arm's length and mix with a twisting motion. If any of them avoid chronic backache, I'd like to know how.

Some sheet-metal workers have to lift heavy materials and tools in positions that strain their backs. House painters are asking for trouble if they stand on ladders and reach out awkwardly with their scrapers and paint brushes. Proper scaffolding, as well as being safer, provides much more comfort for the back.

And speaking of ladders, I mustn't forget to mention firefighting. It's hard to think of a greater challenge to a person's back than climbing up and down a ladder under the most urgent and stressful conditions while toting a heavy fire hose or carrying a fire victim to safety. Firefighters often have to lift other heavy objects as well. One fireman told me how he once had to reach out at arm's length and turn over a rowboat, single-handed, to get at a fire he was fighting.

Even the man who drives the fire engine lets himself in for back problems. He has to manage a huge steering wheel and operate a heavy clutch while bouncing along at high speed.

Flying a helicopter is even harder on the back than driving a fire engine. In flight, the pilot has both feet elevated to operate the rudder pedals, a posture that puts extra stress on the discs. He must keep both arms in action, with engine vibration constantly jarring his spine. One of my patients is a firefighter who moonlights as a helicopter flight instructor. I can't think of a worse combination.

It's a real tribute to the strength of the human system that, although so many jobs produce a high incidence of backache, there is little real damage done to the spine. And vigorous physical conditioning of the muscles of the back and belly can substantially reduce the discomfort.

What about outdoor chores?

Many people develop sore backs doing yard jobs, especially jobs they do only occasionally. Snow shoveling is a prime example. Being seasonal, it's not routine. It involves a lot of lifting, twisting, and turning, all done under cold conditions. And, typically, a householder intent on clearing a sidewalk or driveway won't take the time to warm up to the task. It's an open invitation to back trouble. Powered snow-blowers may be hazardous for other reasons but they're a boon to back pain sufferers.

Can you suggest a specific strategy for people who shovel snow by hand?

Yes – first, dress warmly, particularly over the back. Cold air can tighten the back muscles. If you're about to do a lot of heavy work, run through a short warm-up routine before you go outside. When you shovel snow, lift light loads. Remember: you don't have to clear the whole sidewalk in one shovelful. Carry the snow where you want it, rather than trying to fling it a great distance. And if you're throwing the snow to one side, turn your feet as you do so – don't twist your spine. The job may take a little longer that way, but you'll save yourself a lot of pain.

Some of the same principles apply to grass cutting. Avoid extreme positions, such as bending forward excessively. Work in stages. If your back is sore and the job is likely to take two hours of steady work, spread the task over four or five hours, resting or doing entirely different kinds of jobs in between.

Hedge trimming can be hard on the back, because you often have to hold the clippers at arm's length. Power clippers get the job done faster, of course, but they're also heavier, causing extra strain.

Raking grass or leaves can be another problem. To avoid un-necessary bending or reaching, rake with short strokes, using your arms and shoulders, or moving forward or backward with your legs. Keep your spine fairly erect and as relaxed as possible.

If you are hauling firewood, don't carry an uncomfortably large load. And give the task some variety. For example, you might carry the wood in a relay pattern: first, several trips in from the woodpile to the bottom of the porch steps; then a second sequence, up the steps and into the house. That way, the job becomes less of an endurance test. In many yard jobs, some strain may be unavoidable, but you can reduce it by resting intermittently, if only for a minute or two each time.

I remind you, though, that these chores won't actually harm your back; they'll just make it sore. Going at any task the wrong way may make life unpleasant for you, but it won't actually damage your spine. It can put up with a lot of abuse; you just don't want to push things to the point where it can't take any more without protesting painfully.

Think of it as a sort of bank account: every time you place some strain on your back, you're drawing on its reserves. Every time you rest or perform muscle-strengthening exercises, you're making a "deposit," restoring some resilience to your "back account." That's why it is so important to take those intermittent rest periods between stressful tasks.

What about the indoor chores that most homemakers perform? Can you suggest special strategies for them?

You can easily strain your spine quite unnecessarily doing many ordinary household tasks – vacuuming a carpet, ironing clothes, making beds, lifting objects from high shelves. The most important principle is to find the most comfortable – or, as the case may be, the least awkward – way of doing the job.

If you're running a vacuum cleaner, keep your back in a comfortable position and move your arms and legs. Lunge forward with your legs and reach with your arms while holding your back erect. See yourself demonstrating the grace of a fencing master.

If you're bending over to make a bed, try to bend at the hips and keep your back relaxed or even slightly arched like a ballet dancer's. Or use a knee bend if that's practical. Some people even kneel on the floor while tucking the blankets and sheets under the mattress.

Instead of straining to lift an object from a shelf at arm's length, use a step stool to get close. Remember, that's the most important principle to observe during any kind of lifting or carrying: hold the object as close to your body as you can and keep it there.

At the ironing board, stand with one foot up, on a low box, for instance. If your back is really sore, try ironing sitting down on a stool or a high chair. Change positions frequently. Sit on a stool or even a countertop while you're waiting for that kettle to boil. Move often and give your back a rest once in a while by leaning on your arms to take the weight of your upper body. Standing over the sink is easier when you put one foot on a shelf inside a cupboard.

Any special advice about moving furniture?

The best strategy of all is to use devices, rather than muscle power, whenever you can – a handcart is better than a back for toting a refrigerator, for instance. And with a little ingenuity, you can often improvise. To move a heavy appliance across a smooth floor, for example, you can often tip it onto a thick blanket and then drag it quite easily. If you must use your own power, let your legs or arms help your spine handle the strain.

It sounds to me as though most people face the risk of backache whether they're at home or out on the job. What are the main points to remember if they want to avoid it?

One very important thing is to keep your muscles, especially your stomach muscles, in good shape, through good postural habits and proper exercise.

Look for ways to modify your regular tasks to reduce the strain or risk. Or, in the case of sedentary jobs, find ways to provide variations in your sitting or standing position. Some people who must stand at a counter all day, for instance, might sit occasionally on a high stool.

If you work at a desk or counter, take note that the comfortable height for the work surface is about level with your elbows. Since the same height can't suit everybody, some enlightened employers now provide platforms, adjustable chairs, or varied or adjustable work surfaces, to keep everyone comfortable.

If possible, give your back short rest breaks several times through-out the day.

And, of course, use the back-saving techniques I've described for bending, lifting, handling tools and materials, and so on.

Could you say a little more about lifting? I'm surprised you haven't emphasized that if you have to lift a heavy object off the ground, you should crouch down and do the lifting with your legs, rather than bending over and straining your back.

Well, that's the time-honored advice. But some current evidence suggests that it may not matter whether you lift mainly with your legs or actually bend over and use your back instead. The important thing, as I said earlier, is to "hug" the load so as to avoid lifting it at arm's length. The key is the distance between the load and the spine. The shorter the distance, the shorter the lever arm, in engineering terms, and the smaller the force required in the back muscles to offset the load. And of course that means a lot less pressure on the spine.

Using your legs to lift is fine in most circumstances, but it isn't always possible. You can't do that for instance if you are hauling an outboard motor out of the trunk of a car. Or if you are lifting a large box, you may not be able to squat down and still get your arms around it. Also, if you're especially tired, you're not likely to use the "leg lift" method, because it requires a great deal more energy than just using your back. The body always seems to prefer the most economical way of doing any job.

So, you see, there is no single correct way to lift; it depends on the situation. Try to use your legs and shoulder muscles when you can, let gravity and the object's momentum work for you, and don't forget to hug.

A second important principle for safe lifting is to avoid the twisting action of the upper body I mentioned earlier. Discs don't like to be twisted. If you must turn while lifting, turn with your feet, not with your trunk.

Many people know how to lift properly but ignore what they know. They should keep reminding themselves of what's best for their backs. But let me say it once again: even if you hurt your back while lifting a few more pounds of load than you can handle, you almost never damage it. But for most of us, "hurt" – even though it's not the same as "harm" – is more trouble than we need. Especially if our backs remain sore enough to interfere with daily living for several days.

Would you go so far as to say that some people whose backs bother them on the job should try to find some other line of work?

That's a good suggestion in theory, but it's not that easy these days to find a new job, let alone an alternative type of work.

I feel sorry for people who inadvertently get into jobs their backs simply can't handle, and I feel even sorrier for those who develop back pain after years in one job and can find no way of switching to other work. One of my patients is a middle-aged police officer who had major surgery for spinal stenosis, a condition I will talk about later. After the operation his back was much better but not normal, by any means. His superiors wanted him to get right back into harness, as a uniformed patrol officer, but he dreaded the prospect of having to spend each shift in a cruiser. On patrol, he has to sit for hours at a time on a badly sprung car seat, with the weight of a holster, gun belt, and gun all pulling on his back muscles. In the winter, his back bears the extra weight of a heavy coat. And there is always the chance that apprehending a suspect might require heavy physical exertion.

Well, he went back to work, and for the first few weeks managed to get posted to courtroom duty. But, the last I heard, he was under pressure to return to his regular assignment. He told me that if he resisted much longer, he'd likely be fired. If he went back and couldn't cope, he'd probably be fired anyway.

Another patient of mine had a different problem. He's a radiologist specializing in angiography, the X-ray study of blood vessels. Routinely, he puts on a lead apron that weighs about twelve pounds (5.5 kg) and bends over the X-ray table to inject contrast material into patients' arteries. Because of his backache, he couldn't do that work for more than a few minutes at a time. When I saw him he was already on disability leave and was considering changing his specialty to something less demanding. But that meant throwing away twelve years' experience to start training for something new.

Those are just a couple of examples of occupational problems for which there are no easy solutions.

I can see where a lead apron would cause trouble, but what about some of the commoner items people wear? For instance, I've heard that women shouldn't wear high-heeled shoes. Do you advise your patients to give them up?

No. I consider that unrealistic and somewhat unnecessary. High heels may increase the curve in the small of the back (doctors call it the lumbar lordosis), and this posture can lead to backache. But high heels don't harm the spine – nor, incidentally, do low heels automatically make a woman's back feel better.

If high heels are causing a problem, I suggest several simple strategies that many women already use as a matter of course. Avoid standing for long periods. Or take along a second, more comfortable, pair of shoes and use them intermittently. Or, in a casual situation, walk around in stocking feet.

What do you advise back patients to do when choosing a pair of shoes?

New shoes should feel comfortable almost from the moment you put them on. I tell my patients, "You're not breaking in the shoes; you're breaking down your feet." The height of the heel affects the posture of the spine. The width of the shoe determines the pressure on the toes. When you stand up, your foot widens under the weight of your body, and that's when the fit of the shoe can be determined most accurately.

What about jogging shoes?

My first inclination is to advise back patients not to take up jogging at all. But if jogging is your choice as a recreational sport, I suggest you get jogging shoes that are well-cushioned, to soften the impact on the spine. The heels should be broad to minimize the natural torque action of running – that is, the slight rotation of the leg at the knee.

Could you explain more about "torque action"? If rotation is natural, as you said, why should joggers need shoes with broad heels to prevent it?

If you'd spent your life running all day every day, your knees would develop a tolerance for that increased rotation. But most joggers aren't seasoned runners, and it's easy for them to push their bodies beyond their normal experience.

What is your main objection to jogging?

I don't necessarily object to jogging, although I do feel the joggers I see should be given only one of two choices: they can jog or they can complain. The most important factors are the total mileage (distances under two miles a day generally don't cause trouble) and the running surface. I see nothing wrong with jogging on grass, cinders, or a sprung track. But people are just asking for trouble by jogging on concrete or asphalt – their feet, knees, and backs can't take that kind of punishment.

If you want to give your heart and lungs a regular workout, you can choose one of several exercises that are just as effective as jogging, with less potential for back pain. These include swimming, certain aerobic exercises without a great deal of bouncing up and down, and fast walking – not Olympic-speed walking, just walking briskly. Walking doesn't have the glamour of running, but it's an excellent cardiovascular exercise.

Are there a lot of other recreational sports that may cause wear and tear on your spine?

Most athletic activities don't cause wear and tear; they just aggravate what you have already developed naturally. Every activity causes *some* strain on your back, and your spine has no trouble keeping it under control. The unfortunate cases occur when people go to extremes and actually cause heavy wear on their spines quite needlessly. One patient of mine was a well-built man in his twenties who came to me complaining of severe back pain. And no wonder. He was working out regularly with bar-bells, using routines he had invented, without any understanding of what their effects might be.

For instance, he would take a fifteen-pound (7 kg) weight in each hand, extend his arms at shoulder height, and then swing his whole upper torso back and forth as hard as he could, in violent rotations that must have had his discs pleading for mercy. And he was routinely doing a thousand repetitions every day.

I explained to him that while a healthy back can put up with almost anything, discs hate violent twisting. He'd been asking for trouble – and he got it. His objective had been to keep his mid-section fit and trim. But, as I told him, there are many exercises that will do that without placing all the strain on the discs. Side bends will usually keep anyone's middle-age spread under control. Slow, resisted rotations on an exercise machine can strengthen the waist muscles that protect the discs, and can do so without injuring the spine in the process. Even running or walking can do a lot to tighten the waistline.

I'm not suggesting that this young man's back was ruined for life, but he was inflicting a lot of needless wear and tear for a result that could be achieved in several painless ways.

Is pain a pretty accurate indication that a particular sport is bad for your back?

Not at all. As long as your common sense keeps you from going to extremes, you can consider playing almost any sport you enjoy. If you're a 150-pound, forty-five-year-old male with a disc problem, you will obviously decline to get out onto a field to play serious football against a lineup of 300-pounders. But it's a mistake, in my view, to avoid a friendly game of basketball, or an afternoon of tennis, just because you know your back will start hurting. It's a tradeoff: if you like the activity, that pain is the price you pay for the recreational and social enjoyment you get from the game.

I have a booklet published by a drug company for doctors to hand out to their back patients. It is filled with all sorts of silly advice, the silliest of which is a list of "good" and "bad" exercises. Never mind the fact that what's "bad" for one back patient might be perfectly okay for another, this company plays the whole thing so safe it's laughable. What happened, I'm sure, was that their lawyer said, "Look, we can't afford to have our name on this booklet if there is even the slightest possibility of somebody getting hurt after taking our advice."

The result was that virtually every popular sport appears on the "bad" list: tennis, golf, squash, basketball, volleyball – you name it. The "good" sports column is limited to such innocuous activities as swimming and slow walking. I wondered why they didn't include tiddly-winks, window-shopping, and indoor bird-watching.

The underlying message is that people with back problems aren't allowed to have any fun – which is sheer nonsense.

Do you have your own list of sports that are good or bad for people with back problems?

No, I don't think of them that way. Some sports entail risks even for people with healthy backs – hang-gliding, ski-jumping, sky-diving, boxing, wrestling – not just because they impose a strain on your spine but because they entail the risk of serious injury to other parts of the body, which is a completely different thing.

We have to assume for the purpose of this discussion that you will be careful enough and lucky enough not to get seriously injured in the sport of your choice. With that proviso, I see no need for a list of "safe" and "unsafe" sports. Virtually every sport involves some strain on your back, and virtually every back can stand it.

Then how can I make the choice from among the sports that appeal to me?

It helps to understand that strain on your back may take three distinct forms: placing extra weight on your spinal discs, arching your spine and loading the small joints, and rotating your trunk to produce that twisting effect I described.

Once you're aware of these causes of strain, you don't need medical training to decide which of them are involved in the sport of your choice and whether the satisfaction and fun will be worth the resulting discomfort or pain. Barring accidents, you won't actually harm your back engaging in the popular sports you might choose, and it's ridiculous to avoid any activity just because it may hurt a little at the time or produce some stiffness or soreness the next day.

What sort of activity places extra weight on your spine?

Extra weight can mean either literally taking on an extra burden, as you do in weight-lifting, or producing a pounding action on the discs, for instance by running on a hard surface. Sports that load extra weight on your spine include curling, bowling, horseback riding, dirt biking, hunting, and fishing.

Once you understand the basic mechanics, you can easily figure out how to reduce the hazard, by adopting certain techniques or simply by going at it less vigorously. If you haven't bowled for several weeks, restrict yourself to just a game or two, with intervals of rest. If you go fishing, be careful how you lift that outboard motor from the car trunk, and don't try to manhandle that big canoe ashore all by yourself. When you are hunting in the bush, keep your pack light and let someone else carry out the moose. On horseback or a dirt bike, choose the trail carefully and save your back by making your legs absorb those bounces and jolts.

What are the sports that force you to arch your back?

You arch your back at some time in nearly every popular recreational sport: basketball, tennis, badminton, volleyball, hockey, baseball, skiing, and certain styles of swimming, notably the breaststroke. Arching the back is inherent in the actions of rowing, canoeing, and archery.

Is there anything I can do, then, if I'm determined to play one of those "arching" sports and it makes my back hurt?

If your problem is in the small joints of your spine, arching your back may cause pain. It's impossible to avoid that posture completely, but you can avoid extreme positions by practicing a pelvic tilt to flatten your lower back a little; I'll describe the pelvic tilt in more detail later when we talk about exercises. Rest during the game by bending forward slightly – and resolve to live with the remaining discomfort as part of a fair tradeoff.

I can see where many of the "arching" sports also involve twisting or rotating the upper part of your body.

That's true. Baseball and tennis are two examples. But the worst offenders are squash, racketball, and golf. Compared to those racket sports, golf may seem pretty sedate, but, in fact, a well-executed golf swing places an enormous rotational strain on your spine. Even so, if you play golf you can learn to modify your swing to reduce the strain. Using an exercise machine to practice careful, resisted rotations can strengthen the trunk muscles and help protect the discs from sudden, twisting movements. And, with any sport, you can practice moderation in one way or another, playing less intensely or for shorter periods and taking longer or more frequent rests.

About the "tradeoff" you mentioned – is it just for professionals and ambitious amateurs, or should ordinary people go on playing sports in spite of back pain?

Anybody can make a tradeoff – and many ordinary people do, simply because the enjoyment and satisfaction outweigh the pain. Two of my male patients are among the most enthusiastic jocks I've ever met, but they are not exceptional athletes, just ordinary people who enjoy exercise and friendly competition. One is a forty-nine-year-old with disc trouble. He loves to play hockey. Sometimes, during a tournament, he'll play two or three games in one week. Often, his back pain begins just as he bends forward to lace up his skates, and sometimes it gets so bad he has to leave the game. But he keeps going back for more.

The other fellow, also middle-aged, is an avid windsurfer. I can't think of a sport where the back is arched more acutely; and the weight-loading factor is considerable, too. This man has some problems with wear in his spinal joints that may need surgical attention some day. But you would have to lock him up to keep him off that sailboard.

Both men put up with a fair amount of pain and stiffness in order to participate in the sports they enjoy so much. I can't think of a better tradeoff than that – and, obviously, neither can they.

Could they actually help their backs that way, in the long run, by staying active?

Only in the general sense that they are building up muscular strength that may help protect their spines from unnecessary strain. But, like most competitive or recreational sports, hockey and windsurfing are far from being remedies for back pain. What these two men *are* doing is refusing to let back pain keep them on the sidelines. Both men also make a regular habit of doing specific exercises to strengthen their backs – an entirely different matter, which we will discuss in the final chapter.

The important thing to point out here is that whatever activity you may engage in – from toting a garbage bag to climbing a mountain peak – you can use techniques that will minimize the effects of natural aging on your spine. It's up to you to decide whether a particular activity is worth the stiffness or pain it will produce.

It's also up to you to adopt or devise strategies and make personal choices to ensure that you, not your spine, will determine the quality and style of the life you lead.

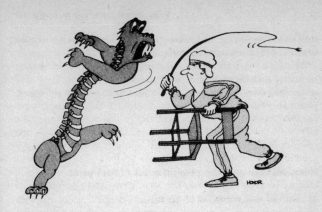

2. TAMING THE BEAST

There is no denying the fact that virtually everyone with a back problem will experience painful episodes from time to time.

I often tell my patients once they're pain free, it would be to their benefit if they could have one more acute episode which they could successfully abort. That way, they would discover for themselves that they are in control. This observation is based on my experience with thousands of patients who have trained themselves to ward off an attack and then actually done so. If they have faced and tamed the beast even once, they no longer have reason to fear it.

One of the great satisfactions of my work is to have a patient come in and say, "I just had a bad attack last week, but I knew what to do, and now I'm fine."

Even before you reach that stage, however, there is one consolation to keep in mind: *without exception, every acute attack eventually subsides*. It may be hard to remember at the time – and even harder to believe – but no pain attack, no matter how severe, will stay with you indefinitely. It will always get better.

What you can usefully remember, too, is that as long as you are taking the right steps to look after your back, no attack will

return you to square one. There is always some residue of gain
from your previous training and exercise.

As long as you are making the proper effort, you will find it
satisfying to look back from time to time, to see how far you've
come. And even more satisfying to realize that the beast is, indeed,
thoroughly tamed – and you are in control.

How would you describe a typical attack of back pain?

As with so many aspects of back pain, people's problems with
acute attacks vary from one individual to another. Pain is the
common feature, but it is not the same type or intensity for everyone,
and it is certainly not constant.

One of the stories I often hear from people who have had
minor attacks is that they are immobilized by the terrible fear
that "something is going wrong" with their backs. I know the
feeling. When it comes over me, I know instinctively that if I try
to move I am going to trigger some pain. For all practical purposes,
I feel trapped in one position.

In other words, you are paralyzed by your back pain?

Not actually. Paralysis is a very exact term denoting the loss of
muscle power due to a disruption of the normal nerve impulses.
What we're talking about here is a powerful psychological inhibition
against movement. Your body "knows" that movement will cause
pain and refuses to let you try it.

The trick, then, is to assume and remain in the most soothing
rest position you can find. There is no single correct position.
I remember one patient who was comfortable only on his hands
and knees, and he even stayed in bed that way. You should
experiment gently until you find a position that works for you.
Most rest positions remove the loading effect of gravity and restore
the neutral curve of the spine. If you are able to do that, you
can, in most cases, eliminate the pain almost completely.

I think some people who have had severe attacks will find that hard to believe.

I'm sure they will. My comments apply to typical attacks, but the amount and character of the pain can range across a wide spectrum. At one extreme, the pain is immediate and so severe that the person may actually fall to the floor. The severity depends on several factors, including the source of the pain, the degree of muscle spasm, and the amount of fear.

But even in the worst attacks, the pain is typically intermittent. If a patient describes back pain as constant – twenty-four hours a day without change – and if the physical examination shows evidence of nothing but natural wear and tear, I can be sure the pain is being aggravated by the person's emotional responses.

What's the first thing a person should know about coping with an acute attack?

Timing is critical. The sooner you can take action the better, because the longer the muscles remain cramped, the more they become irritated and likely to continue in spasm. In time, they begin to retain fluid. And that extra fluid – medically it's called edema – swells the muscles, increases the muscles' irritability, and creates more pain.

Are you saying that back pain is simply a spasm of the back muscles?

Not precisely. But usually the most important pain-producing factor in an acute attack is the accompanying muscle spasm. You want to help the muscle relax as quickly as possible. Sometimes all it takes is a little bit of positioning and gentle stretching, much like getting out of bed to walk off that cramp you get in the calf of your leg. Sometimes aborting the acute attack can be as simple as sitting down and hugging your knees to your chest. Or sometimes squatting can provide the relief you need.

Or you could try doing what I sometimes do. When I have an attack, I lie on the floor with my feet and calves resting on the seat of a chair and my body close underneath, so that my knees are right above my chest. If you had a side view of me in that position, I'd look like the letter "Z." Then I place a thin cushion under my buttocks, to raise my hips slightly. This position takes the tension out of my back.

But in some settings, don't you feel pretty foolish suddenly getting down and lying on the floor like that?

Of course I do, so I try to get away where I'm not the center of attention. But it's a tradeoff: better that than looking foolish by being off with a bad back for the next few weeks.

How important is bed rest in the acute attack?

Very important, and as soon as possible. If your attack occurs at work, you may be in the kind of job where you can't just get up and leave. But as soon as it's practical, get home and get off your feet, to stop gravity from pressing down onto those sore joints or discs, because that pressure can trigger muscle spasms. Stay put, even for a few days, until the acute phase has subsided.

Any advice about the best way to lie in bed?

As I have said, there is no one best way. Adopt whatever position feels most comfortable. If the pain has been bad on forward bending, try lying on your stomach, as a temporary measure. If your back pain originates from a disc, even ten or fifteen minutes of lying on your stomach and arching your back slightly can make all the difference in getting rid of that spasm.

When your back pain originates in the spinal facet joints and arching backward increases your discomfort and pain, you should obviously get yourself into a position where you are hunched forward, to take the stress off those sore joints. Curl up in the fetal position with a pillow between your knees. Most people prefer a fat pillow, but try several to find the size you like best. Or lie on your back or your side and use the pelvic tilt, gently thrusting your hips forward to reduce the arch in your back. Whatever position you use, the important thing is to stay in bed and get up as little as possible.

What do you do next?

I try to relieve the pain through the use of a counter-irritant. Ice seems to work better for me at the moment, but heat and cold are both counter-irritants, and so they're both capable of reducing the pain. You should discover for yourself which one works best for you. Sometimes even alternating an ice pack and a hot-water bottle can be effective.

What about a hot bath, then, or a cold shower?

A cold shower would certainly take your mind off your back pain, but too much concentrated cold can actually increase the muscle spasm and increase your problem. I suggest you try a hot shower instead. Standing in the shower with one foot up on a ledge or low stool may be just the thing to relax your back. The sitting posture in a bathtub may put too much strain on your spine and offset the benefit of the heat. Also, a lot of people with bad backs find that getting in and out of a bathtub is so uncomfortable that the benefits aren't worth the effort.

People who have access to more modern conveniences will find that a whirlpool bath or a hot-tub can provide all the benefits of a hot bath without requiring you to curl up in a way that might put a needless load on your discs. Being able to stretch out in a hot-tub or lie with your back to the jet in a whirlpool is certainly excellent emergency treatment, if you have one of those facilities at hand.

Whatever form of bathing you choose, remember that you aren't your normal self, and if possible you should have someone there to help you in and out of the shower or tub, to avoid an accident.

Are there other effective counter-irritants besides heat and cold?

Yes. Liniment often provides relief, although you should recognize that neither the liniment nor the heat it produces actually reaches the muscle. By causing a burning sensation on the skin, liniment helps block the pain signals from deeper inside the body.

What other remedies are worth trying?

Gentle stretching often helps. The order of action is: rest your back, ice it (or heat it), and then stretch it. By stretching I mean just moving your back gently, in the directions that are comfortable. If bending in one direction causes pain, don't bend that way; try the other direction. If both directions hurt, wait a few hours before trying again.

You may actually produce comfort with gentle, repetitive movement in the direction that causes pain. In other words, start off by doing the things that are least painful. Then when you've recovered some mobility, cautiously try doing the things that hurt. For example, if forward bending hurts, gently bend forward to the point of discomfort and then stop. Then repeat that movement several times. If the movement is making the pain worse, don't persist. But if it isn't any worse, or if you begin to notice some slight improvement, keep it up. Spend a few minutes gently – and I emphasize gently – repeating the movement. Rest for a while, then try it again later on. Do this perhaps eight or ten times a day for a few days.

What about medication?

Having done all the right things during the first stage of your attack – and those are by far the most important counter-measures you can take – you may gain additional benefit from a relaxant or an anti-inflammatory drug. If your doctor is already familiar with your back problem, you can probably arrange by telephone to have one of these medications prescribed for you on an emergency basis. But be aware that they don't always work. There's just no guarantee. I find there is about a fifty-fifty chance of relief, whether you are taking anti-inflammatories or muscle relaxants. And, by the way, the drugs aren't just *back* muscle relaxants – they relax your whole body. I usually refer to them as "people relaxants."

What about pain killers?

Pain killers may help you get over the worst of it, although they can be surprisingly ineffective with acute back pain. Remember, they do nothing to alter the actual mechanism of the spasm. They simply dull your perception of pain. That effect may be welcome, but it might be unwise for you to take a strong medication in some circumstances. It could present a risk, for instance, if you took something at work and ·then tried to drive home. In that situation, you're better off just toughing things out until you're safely through the door.

What about a good belt of brandy - or whatever?

Alcohol can be helpful, if you're normally a moderate drinker. I'd hate to think that anyone would use a pain attack as an excuse to go home and get drunk. But a couple of drinks, in a controlled situation, and combined with bed rest, may help to relieve the tension and the anxiety that go along with the spasm.

Is it a matter of choosing between alcohol and medication? Or is it okay to take both?

It's usually a good idea to make it one or the other and not mix the two. On their own, anti-inflammatories and alcohol are both inclined to upset your stomach. So a dose of each could cause stomach problems you don't need, especially when you're already in pain. If you're taking strong pain relievers or relaxants, they'll cloud your thinking and make you drowsy, and alcohol will only accentuate that effect. That's not necessarily a bad thing, if it helps you sleep. But I am always concerned about the risk of becoming dependent on alcohol or any other addictive substance.

How long does an acute attack usually last?

Most attacks originating in the facet joints will be gone within a few days – two weeks at the most. The pain may be replaced by a dull ache or discomfort that may last for several weeks, but the acute episode is usually gone within a matter of days.

Do some attacks last longer?

Yes. If you have an attack of pain from a bulging disc, it will probably last four or five weeks. And it's a different kind of attack. Not everyone responds in exactly the same way, of course, but generally speaking disc pain tends to come on more slowly than facet pain. Often patients with disc problems will tell me, "I did something to my back in the morning, and by that night it was much worse. By the next day I couldn't move."

What's the shortest period I can hope for?

Just minutes to hours. If you act quickly and manage to beat it, you could be out of the acute attack before the day is through. At best you will have truly minimized it. It is well worth developing the skills to get around those painful episodes and continue to function normally.

But remember what I said earlier: *without exception, every single acute episode will end.* Furthermore, the original source of trouble will resolve. With time, the body repairs worn joints and bulging discs, and only the muscle pain remains to be treated.

I've heard of backache sufferers who got relief by having chiropractors manipulate their spines. Is that worth trying?

By all means, as long as your problem has been accurately diagnosed and you know that your low-back pain is originating in a facet joint or a disc. In that case, manipulation is safe and may provide relief from acute muscle spasm. But if your problem is caused by direct nerve pressure, manipulation can actually make matters worse.

What are the chances that nerve pressure is the source of my pain?

Irritation and pain caused by something pressing directly on the nerve occur in only about 10 percent of all cases of common backache. That statistic alone means low-back manipulation is usually safe. And when properly employed, the treatment should bring prompt relief. Manipulation is not one of those routines where you have to feel worse before you feel better.

Would you recommend seeing a chiropractor?

I don't object to your going to a chiropractor for treatment of an attack of back pain, as long as your condition is properly defined before any manipulation is attempted.

Do I need a doctor to diagnose my problem? Can't a chiropractor do that?

He will certainly try. Some chiropractors are good diagnosticians; many others are not. I'd want to feel confident that my chiropractor could detect nerve pressure and, if he found it, would not attempt manipulation. If you're not that confident about a chiropractor's diagnostic abilities, I'd suggest you get a second opinion before proceeding. I am not opposed to chiropractic treatment, but I do have certain reservations, which I will discuss later.

Is a chiropractor the only one who can provide relief by manipulation?

No. In my own practice I usually refer patients to trained physical therapists (or, as we say in Canada, physiotherapists), who are well qualified to perform manipulation. A massage therapist can also provide temporary relief by relaxing the muscle spasm, to get you through that crucial first stage.

What is the attack like if the pain is caused by direct nerve irritation?

There may be a sudden onset of pain, and typically it will be felt more in the leg than in the back. The leg pain may last for a considerable length of time and even be associated with weakness in certain groups of muscles.

If the pain runs into my leg, does that mean I must have a pinched nerve?

No, I didn't say that. All types of back pain can radiate into the leg, and most do. But you can use this test: say to yourself, "I am allowed to complain of only one pain. Which one will it be – the pain in my leg or the pain in my back?" If you choose the leg, there is a good chance that the pain is caused by nerve irritation. If you choose your back or your buttocks, you're probably in the

90 percent group – the people who have either facet or disc pain. You could try one other test to determine the cause of the pain in your leg. Pain in the toes is generally associated with direct nerve pressure. But be careful: we're talking here only about *leg pain* – not the numbness or tingling feelings that so often accompany an attack.

When you describe a disc pain attack as lasting for weeks, are you saying the person will be completely immobilized that whole time?

No. What it means is that after you've come to terms with the initial episode, you will have to rely heavily for some time on all the skills I hope you have learned, or will learn from this book, for dealing with your back. And, depending on the particular situation, I might recommend using a brace.

But aren't you on record somewhere as saying braces aren't a good idea?

Not exactly. I've always maintained that a brace is no substitute for muscle control and exercise. But in the short term, right after an acute attack, a brace may be the only thing that will get you up and around.

And once you are mobile, you should use all those tricks we've talked about here and in Chapter 1. Move slowly with care and grace. Don't make any sudden movements. Use the right seating. Make use of a foot-rest, and so on.

Is this one of those situations where the person's attitude is also important?

Definitely. Fear is your worst enemy. If you're constantly afraid of having another attack, or if you're worried that the present attack will never end, you're bound to be tense. And that tension, of course, will perpetuate the very spasm that is causing the pain. Once you know how to cope with an attack, and once you realize it will subside, you have no reason to be afraid, and you stand a far better chance of recovering quickly.

That sounds very positive – as long as the person has begun a proper program of back care. But what about people who haven't started?

Well, if you've just had an acute attack of pain, this is not the time to begin a long-range program of back care, including daily exercises. But perhaps the attack will serve as your motivation to get started as soon as you're back to normal. That's the best preventive medicine there is for bad backs.

Will regular exercise actually guarantee that you'll never have another attack?

There are no guarantees. Even the best automobile drivers have accidents. But certainly with the right exercise program you will substantially increase the odds in your favor.

3. WHY BACKS GET SORE

When I first wrote about the common causes of backache, I focused on the three principal sources of the pain: a worn facet joint, a bulging disc, and a pinched nerve. Recently, increasing numbers of back patients have been asking about a "new" condition called spinal stenosis, as though it were something doctors had just discovered.

In fact, the importance of an abnormally narrow spinal canal as a cause of pain has been recognized, at least by back specialists, for a generation or more. Its relationship to bulging discs was described in 1953 by Schlesinger and Taveras. In 1954 a Dutch surgeon named Verbiest made the significant observation that structural narrowing of the spinal canal alone could produce nerve-root compression.

In *The Back Doctor*, first published in 1980, I chose not to discuss spinal stenosis as an independent entity but to consider it merely a variation of the pinched nerve syndrome, which indeed it is. Since then, however, advancing medical knowledge and public concern have combined to convince me that spinal stenosis warrants separate classification, partly because of its distinctive characteristics and partly because the very act of singling it out in this way should help to make it more widely understood.

As a result, readers familiar with the contents of *The Back Doctor* may be especially interested to discover that, in this chapter, as I review and elaborate on the conditions responsible for common back pain, I refer not just to the three basic causes described in my first book, but to four. I hope that people who are anxious to know more about spinal stenosis will find their questions answered clearly and completely.

What, exactly, causes a person's back to ache?

There are dozens of possible causes, but let's begin by talking about the causes of almost 90 percent of all cases of common backache, which is the affliction most people will want to know about. The basic problem can be summed up in three simple words: wear and tear, and age.

Wear and tear occurs in various forms over the years, often through nothing more than ordinary everyday activity. It affects the two principal parts of your spine: the little drum-shaped bones called vertebrae and the small, oval pads that separate and cushion them, called discs. Because of the way your spine is constructed, the vertebrae and discs in the lower part of your back carry the heaviest loads and are consequently subjected to the most wear and tear.

Each drum-shaped vertebra has a tunnel along its posterior edge and three wing-like parts protruding outward around that tunnel. A vertebra also has four specialized projections – two pointing upward and two downward – capped with cartilage: a smooth, slippery substance that allows easy movement. Each pair of upward projections interlocks with the pair of downward projections on the adjacent vertebra, forming two knuckle-sized joints called spinal facet joints, or simply facets. These joints are able to bear some of your body's weight, but their main function is to control movement, so that you won't bend or twist your back further than it should go.

Sometimes, as a person ages, a disc will dry out and flatten so much that the two joint surfaces above it will bear down and jam against the two joint surfaces below. That extra pressure within the two facet joints begins to wear away the cartilage covering the bones. This action roughens the surfaces and leads to pain in the joints, a very common cause of backache I call Type One back pain.

Type Two originates in the discs, which normally contain a jelly that helps them serve as cushions, not merely "spacers" between vertebrae. A healthy disc is an excellent hydraulic shock-absorber, although it does not contain any free liquid but rather a fluid-retaining gel. You couldn't puncture a disc with a needle and expect it to leak.

In a young disc, that soft nucleus functions to protect the spine. As a person reaches the mid-teens, the nucleus starts to slowly dry out. Through the years, the disc, losing some of its "cushiony" quality, flattens down in the center and bulges out around the edges. Imagine a round air-cushion half full of air. If you placed it on the floor and stepped on the center of it, the edges of the cushion would bulge out and might even pop open. That's about what happens with a bulging disc. As the shell of the disc spreads beyond its normal diameter, it stretches and frays. The central jelly, now rather hard and lumpy, may be pushed out through a split in the shell.

The outer portion of the disc is pain-sensitive, and if part of it bulges too far out of shape or tears, you will feel Type Two pain.

I think many people believe almost all backache comes from a pinched nerve.

Many people do believe that, while, in fact, Types One and Two are far more common. The pinched nerve is the cause of backache in only one out of every ten patients I see.

Many people also believe that backache caused by a pinched nerve is inevitably more severe than backache from the other two common causes. But that's not necessarily true either. The intensity of pain depends on the severity of local muscle spasm, a feature common to all three types; the amount of inflammation present; the degree of wear in the facet or disc; and the patient's individual response to pain. That last factor is something I will talk more about later.

In Type Three pain, a nerve is being pressed or irritated by a bulging disc, or, when the disc ruptures, by some of the nucleus that has squeezed out through a tear in the shell. This pinching generally occurs at a point where the nerve passes over the back corner of the disc on its way out of the spinal canal. If the disc ruptures, there are only two likely causes of nerve pain: the direct pressure I just mentioned, and an inflammatory reaction in the nerve caused by the jelly from inside the disc – one of nature's unwanted chemical spills.

Discs, however, are not the only source of pressure on the nerves. Nerve irritation is also a part of Type Four back pain, spinal stenosis.

As I mentioned, your spine has a passage called the spinal canal, which runs down through the back of each vertebra. It contains an elaborate system of nerve tissue known as the spinal cord, which is actually an extension of your brain. The spinal cord ends just below the level of your twelfth rib, and the spinal canal in the low back contains nothing but the nerves that run on down to the legs. This complex tangle has the name *cauda equina* or "horse's tail." A pair of nerves from the cord or from the *cauda equina* leaves the canal at every level through small openings on either side of the spine between adjacent vertebrae.

In some people's spines one or more of those openings or part of the lower canal itself is abnormally narrow – too narrow for the *cauda equina* or the roots to pass through comfortably. Like a shoe that's too tight for your foot, the narrow passage exerts pressure on the nerves. That condition is what we call spinal stenosis.

Is there some way for me to determine on my own whether my problem is common backache?

Yes, you can assess your own symptoms and conduct certain tests, which I'll describe in a moment. But first, it's important to make sure your pain is originating in your back. Pain along the spine doesn't always come from the back. Kidney pain, for example, is usually felt in the low back and in one flank and can be extremely severe. Another frequent source of confusion is pain in the hip, so you may want to try this little test:

Lie on your back and draw one knee up to your chest. Does that cause pain in your groin? If so, you may have hip trouble.

Now keep your knee bent and gently turn your lower leg outward. If that also causes pain in your groin and perhaps down
the front of your thigh to your knee, the cause, again, may be
in your hip. If neither movement causes pain, your hip is probably not to blame.

Is there a test to rule out injury to the back?

You don't need a test for that. If your back has been injured severely
enough to cause serious structural damage, you will remember
the incident: an airplane crash, a fall off a building, a major sports
accident, that kind of thing. A healthy back is too rugged to be
injured by minor bumping or an injudicious bit of bending or
stretching.

Then what about disease as a cause of my back pain?

First, most diseases causing back pain also produce symptoms
in so many parts of your body that you wouldn't consider yourself
a backache victim, and you wouldn't be looking for answers in
a book about backs.

Second, you can be fairly certain that your problem is not caused
by a disease of the spine if you can answer "yes" to four questions:

1. Does your back feel better after a good rest?
2. Even if you have recurring attacks in rapid succession, do
you usually recover from each acute episode within a few weeks?
3. When your back is bothering you, are you free of other symptoms: weight loss, skin rashes, fever, joint pain in your fingers,
toes, hips, or knees?
4. Considering your age and physical condition, once the pain
has subsided, does the movement in your back return to normal?
Remember to take into account the fact that after a few weeks
of rest and inactivity, most backs will stiffen up. You may require
a little time and effort to regain your normal flexibility.

"Yes" answers to all four questions virtually ensure that your
back pain is not caused by any disease. Even one or two "no"
answers are not definite indication of a specific illness. Statistically,
it is still far more likely that your problem is common backache –
that is, Type One, Two, Three, or Four.

What are the symptoms of Type One and Type Two back pain?

If you have typical Type One pain, your description might go like this [with variations described in square brackets]:

Each attack begins with a minor incident or nothing at all. In my last incident, I simply bent over to pick up the lawn rake [golf ball, small grandchild]. Instantly, I had a flash of sharp pain in my back, which almost took my breath away. I couldn't move. The pain was worse when I tried to stand up straight, and it eased off a little when I bent forward.

My pain was mainly in my low back, although there was [sometimes but not necessarily] pain in my buttocks and down the back of my leg[s] as far as the knee[s]. I had no pain in my lower legs or feet. If you asked me to pinpoint my problem, I would say the most painful area was the top of my buttocks. I've had other attacks where the pain wasn't so severe but it always starts suddenly and stops me from going on with what I am doing. I know that if I try to arch my back the pain will get worse.

I get the same problem about two or three times a year. If I rest for a few days and don't aggravate the pain, it goes away completely within two weeks [as soon as four or five days]. Usually I can do anything I want between attacks and feel no pain [but I'm always aware of some discomfort that makes me a little nervous].

If you have typical Type Two pain, you might describe your problem this way:

My first attack began when I slipped on a patch of ice, twisted my back but didn't fall [when I found myself holding the whole 200-pound box after my partner suddenly let go].

Like the Type One patient, I've had other attacks following some minor lifting [sudden twists, hockey game, golf swing] but my symptoms are not quite the same. I feel something go [give, pull] in my back. I wouldn't describe it as pain but I know I've done something. At first it's just discomfort. The pain builds up over several hours [a day or two] until it is really severe. It recedes within a few weeks after that, but it doesn't disappear. Instead, it lingers on. One time it was just a nagging backache [another time it was really intense].

TYPE ONE (FACET JOINT PAIN)

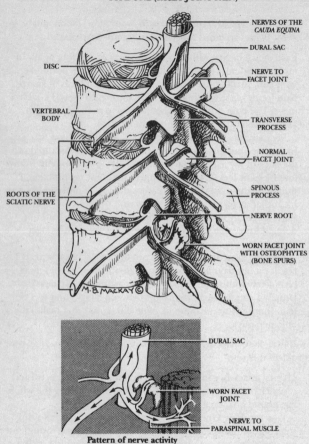

NERVES OF THE *CAUDA EQUINA*

DURAL SAC

NERVE TO FACET JOINT

TRANSVERSE PROCESS

NORMAL FACET JOINT

SPINOUS PROCESS

NERVE ROOT

WORN FACET JOINT WITH OSTEOPHYTES (BONE SPURS)

DISC

VERTEBRAL BODY

ROOTS OF THE SCIATIC NERVE

M. B. MACKAY ©

DURAL SAC

WORN FACET JOINT

NERVE TO PARASPINAL MUSCLE

Pattern of nerve activity from an irritated facet joint

The Type One patient said it hurt to bend backward and felt good to bend forward. I have exactly the opposite problem, and so when I'm active again after an attack, I stand up as straight as I can, and I avoid bending forward or lifting anything.

My pain is mainly in my low back, but I can feel it as well in my buttocks and upper legs — pretty much, I gather, the same as the Type One pain.

The worst part of my problem is that, although an acute attack will be gone in four or five weeks [two or three weeks], it can take me as long as three months [six months] to recover completely.

If you are one of the unfortunates who have a combination of Type One *and* Type Two, you might add this comment:

I have kept a record of my attacks and their duration, and I find that not all my attacks begin the same way or last the same amount of time. I have had acute, short-term attacks interspersed with longer-lasting ones.

Is the problem more serious if it combines Type One with Type Two?

No. But, compared to either type alone, the source of the pain is harder to locate. It's important to note that the wear of normal aging takes place in joints and discs alike, so both areas are usually affected even though only one may cause trouble.

If these descriptions have left you uncertain whether you have Type One or Type Two pain, you might like to perform a few simple tests, which will do you no harm, although they may cause momentary discomfort. Of course I don't recommend that you undertake any testing of this kind while you are still in acute pain. Wait until the attack begins to subside and you feel confident about making unfamiliar movements.

Type One pain increases when you arch backwards to look up. The pain is felt mainly in the back and it radiates downward no further than the knees.

Type Two pain is worse when you bend forward and, again, it is back not leg pain that discourages further movement.

These are positive tests. When one of them produces typical

TYPE TWO (DISC PAIN)

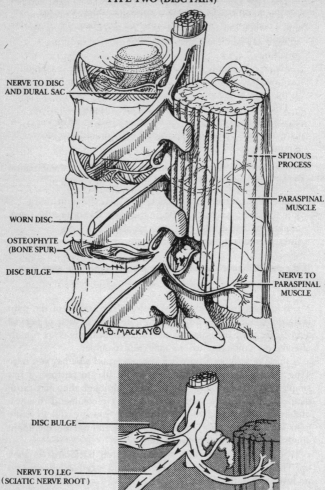

NERVE TO DISC
AND DURAL SAC

SPINOUS
PROCESS

PARASPINAL
MUSCLE

WORN DISC

OSTEOPHYTE
(BONE SPUR)

DISC BULGE

NERVE TO
PARASPINAL
MUSCLE

M.B. MACKAY©

DISC BULGE

NERVE TO LEG
(SCIATIC NERVE ROOT)

**Pattern of nerve activity
from a bulging disc**

pain, we know immediately where the problem lies. A negative test helps confirm that a certain condition does *not* exist. This next test is designed to help you rule out the possibility that your problem is Type Three, a pinched nerve.

As you lie on your back, try to lift one leg with the knee straight. If you can't lift your leg alone, have someone help, gently. Lifting your leg may increase your back pain, but this is not significant, since this movement can aggravate either Type One or Type Two discomfort. The pain to check for is pain radiating down the leg, particularly below the knee and into the foot and toes. If it's Type Three, the pain should occur before the leg is lifted two-thirds of the way to the vertical. Pain occurring after the leg is lifted above that height is generally the result of tight muscles and poor flexibility.

If this test is negative – that is, if you can accomplish the two-thirds lift without pain radiating into your leg – you can conclude with fair certainty that you do not have Type Three pain, and that, as a victim of common backache, your problem must be Type One, Type Two, or a combination of both.

The back pain in Type Four trouble is either from the joints (Type One) or from the discs (Type Two). Although the spinal stenosis may produce pressure on a nerve, the pattern of leg pain differs considerably from Type Three.

What are the symptoms if my problem is Type Three, that is a nerve pinched by a bulging disc?

For a quick grasp of Type Three symptoms, refer back to the description of Type Two. All the symptoms you see there apply to Type Three; but there is one substantial difference. A typical Type Three patient might describe it this way:

My problem is not really my back but my leg. My leg pain is far worse than my back pain, and it doesn't stop at my knees; it radiates into my lower legs [and in some cases, into my feet and toes].

TYPE THREE (PINCHED NERVE)

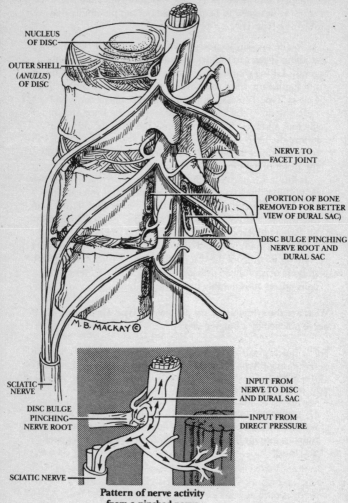

NUCLEUS OF DISC

OUTER SHELL (*ANULUS*) OF DISC

NERVE TO FACET JOINT

(PORTION OF BONE REMOVED FOR BETTER VIEW OF DURAL SAC)

DISC BULGE PINCHING NERVE ROOT AND DURAL SAC

M. B. MACKAY ©

SCIATIC NERVE

DISC BULGE PINCHING NERVE ROOT

INPUT FROM NERVE TO DISC AND DURAL SAC

INPUT FROM DIRECT PRESSURE

SCIATIC NERVE

Pattern of nerve activity from a pinched nerve

Besides straight-leg raising, what other tests can I do to check for Type Three trouble?

Pressure on a nerve usually causes irritation but no loss of normal function. In rare instances when the nerve does lose its ability to conduct messages in an orderly fashion, there are three groups of tests we conduct: for muscle power, reflexes, and sensory ability. The examinations, in order of their reliability and significance, are:

A two-part test for muscle power.
   Part 1: Stand erect and try to raise yourself into a tip-toe position, that is by raising your heels so you're standing on the balls of your feet. Raise and lower yourself ten times this way, on both feet at once and then on each foot separately. The pain may restrict your movement, but if your muscle power is normal you should nevertheless be able to perform this action.
   Part 2: Stand with your feet comfortably apart. Now raise your toes and arches as high off the floor as you can and see whether you can walk that way, with your weight entirely on your heels. It's not a comfortable position at the best of times, but, disregarding the way it may aggravate your back pain, you should able to walk as well this way now as you ever could.

If you passed both parts of the test, your nerve activity to the muscles is probably normal.

A test of your knee and ankle reflexes. What you are trying to find out here is not whether your reflexes are strong or weak but whether they have been changed by your spinal problem. It's significant, for instance, if you find that your once-strong reflexes are now noticeably weaker, or if they have become weaker in one leg than in the other. If your reflexes are normal, your back condition has not affected the function in the nerves that supply the reflex action.
   Knee reflex test: Sit in a chair of normal height and dangle one knee over the other. With a heavy object (such as a moderately thick book), tap the exposed knee sharply but not too severely in the soft area below the kneecap. (Or have someone do the tapping for you.) If the tapping is done properly and your reflex is normal, your leg will kick upward in a sudden,

involuntary motion. If you do not get that reaction the first
time, try several taps before drawing any conclusions. Now
switch to repeat the test on the other knee. If both legs react
with the same involuntary kick, the nerve that supplies that
reflex is probably normal.

Ankle reflex test: Sit down in an ordinary chair, remove your
shoes, and lay the side of one calf over the other knee so that
the ankle and foot project out to one side. Now, in the same
sort of action you used on your knee, rap your Achilles'
tendon – that thick tendon at the back of your ankle, right
above the heel. If you conduct the test correctly, your foot
should jerk downwards. Since this is a harder test to conduct
on yourself than the knee reflex test, you may prefer to have
someone test your ankle reflexes for you. In that case, you can
adopt a different position: kneel on the chair with your ankles
hanging free and have the other person tap gently on one
tendon and then the other. Once several reactions have
occurred, consider whether they are more or less the same for
both ankles. If so, it is unlikely your nerve function in that area
is impaired.

A test of your legs' sensory ability: The objective here is to
determine whether certain parts of your legs or feet have lost
sensation. You are trying to discover whether you still have the
ability to feel the brief flash of pain you normally get from a
pinprick in the skin. Note that this test ranks third in order of
significance and reliability. That's because the area of skin
served by a single nerve is quite variable and because only you
can report on the finding. Your muscular performance and
your reflexes could be observed by others as well as yourself,
but no companion or doctor – even someone who conducts the
test for you – can record the extent of the pain you feel (or
don't feel).

For this test, bare your feet and lower legs, equip yourself
with a safety pin, and sit down. Now reach down and use the
open safety pin in a short, jabbing motion to test three areas
on your feet and legs. First, prick the top of the big toe and
along the inner side of the foot. Now prick the opposite side of
the same foot, from the little toe down the outside edge. Third,
prick a spot anywhere on the calf along the inside of the leg.

Now repeat this procedure on the other foot and leg. If every one of these pinpricks produces typical pain, there's nothing wrong with the nerves' ability to conduct normal impulses from the skin.

If the results of these three groups of tests have all been negative, you have ruled out nerve damage caused by Type Three or Type Four back trouble. Your problem, in all likelihood, is Type One or Type Two pain or, at the very most, Type Three pain with only nerve-root irritation.

I guess that brings us back to Type Four pain – spinal stenosis. How does it develop?

As I said earlier, spinal stenosis is a condition in which the passage containing the large collection of nerves at the bottom of the spine, the *cauda equina*, is abnormally narrow. "Stenosis" just means "narrowing." It's a condition that can be either congenital or acquired.

In a congenital case, the person is born with a small spinal canal that is triangular in cross section instead of the normal five-sided shape. This abnormal size and shape may exist in just a short segment or it may extend throughout the whole lumbar canal. The condition will remain undetected unless the amount of narrowing is enough for the nerves to start feeling the squeeze.

Acquired spinal stenosis will develop when the volume of the spinal canal is reduced by a chronically bulging disc or the normal extra growth of bone that occurs in the spine with age. Of course, stenosis may occur through a combination of congenital and acquired causes – a narrow canal made even narrower by a bulging disc or new bone.

Spinal stenosis sounds like a very serious problem.

Actually the stenosis, in itself, is not the problem. Having a narrow spinal canal is no more painful than, say, having narrow feet. The problem arises when the lack of space interferes with the normal functioning of a nerve. Every symptomatic case of spinal stenosis involves pressure on a nerve, and so in a broad sense, it's like Type Three back pain. But the nature of that pressure is different, and so are the symptoms.

TYPE FOUR (SPINAL STENOSIS)

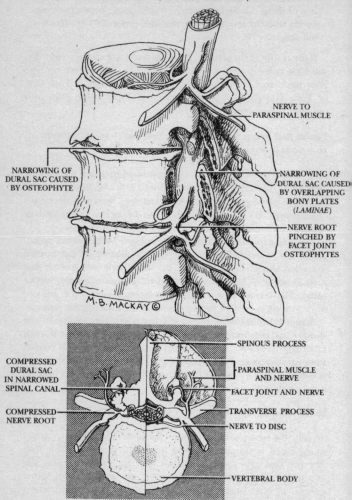

NERVE TO PARASPINAL MUSCLE

NARROWING OF DURAL SAC CAUSED BY OSTEOPHYTE

NARROWING OF DURAL SAC CAUSED BY OVERLAPPING BONY PLATES (*LAMINAE*)

NERVE ROOT PINCHED BY FACET JOINT OSTEOPHYTES

M.B. MACKAY©

COMPRESSED DURAL SAC IN NARROWED SPINAL CANAL

COMPRESSED NERVE ROOT

SPINOUS PROCESS

PARASPINAL MUSCLE AND NERVE

FACET JOINT AND NERVE

TRANSVERSE PROCESS

NERVE TO DISC

VERTEBRAL BODY

Cross section of spinal column with stenosis

Cross section of normal spinal column

In what way are stenosis symptoms different?

Without enough room in the spinal canal, the nerves of the *cauda equina* can't get the extra nourishment they need to supply active muscles. This additional energy normally comes from an increase in the blood supply to the nerves, and a tight fit prevents the blood vessels from expanding to carry the load. At rest, the system manages to keep up with the demand, but as soon as the leg muscles start to work, the nerves are in trouble. In what I call the language of Doctor, this condition is known as *cauda equina* claudication. It occurs only when the narrowing or stenosis is sufficient to interfere with the blood supply to the "horse's tail" or to exiting nerve roots.

If you have typical Type Four pain you might describe your problem this way:

> My back isn't really my problem, it's my legs. And they only cause trouble when I walk. After about ten minutes [a quarter mile, two blocks, a walk down the mall] they get all rubbery [dead, heavy, cold, numb] and I have to stop. If I can sit down for a few [ten to twenty] minutes, my legs feel better, and I can start walking again.
>
> I've noticed I can get relief faster if I sit with one leg drawn up [body bent forward, leaning to one side].
>
> I've tried the Type One, Two, and Three tests. My back hurts more if I bend backward [forward, or doesn't hurt at all]. The rest of the tests indicated no problems.

If the pain is caused by stenosis, does it ever come on as a sudden attack?

No. In cases where the disc is the culprit, the stenosis develops gradually as the disc bulges and begins taking up space in the nerve canal. Unlike the fairly sudden, acute bulging-disc conditions I call Type Two and Type Three pain, this is a slow and subtle impingement on the nerve. Consequently, the person doesn't experience the acute onset of pain that comes with a ruptured disc or the chemical reaction that occurs when the jelly escapes. Instead, the pain develops gradually over time.

In the other form of acquired stenosis, where bony growth is to blame, the narrowing often develops from nature's attempt to overcome facet, or Type One, pain. As you'll remember, I described how the flattening of a disc forces the pair of facet joints to come under increasing pressure. At first, the slippery cartilage surfaces are worn away, producing facet pain. Eventually they become jammed so tightly together that the rubbing stops. And now that the joint is stiff, there is less pain because there's less movement. At that stage, the body begins reshaping the bones of the spine to suit the new conditions.

The body reshapes the spine? How?

Two ways. First, by forming little bony projections or spurs called osteophytes, which help stabilize the joints and disc spaces; osteophytes can do this by growing out from adjacent vertebrae and forming a bridge of bone, which fuses the joint or encloses the disc. And second, the body reshapes the spine by removing other parts of the bone to leave ample room for the exiting nerve roots. When this process is complete, the affected segment of the spine is fused just as securely as it would be if the fusion had been performed by the finest surgeon in the world. The joint is now truly pain-free – but it has also ceased being a joint.

Does this stiffening of the joints and discs immobilize the spine?

No. The amount of stiffness that occurs with fusing one or two levels of the spine is not as serious as you might imagine, and there are certainly many people with stiff backs who can move well enough to participate in a number of sports. You won't be as flexible at sixty as you were at sixteen, but that needn't stop you from leading an active life.

What do osteophytes look like?

Osteophytes have many shapes. Some are just bony lumps that tend to form around worn joints. You can see them often in old people's fingers, in the joints nearest the fingertips. Those cartoons of witches with knobby fingers are exaggerations of a real condition that affects older people as osteophytes form around various joints of their bodies.

Then having those little spurs – osteophytes – in your spine is normal for most people?

Yes. Their growth is normal, part of aging, and the body's regular process of repairing itself.

Do osteophytes ever hurt?

Not usually. People often get upset when their doctors point out this condition on their X-rays. They assume that these bone spurs (which are sometimes described incorrectly as calcium deposits) are a cause of pain – but this is not so. In the early stages when there are periods of rapid growth, osteophytes can be tender, but they don't cause pain.

Then osteophytes don't have to be removed?

Not unless they are causing trouble. More often, they're serving a good purpose. By enlarging the surfaces of the joint, the bone spurs reduce the load on any single point and help to decrease Type One pain.

Spurs also form around the edges of dried-out discs, protecting them from being squashed further. They poke out from the sides of the vertebral bodies like little fingers. In some cases they extend up or down, partly enclosing the disc space and bringing one vertebra into contact with its neighbor, creating a certain amount of stability.

But osteophytes in the spine do cause trouble sometimes?

Yes – they sometimes bring on Type Four back pain. Once in a while a spur that has developed to protect a joint from increased pressure will perform a disservice instead by growing into the spinal canal and squeezing against the nerve root that exits just beside the joint. Doctors refer to this condition as bony entrapment.

Is there any way I can test myself for Type Four pain?

As we've seen, Type Four pain is due to nerve compression similar to Type Three but without the acute onset and chemical reaction. For this reason the tests for muscle power, reflexes, and sensation are usually normal in Type Four trouble *except* when the nerves are working hard and running short of blood. If you suspect you have this type of back problem, go for a walk or do whatever you normally do to bring on the pain. Then, as the attack subsides, perform all the Type Three test maneuvers. This is called a provocative test. If there is any loss of normal nerve conduction – and usually there is *not* – it will be brought out under stress.

Pain may be produced on backward bending (indicating Type One backache) or on forward bending (indicating Type Two). Both types are possible, but pain on arching backward is more common for people suffering with spinal stenosis.

Can spinal stenosis be cured by surgery?

Often it can, in an operation that removes the protruding bone or chronically bulging disc and relieves pressure on the nerve. The operation is called a spinal decompression. As you might suppose, surgery is likely to produce the best results when the narrowing is limited to one or two levels. The more levels involved, the more difficult the surgery and the less likely we are to have a good long-term result.

It's important for patients to understand that we operate because there is nerve-root compression, not simply because we detect a narrow passage.

What if surgery isn't feasible for a person with spinal stenosis – I mean, with nerve-root compression? Are there other kinds of treatment?

Certainly. The right exercises can help a lot. So can better postural habits. But even if surgery is recommended, a person with spinal stenosis should first get started on an exercise program. In most cases patients need flexion (that is, forward bending) exercises; although extension (backward bending) exercises sometimes help. Proper posture is important because it helps keep the spinal canal in the best possible alignment to offer the nerves all the room available.

At the time spinal stenosis is diagnosed as the cause of pressure on the *cauda equina*, or on individual nerve roots, the doctor has no way of assessing the possible benefit to be gained from exercise. Exercise alone may be a sufficient remedy. On the other hand, the doctor and patient may find that in spite of their best efforts, the narrowing is so extreme that relief is possible only through a spinal decompression. Even so, the exercise can do no harm, and obviously it's advisable to try for the maximum benefit without surgery.

Is there a danger, though, of putting off the surgery until it's too late?

No. As long as your condition isn't noticeably getting worse, surgery can be done at any time. The doctor's classic line, "If only you'd come to see me sooner I could have helped you," doesn't apply here. Obviously, if you're having severe pain you'll want to get rid of it as soon as you can. But if there's a good reason for delaying surgery, you can safely pick a time that suits you.

Recently I examined a man with severe spinal stenosis at two levels. In his case, surgery is definitely called for. But he's a busy man. He runs his own one-man company, supplying artificial flowers to florists. It's a seasonal business, and if he stops working during a peak period his company could go under.

The poor man can hardly get in and out of his truck, and so he is torn between the need to keep working and the need for surgery. His question is: "If I wait until next fall, will I have waited too long?"

Fortunately, I could tell him there is no harm in waiting. Since his condition shows no signs of growing worse, there is no reason why the operation can't be delayed for a few months. And in the interim he can try some exercises that might help reduce the pain.

Can surgery relieve Type Four pain even if the person is well on in years?

Oh, yes, it often can. One of my patients is a man in his mid-seventies whose stenosis was preventing him from pursuing his favorite pastime, square dancing. Whenever he danced he got pain in his legs and had to stop. I put him on a program of flexion exercises, and when I found that surgery was feasible I carried out a standard spinal decompression. Six months later he came back and told me with great satisfaction that he could now square dance two sets per evening. In his prime he would dance three sets, but now he was delighted to manage two. Whether stenosis patients have surgery or not, they must realize they are faced with an anatomical problem which may be improved upon but which in some cases cannot be fully corrected, and so they must settle for a few compromises.

Now that you have described the four types, have we covered all the sources of common backache?

No, but we have covered the primary causes. There are several important secondary factors, such as muscle spasm, segmental instability, torsion injury, and minor trauma. They are considered secondary not because they are less painful but because they usually arise from one of the primary causes.

How do muscle spasms fit into this pattern of common backache?

Spasms are very common but they are almost always caused by one of the four primary problems. When part of your spine is irritated or under tension, the muscles at the scene become alerted to the fact that a joint or a disc is in trouble and they tense up to protect the area while it is healing. Their reaction is often sudden and sharp, as it is, for instance, if you sprain a spinal joint. Unfortunately, those muscles may tense up so much that they become painful themselves. You recognize the reaction as a spasm or cramp, and it's the commonest way for muscles to become a source of back pain.

If a muscle is in spasm, it draws extra blood, thereby raising its own temperature. As we'll see later in our discussion of diagnostic tools, this extra heat can be readily detected by a technique called thermography.

When you speak of tension in this case, I presume you mean physical tension.

Not necessarily. Emotional tension can also cause muscle spasm. That's one reason why the psychological factor is often an important component of back pain. You may send one or several muscles into spasm either by tensing up *in fear* of physical back pain, or by tensing up *in response* to it. Either way, your emotions have triggered new or additional pain that otherwise would not have occurred. And as long as you keep reacting that way, you have a self-perpetuating problem.

Then how do you ever get over it?

The answer is easy to say and hard to do: relax. That's one reason why a short period of rest is so important early in an acute attack. But, however you treat it, sooner or later, the tension and pain will disappear as the underlying cause resolves and the muscle spasm relaxes.

What is segmental instability – and is it as frightening as it sounds?

It's hardly what you would call a desirable condition, but it isn't grounds for panic. A literal reading of the phrase tells you pretty much what's involved: a segment of the spine (and by that I mean the disc and facet joints that separate a pair of vertebrae) has a little too much play in it and is therefore unstable. It doesn't mean that your spine is about to collapse in a heap.

In practical terms, you may have trouble straightening up after bending forward. Instead of returning to an erect position in the normal way, you find yourself hitching to one side as you straighten up, as if you were coming up around an invisible post. When a normal spine straightens up, it unwinds from the bottom up in a precise sequence, so that the load – that is, the weight of your body – is transmitted in the most efficient way possible. When a segment of the spine is unstable, the system can't follow that sequence, and the load has to be handled in another, less efficient way.

What causes a segment to become unstable?

Usually it's just the wear and tear of aging in the low back. As a disc dries, squashes down, and bulges out, it loses its firm cushion effect and allows an abnormal degree of movement between the vertebrae above and below it. The facets must accept a greater amount of movement, and that strains the joint coverings. All this produces a little hitch as the spine attempts to move. Again, I stress that the abnormal movement is so slight that nothing will slip out of place, but it is enough to alter the way your spine behaves.

Is segmental instability painful?

Usually it is, and the pain may be different from simple facet or disc pain. Typically it takes the form of sudden sharp jabs, occurring when the person twists suddenly or straightens up from a forward-bent position. The pain is not necessarily felt at the site of the trouble. It often radiates into the top of the buttocks. The actual location of the problem can sometimes be determined by pressing sideways on the bony projections that you can feel along the spine under the surface of the skin. The area of instability may be tender, if not sore. Of course, local muscle spasm can give the same pattern of tenderness in the back, and for that reason the examination is of limited value.

Is there a satisfactory remedy for segmental instability?

Occasionally exercise to strengthen the muscles along the spine can give good relief. For greater degrees of instability the solution may be an operation in which the two adjacent vertebrae are fused together so that they function as a jointless unit. This operation has a high success ratio when the instability is found in only one segment. If several levels are unstable, surgery is more difficult and less likely to succeed.

A friend's young daughter went through a screening program at school and was found to have scoliosis. Naturally, her parents are quite upset.

The term scoliosis refers to an abnormal, side-to-side curve of the spine. Viewed from behind, the back should appear a straight line. The S-shaped curve of scoliosis can result from several conditions: abnormalities of spinal growth, certain neuro-muscular diseases, the extreme effects of wear and tear, and even, temporarily, the severe muscle spasm that can accompany Type Two or Type Three back pain. The term scoliosis, however, describes only the presence of the curve and says nothing about the cause.

I can understand how that girl's parents feel, but chances are they have nothing to worry about. Idiopathic scoliosis (the kind that results from abnormal growth in the spine) is found in about 5 percent of all children, and most cases are so mild that they require no medical attention whatever. Slight curves cause no complications or pain and are scarcely noticeable except to a physician or a nurse who is looking specifically for this condition. Parents are likely to notice only when they see their child wearing a bathing-suit or getting fitted in a clothing store.

Even most of the severe curves are no cause for alarm. They are usually painless, and they can be remedied in several ways if they are detected early. And, these days, most cases *are* detected early, either by family physicians or through scoliosis screening in our schools.

What causes idiopathic scoliosis?

The word "idiopathic," in Doctor, means "without cause." We know a lot about the condition but we don't know exactly why it happens. It is by far the commonest form of scoliosis – the type the public health people look for during the school screening programs. It develops around the age of puberty and is found more often in girls than in boys. For some unknown reason it almost always causes the upper spine to curve to the left. The curve is often associated with a rotation of the spine pushing the ribs backward on the right side of the chest and producing the typical hump. A child's susceptibility to the condition is related to hereditary factors, but researchers have yet to come up with ways of predicting or preventing it.

I've heard that scoliosis causes back pain. Isn't that true?

Surprisingly, idiopathic scoliosis doesn't usually cause pain. The incidence of common backache among people with scoliosis is about the same as for the population at large. And so when people with scoliosis come to me complaining of back pain, I explain that they have two problems: the back pain and the curvature, and each must be treated separately.

What's the treatment for scoliosis?

In most cases, none. Generally the curvature of the spine is so slight that people don't even know they have scoliosis unless it is detected by someone else. Those mild cases cause no difficulties of any kind – even in appearance.

A few youngsters have scoliosis that progresses rapidly during their teens, and they require treatment. Usually they wear braces during their growing years, to keep their spines in proper alignment, much the way you brace a plant to help it grow straight. If bracing is not sufficient, surgery may be required to straighten the back.

For the small percentage of patients who must undergo surgical correction, the process can be arduous. Occasionally, more than one operation is required, and the time in hospital can extend over many weeks. After surgery, the patient is usually required to wear a custom-fitted brace for several months until the fusion is complete. Although major surgery of this type is painful and the effect of repeated hospitalizations can disrupt a normal childhood, the end result with current operative techniques is generally excellent.

Does a scoliotic curve keep getting worse throughout a person's life?

Not very often. If the curve is slight or moderate, it stops progressing, even without medical intervention, once the person is fully grown. Sometimes a severe curve will continue to progress after maturity and require fusion; a brace is no use at that stage.

Some of the fear about scoliosis has arisen because of stories concerning the unusual extreme case that was neglected until it distorted the person's whole body. Or the fear may reflect someone's brief encounter with a child in the midst of a series of intimidating operations or suffering post-surgical complications. But thanks to our increased awareness and surgical skill, such cases are rare these days.

If idiopathic scoliosis is detected at an early stage, as happened with your friend's daughter, there is usually nothing to worry about. She probably won't need treatment of any kind. At most, she will need to have the curve corrected by bracing or, far less likely, by surgery. But one way or another, with modern management, she has little to fear from scoliosis.

You said earlier that some types of injuries are also considered secondary causes of backache. What types did you mean?

I make a distinction between two degrees of injury: on the one hand, a violent physical disruption of the spine – the kind of injury you might suffer in a high-speed automobile crash or by diving head first into a shallow swimming pool – and on the other hand, the degree of everyday strain that will bring on a pain attack because a facet joint or disc has already been made vulnerable through wear and tear. I consider this latter kind of injury to be a secondary factor because it arises out of one of those primary causes of common backache.

Although I keep pointing out that there's an important difference between "hurt," which suggests merely irritation resulting in temporary pain, and "harm," which indicates actual damage, sometimes it's hard for the back pain sufferer to tell them apart. If you walk barefoot on a beach and stub your toe on a rock, you may or may not consider it a serious injury. Even though it's terribly painful you know it's "just a stubbed toe" that will heal itself. Yet there may be an element of physical damage that can lead to annoying, long-term problems. The same principle applies when you sprain a facet joint.

But how would a sprain occur in a facet joint? People don't go around stubbing their spines.

You can wrench a spinal joint and cause an acute sprain by twisting your back violently or picking up a heavy load. The resulting Type One pain may come and go for months. Even though you have not damaged the joint, and it will eventually heal, it may cause you pain for so long that you come to believe the injury is permanent.

It's worth remembering that, compared to the joints in your

fingers or toes, a facet joint can withstand a considerable amount of punishment.

But with a spinal joint sprain, there is also a heavy emotional factor you don't usually find with, say, a sprained ankle. Because they don't understand much about their spines, many people are fearful of having anything happen "back there" and, often, they're terrified of permanent disability. Recognizing the emotional component, you can see how a relatively minor facet joint sprain can quickly become magnified into a major attack of back pain.

If the strain is severe enough, however, the joint may never recover fully from the damage and may remain slightly more susceptible to a new strain or injury, just as you might live out your life with a "trick knee" or weak ankle that was injured years before.

Does that mean that an old injury you've all but forgotten can remain dormant for years and then suddenly flare up in an attack of back pain?

No – that simply doesn't happen. If you're one of those people who have an old problem that flares up every so often, you'll obviously remain aware of it. But if it has healed enough for you to have forgotten about it, you can be sure it's not lurking there, waiting to give you an unpleasant surprise. If you suddenly get an unexpected attack of back pain, you shouldn't blame some old, long-ignored accident. The likeliest explanation is the "last straw" syndrome: you have placed an unaccustomed strain on some part of your spine that has been gradually weakened by natural wear and tear.

But let's not make it sound any worse than it is. Although sprains can be very painful, they are rarely permanent, and even the few that persist indefinitely will produce only temporary episodes of pain, not permanent disability. And the symptoms can often be reduced further by simple care and exercise.

What is a torsion injury?

Torsion and torque are terms borrowed from physics, both meaning rotation or, simply, twisting. In its extreme form, it's the most damaging of all back movements.

Then shouldn't extreme twisting be considered just another form of trauma, rather than a separate cause of back pain?

Yes, if the twisting happens to a healthy back. As you remember, that's what was happening to the young weight-lifter I described in Chapter 1, who was twisting his back so violently doing his "home-made" exercises. But for most of us the torsion affects discs that have already begun to dry out and fray a little.

Exactly how does torsion injure my spine?

If you twist your spine hard enough and often enough, some of the radial-ply fibers in the shells of the discs become slack. Gradually the discs lose their normal resistance to rotation. The more you twist, the easier it becomes for you to stretch those fibers still further. If the excessive rotation continues, the fibers will weaken and may eventually tear. This kind of torque shouldn't be confused with a controlled rotation exercise that can strengthen the trunk muscles and actually protect the discs from injury.

The damage can be more extensive if you combine torsion and load; that is, if you twist your back while some extra weight is bearing down on your spine. For example, if you're working in a warehouse where you must twist to lift heavy cartons from a shelf and place them on a conveyor belt. If you do that long enough by rotating the upper part of your body, instead of using your feet to turn around, you are combining torsion and load in a way that can injure your spine.

What actually happens to your spine when, to use your example, you twist your body while lifting that heavy box?

To understand that you need to know a little more spinal anatomy. The outer shell of the disc is not attached directly to the bone of the vertebra. Rather, it is attached by means of a fibrous cartilage plate known as the end plate. The end plate adheres directly to the flat surface of the bone. When your spine is subjected to extreme torsion under load, a small fragment of the end plate can be ripped right off the vertebra, creating a form of Type Two back pain.

What can be done for a person whose back is injured in this way?

Although the problem involves an end-plate rupture, the result is just another form of disc bulge. If the protruding portion of the end plate and disc wall are close to a nerve root we may have Type Three problems. In either case, most of these people will get better with rest and proper exercise. Very few will need surgery.

The damage can also lead to segmental instability, and we have already talked about the treatment for that.

How do you reconcile your description of common backache with the back problems we all hear about, such as "slipped disc," or "herniated disc" or "disintegrating disc" or "degenerative disc disease"?

I don't try to reconcile them. I concentrate instead on trying to get across the message that many terms you hear used to describe back problems are misnomers, and others are just fancy or long-winded terms for conditions that can be described more sensibly in ordinary language. A herniated disc, for instance, is just a ruptured disc that went to college.

Another part of the confusion arises from the fact that there is an indistinct progression from a disc that is mildly bulging to one that is herniated. From physical examination, it's impossible to tell whether the disc has bulged almost to the breaking point or has actually begun to rupture. There are no changes in the Type Two symptoms. As we've already seen, Type Three pain (pressure on a nerve) can result from a disc that merely bulges or from one where the nucleus has begun to escape.

Among the misnomers, "disintegrating disc" is a fraudulent term. Discs may dry out a little with age but they don't disintegrate. The notorious "slipped disc" is the most pervasive and demoralizing misnomer of all. I wish I had a dollar for every time I've had to explain to someone that there is no such thing. The fibrous outer shells of the discs are so firmly embedded in the cartilage of the end plate that they can't possibly slip out of place. Even if you got struck in the back by a speeding bus, the impact could break the vertebrae without dislodging the discs. That's how firmly the discs are positioned.

The "slipped disc" is just one of those figures of speech that persist as folklore. Some doctors use it although they know how inaccurate and misleading it can be. It's not something they readily admit doing, however. Often when I speak to medical audiences I ask for a show of hands to see how many of my listeners use the term "slipped disc" when discussing backs with their patients. Nobody ever raises a hand. Several years ago, while working in an out-patient department, I overheard the orthopedic surgeon in the next cubicle telling his patient that she had a slipped disc. I felt a strong urge to leap into the room and accuse him of being the one who's going around North America spreading all this misunderstanding.

"Degenerative disc disease" is another phrase that invites confusion. Some doctors use the term – mostly, I suspect, because it abbreviates conveniently as "DDD" in the notes they write for patients' files. All that DDD means, really, is wear and tear. I object to the use of a pretentious word like "degenerative" instead of "wearing out," but I am far more upset by the use of the word "disease." By any reasonable definition, wear and tear is not a disease, whether it occurs in a facet joint during the normal use of your spine, or in the palm of your hand during a tug-of-war contest. ("Stop the tug-of-war and call the doctor, Ma! I've got degenerating palm disease!")

I dislike the term not only because it overstates the seriousness of simple aging but also because it's likely to send patients off in search of a cure – and we're not talking about a curable affliction. We're talking about a condition that has to be managed over a long period to prevent avoidable wear and to give nature time to contribute to the healing process.

But surely a lot of terms we hear aren't just folklore or fancy phrases. Arthritis, for instance – isn't it a disease that often attacks the spine?

No, arthritis is not a disease, either. It's just a description meaning "inflamed joint." It says nothing about why the inflammation has occurred. And, as you no doubt realize, a joint can become inflamed for many different reasons.

Let's assume that I am hurrying out of a room and I accidentally slam the door on my thumb. Immediately the joint of my thumb becomes swollen and sore. Does that make me an arthritis sufferer? Most people would say no, but the correct answer is yes. Technically, any time one or more of my joints are inflamed I have arthritis.

The term arthritis, then, doesn't convey much useful meaning unless it's accompanied by an adjective or phrase indicating what caused it. The type of arthritis that comes from injuring a joint is called traumatic arthritis. The inflammation that develops in the facet joints of the spine as a result of the natural wear and tear of aging is called osteoarthritis. And, as you might suppose, the word "arthritis" is used with various other adjectives to denote joint inflammation from various other causes.

For that reason, you can't expect to get a helpful answer if you go to your doctor and say, "I've got arthritis – what should I do about it?" All you are telling him, at the very most, is that you have an inflamed joint, or, more likely, just that you have a sore joint. Without knowing *why* the joint is sore, the doctor has no information on which to prescribe treatment. He must determine the cause of your arthritis before he can help you.

But doesn't the arthritis society run ads on television and in the newspapers suggesting that arthritis is a terrible disease for which they are trying to find a cure?

That's right. I remember one of their TV commercials. It showed people's hands with the joints grotesquely deformed by rheumatoid disease. But the message was: "Beware of arthritis."

Isn't that a form of misleading advertising?

Yes, but I suppose they would argue that all they have done is leave out the qualifying adjective to keep the message clear and simple, since the public really doesn't care whether they are seeing rheumatoid arthritis, osteoarthritis, traumatic arthritis, or any other kind, for that matter. After all, a commercial is supposed to be an attention-getter, not a scientific lesson. And it *is* all in a good cause, since the society is trying to find a way to prevent or cure diseases that cause joints to become inflamed. Nobody can quarrel with an aim like that, but the unfortunate side effect is that the word arthritis becomes impressed in many people's minds as the name of a serious disease instead of what it is – merely a description of an inflamed joint.

Matters are only made worse by the fact that many doctors use the word casually and incorrectly to describe a wide range of conditions that can produce sore joints – the well-known "touch of arthritis."

In fact, the notion of arthritis as a disease is so thoroughly entrenched in our thinking that some back patients refuse to believe that their inflamed joints are the result of nothing more than wear and tear. In their view, wear and tear may be something that happens to other patients' backs, but their own problem is the "disease" they know as arthritis. And that's a shame, because as long as they see their condition that way, they are unlikely to be interested in the simple preventive measures that can help them.

Then you're not objecting just because some people don't use certain words according to the definitions in some medical dictionary.

Certainly not. I object in general to the misuse of a word like arthritis for two very practical reasons. First, because the misused word often displaces a term that could tell you something useful; and, second, because it often conveys a false impression in a patient's mind. A patient will ask me, "If I have arthritis in my shoulder, will it spread to my spine?" Obviously, the person is thinking of arthritis as a disease capable of moving around the body, wreaking pain and destruction wherever it goes. But now that you understand what arthritis really means, you can see that although the concern is valid, the question is meaningless. Any possible spread depends on the underlying cause of the problem and not on the mere presence of an inflamed joint.

I am just as critical, by the way, when medical people confuse their patients by speaking the language of Doctor – deliberately ignoring perfectly useful everyday words in favor of pretentious medical terms. A physician addicted to speaking Doctor may tell a patient, for instance, that he has "a myofascial sprain" when he could simply say "a pulled muscle."

I'm beginning to suspect that Doctor as a language is even more contagious than many of the afflictions it describes. I was sitting down for a haircut the other day when my barber suddenly announced that I had *alopecia areata*. The very idea would have paralyzed me with fright if I hadn't happened to know that *alopecia areata*, in simple English, is a bald spot. And in fact it wasn't even *that* – it was only a cut from a minor mishap several weeks earlier. I should have countered him by saying he'd been standing around in his shop so long that he'd developed a bad case of *pes planus* – that's Doctor for flat feet.

Some technical terms are necessary, of course, because they have no equivalents in ordinary language. But many terms you hear add little, and doctors would be performing a great service by abandoning them when they're talking to their patients.

How can a patient tell, then, which terms are significant and which are just fancy ways of saying ordinary things?

Any time your doctor uses a term you don't understand, ask what it means. Never be ashamed to admit you don't know some medical word or phrase. Medical people don't know them all either, and many of them speak poor Doctor.

The word sciatica is a good example. Sciatica means acute leg pain caused by direct pressure on a nerve. But by sloppy usage it has come to mean any leg pain associated with back trouble. And, as I have mentioned, leg pain is a symptom of all four types of common backache, whereas only Type Three produces true sciatica. And so if I merely tell another doctor that a patient has sciatica I may be using the word correctly, but the other doctor can easily misunderstand the meaning.

We've talked a lot about common backache, but there must be specific diseases that cause pain in the back.

Yes, and there are two in particular that ought to be mentioned here. One is ankylosing spondylitis; the other is rheumatoid disease.

Ankylosing spondylitis is primarily a young man's disease, with very distinctive characteristics. These include a visible flattening of the surface of the low back, loss of chest movement, progressive stiffness in the joints of the spine, and, in about half of all cases, stiffness in the hips or knees. The spinal stiffness is particularly noticeable first thing in the morning, and it is greatly relieved by exercise or almost any form of physical activity. If you think I have just described your symptoms, ask your doctor for an examination. There are some X-rays and blood tests which can rule out this and several other diseases that affect the back.

Rheumatoid disease is a condition in which the body reacts against itself, behaving as though it were coping with a foreign substance. It's a process that can affect many parts of the body including the nervous system, the internal organs, the skin, and, of course, the joints. If the joints are affected they become inflamed and eventually damaged. This aspect of the disease is called rheumatoid arthritis.

Obviously, it can be a serious affliction at its worst, but the great majority of patients with rheumatoid disease do very well. And to keep it in perspective: only 2 percent of the population have the disease, and only 10 percent of *those* people have severe joint problems. What those percentages mean, then, is that only two people out of a thousand suffer severe joint problems from rheumatoid arthritis. In contrast, about 800 out of every thousand people, at some time in their lives, suffer from common backache.

Then only a tiny fraction of all back pain sufferers have arthritis caused by rheumatoid disease?

Exactly. But can you imagine how many of them saw that TV commercial depicting rheumatoid arthritis – and how upset and frightened they would have been if their doctors told them later that they had a "touch of arthritis" in their spines?

Yet we know from statistics that most of those people have nothing more than a minor case of Type One or Type Two back pain. Their backs are hurting simply because the facet joints are worn. That's the extent of their arthritis.

Then you're not just quibbling when you insist on correct usage of terms like arthritis.

Far from it. A talented writer once said, "The difference between the *right* word and the *almost-right* word is like the difference between a lightning bolt and a lightning bug."

As a back patient, do yourself a favor: don't be frightened by words. Those lightning bolts you're worrying about may well turn out to be nothing more than lightning bugs.

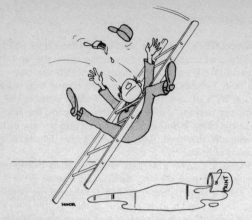

4. "WHIPLASH" AND OTHER FOLKLORE

As an author, lecturer, and physician, I have seldom passed up an opportunity to poke fun at the idea of the "slipped disc." It's one of the great fallacies of our time, and I like to think my efforts have helped reduce popular belief in this frightening and erroneous phrase. Unfortunately, it's only one of several common and misleading expressions that create a lot of unnecessary apprehension and fear.

This chapter is devoted to three such misunderstood terms. One is that special favorite of the legal profession: whiplash.

The other two are the broken neck and the broken back. Both are injuries that can, of course, be extremely serious. But, contrary to popular impression, they do not automatically consign their victims to paralysis or death. Right at this moment there are people walking around with broken backs who'll tell you they have nothing ailing them but a few stiff muscles. And I've seen many patients with broken necks who have recovered and now have no neck pain at all.

Is it true that whiplash is one of the most serious ailments you can have?

You have just expressed a basic misconception shared by many people. However, *whiplash is not an ailment or physical injury at all but an action* that occurs to the neck under certain specific conditions and may or may not cause injury.

The commonest situation, as you probably know, is a traffic accident where the victim is riding in a car that is struck from the rear. Being rear-ended by another car is not the same as being in the car that does the rear-ending. They involve two entirely different forms of impact, and they propel you in distinctly different ways.

If you are in a high-speed accident where your car rear-ends another vehicle or crashes into some other obstacle, your body may be restrained but your head is thrown forward. It can't bob forward very far before your chin hits your chest. That may hurt a lot. It may bruise your chin and wrench your back muscles. But the action is limited, and because your neck is protected from further movement, there is no whiplash effect.

Now consider what happens if you're in the car that gets rear-ended in a high-speed collision. Let's assume your car seat is not equipped with a head-rest. When the vehicle behind you smashes into your car, your whole body, from the shoulders down, is suddenly propelled forward. Your head, having nothing in back of it, gets left behind. In this situation, there is no equivalent of your chin striking your chest, and so your head snaps backward as far as it can go. (Some victims recall having their heads thrown back so far that for a split second they actually caught an upside-down glimpse of the car's rear window.) An instant after this violent backward motion, your head recoils forward with almost equal force.

Your neck, which lacks the protective structure of your middle and lower spine, has just been subjected to whiplash. And, of course, the more violently your head is thrown backward and forward in that lashing motion, the greater the strain on the muscles, ligaments, and joints in your neck. That's why a rear-end collision poses a greater threat to your neck than colliding head-on.

Is it true that once you've suffered from whiplash your neck will never be normal again?

That depends on the nature and extent of the injury. If it's really severe, the ligaments that stabilize the bones in your neck could be torn, some joints in your upper spine could be severely sprained, or several vertebrae could be fractured. But if you're in a low-speed rear-end collision where that whiplashing action is minimal, you may sustain only minor injuries or no injuries at all.

I'm beginning to see why you say whiplash is not actually an ailment or physical injury.

It's one of those words that confuses an issue. Although you may *experience* whiplash, there is no such thing as *having* whiplash in the sense of having a sore joint or a sprained ligament in your neck. Whiplash, in other words, is just a way of getting hurt. There are lots of ways to get hurt, as we all know. You can slip on an icy sidewalk or walk into a brick wall or fall off a ladder.

If I called you up on the phone and told you I fell off a ladder last weekend, you'd wonder whether I merely skinned a knee or was lying in a hospital with two broken legs and several cracked ribs. You'd ask, "Were you badly hurt?" You wouldn't say, "Oh, what a terrible thing! You've got ladderfall! My Uncle George, the house painter, got ladderfall once, and he almost died!"

Yet people talk that way about whiplash, not realizing that, like "ladderfall," it's a term that describes a possibly injurious action but says nothing about the actual damage – if any. That's why it's meaningless to say, "I've got whiplash – will I ever be normal again?" Or, "What's the treatment for whiplash?" The answers depend on what injuries occurred and how serious they are.

You may be technically right, but my sister's doctor told her she had whiplash – and her lawyer even proved it in court.

That doesn't surprise me. Lawyers misuse the term all the time, and so do some doctors. A woman who had been in a car accident years earlier came to see me about neck pain. In the course of relating her medical background, she made a point of repeating something she was told right after the accident. A young doctor (fresh out of medical school, I suspect) examined her neck and announced that she had the worst case of whiplash he had ever seen.

Never mind that probably this young doctor had never before examined a patient with acute neck pain. Since he was not present at the accident he could not have *seen* her whiplash – only its result. Yet a frightening comment like that, especially from a medical person, can seriously inhibit recovery. This woman honestly believed she had "the worst case of whiplash" in the annals of medicine. There was nothing I could say to convince her she would some day get well.

In contrast to that young doctor, others go to the opposite extreme. Instead of simply rejecting whiplash as a diagnosis and explaining that it's a mechanical action, some doctors deny that there's any such thing at all. And so the patient hears that opinion from the doctor, only to hear it contradicted by his lawyer, who probably sees "whiplash" as a magic word worth several thousand dollars in court. And, of course, when it suits their argument in litigation, lawyers can make a whiplash injury sound far worse than it is.

Lawyers also apply the term far too broadly, sometimes using it to mean a neck injury of any kind. Obviously, they savor the sound of the word. I have to admit "whiplash" sounds a lot more dramatic and damaging than "sprain" or even "torn ligament." Unfortunately, there are some doctors who do not hesitate to use the term when testifying in court. It's not hard to guess which witness the jury would find more convincing – the specialist who details the horrors of whiplash or the one who drones on about minor soft-tissue injury.

Some lawyers codify this misconception further by putting price tags on this non-existent diagnosis. I've heard them talk about a client having "a five-thousand-dollar whipper" ("whipper" being Lawyer for a whiplash injury). In this example, five thousand dollars does not refer, as you might assume, to the patient's medical costs. It's the amount the lawyer calculates the "whiplash" might generate in settling a court case. And I can hardly blame anyone for reasoning that if whiplash is worth that kind of money in a court of law, it must surely be a real and serious condition.

Do head-rests on car seats help prevent the whiplash effect?

The good ones do, but most head-rests are poorly ,designed or incorrectly positioned. They are almost always too low. A head-rest is useless behind your neck. To provide the support needed to prevent the whiplash action, it must be behind your head.

I suggest that all car owners check their head-rests to see that they're high enough. If a head-rest is too low and cannot be adjusted, it should be replaced. That may be costly, but it will be well worth the money if it can prevent a serious neck injury. In certain circumstances, a properly installed head-rest can prove as important to safety as a seat belt. And while we're on the subject, I can testify from professional experience that seat belts save lives and prevent many serious injuries, and I urge every driver and passenger to use them.

You've explained what whiplash is but you haven't said much about the injuries it can cause. Can whiplash break a person's neck?

Yes – although, as I said earlier, a broken neck is not necessarily fatal or crippling. When your head is whiplashed back and forth, the ligament along the front of the spinal column may be torn. If it tears loose, it may take with it a little bit of bone from the front of a vertebra. And, technically, that's a broken neck – a fracture in this case caused by whiplash. (I never use those terms without reminding people that there is no difference between a break and a fracture or a crack. They all mean the same thing.)

People worry a lot about broken necks and broken backs, and I don't blame them. According to popular mythology, a broken back will paralyze you for life and a broken neck will kill you. These notions are not entirely fictional, of course. They're based on true stories of very serious mishaps – people diving into shallow pools or getting their necks snapped in skiing accidents. But for every life-threatening case there are hundreds of cases of broken vertebrae that are almost inconsequential.

I've seen patients who had broken necks and didn't even know it. And yet in each instance the break was there to be seen by X-ray. The person didn't realize it was a fracture because it hurt no more than a muscle spasm would. Perhaps the break occurred because bone had grown abnormally thin, as it does with the osteoporosis found in older people. In such cases, the only symptom may be a bit of temporary neck pain.

It must be touchy to tell a patient, "You've got a broken neck."

In cases like that, I'm very careful about what I say – or, more precisely, how I say it. I want people to realize that a broken neck is not necessarily a serious problem. And, knowing what the typical view is, I'm wary of causing needless alarm. Unless the question comes up directly, I tend not to use the term "broken neck." Instead, I would describe the problem in more specific terms, by saying something like, "There's a small crack in one vertebra. . ."

I gather that even when it is very painful, a broken neck is unlikely to be life-threatening.

Yes, that's true. One good example is an injury known as clay shoveler's fracture, which occurs in the lowest of the seven vertebrae in your neck. That's the bone that forms a little bump at the point where, so to speak, your neck joins your back.

Clay shoveler's fracture is exactly what it sounds like: an injury that occurs when someone digs into clay or other hard ground. He stabs the point of the shovel into the soil but it doesn't give. The shovel stops dead, sending a jolt up through the person's arms and shoulders. His back muscles react with such tension that they tear away a wing-like part of the vertebra called the "spinous process."

I know that sounds horrible, and certainly it's painful, but it's not as damaging as you might suppose. It doesn't affect the function of the neck or the nerves. It's a broken neck in the true sense of the term but it has no serious consequences.

How do you treat a clay shoveler's fracture?

There's no need to treat it. The spinous process heals by itself. The victim is in pain and won't feel like using a shovel for a few months. But otherwise he is okay.

My main point is that there are many forms of broken necks and broken backs that you don't often hear about because they aren't dramatic or dangerous.

Let's talk about the serious cases.

All right, but they, too, need to be kept in perspective. A broken neck can be very serious. If a bone in your neck is fractured and dislocated, it may move and cut the spinal cord. And if that cut occurs above the level of the nerves that control the diaphragm, you stop breathing and die.

But the human body can survive some devastating injuries and eventually mend itself. I had one patient who suffered a broken neck in a car accident. The car ran off the road into a deep ditch, rolling over several times. The man doesn't know exactly what happened but he remembers having to lift his head by his hair; he couldn't raise it any other way. He had broken the vertebra near the top of the neck that permits the head to rotate from side to side. The broken bone had shifted slightly out of place, but luckily there was no damage to the spinal cord, and his nervous system was functioning normally.

For treatment, he was fitted with an outfit called a halo vest, which is now standard equipment for such cases. The halo is fastened to the skull with specially designed screws, and mounted on metal posts, which are attached to a shoulder harness and incorporated into a plastic vest. The idea, of course, is to immobilize the neck until it mends.

This fellow wore that outfit for about four months. He wasn't comfortable but he was up and around. Certainly it was better than the old-style treatment, which would have kept him flat on a turning frame for the same time, in traction provided by a pair of skull tongs.

After the prescribed time, the halo vest was removed. The fracture had healed, and the man's neck was normal again. I mention this case not because the recovery was exceptional – it wasn't – but because the outcome is typical of what patients with this sort of serious injury can expect.

You did say earlier, though, that the neck lacks the protective structure of the middle and lower spine. Does that mean my neck is more vulnerable than my back?

Yes, it is. Your neck contains seven vertebrae interspersed with discs. These are the cervical vertebrae, and they are designated (from the top down) as C_1 through C_7. The C_1 is called the atlas, named for the Titan from Greek mythology who bore the earth on his back and the heavens on his shoulders.

The atlas is unlike any other vertebra in your spine. A ring-shaped bone with flat surfaces, top and bottom, it balances two small prominences extending from the base of the skull. The atlas is joined to the second (or C_2) vertebra, called the axis, which has a peg known as the "odontoid process" that sticks up through the front of the C_1 ring and is held in place by very strong ligaments. This peg-in-a-hole arrangement permits you to rotate your head from side to side. (The odontoid was the part that got broken in the case of the car accident victim I mentioned; you can understand why he had trouble lifting or turning his head.)

Passing down behind that "tooth" is the spinal cord, which comes out of a hole in the skull, passes through the ring of C_1 and through the hole behind the odontoid process of C_2.

The other five neck bones (C_3 through C_7) are much like the vertebrae in the lower back, except that they are smaller, and the holes forming the spinal canal, for the spinal cord, are proportionately larger.

The facet joints in the neck, instead of being L-shaped like those in the low back, are flat, like clutch plates in a car. Because of their shape, your neck vertebrae don't interlock the way the vertebrae do in your lumbar spine. They rely instead on joint capsules and ligaments to hold them in place.

Like any movable joint, a facet joint can be dislocated. Dislocation is the complete separation of one joint surface from another. Because of their structure, neck joints are more likely to be dislocated than low back joints. In the low back, you'll never find a dislocation unless one or more bones are broken. In your neck, it's possible to have a dislocation without a fracture.

I gather that cases of broken backs run the same gamut as broken necks, from minor to serious.

Yes, they do. As you can appreciate by now, the concept of the broken back is far too broad and vague to have any real meaning. We think of broken backs as occurring in horrendous traffic collisions or falls from tall buildings. These injuries do occur, of course, and can be fatal or leave permanent and serious disability. But a broken back can be the result of something as mild and simple as a sneeze in the case of a person with osteoporosis. The sneeze – or, more precisely, the pressure that a sneeze exerts on the spine – can crush a vertebra slightly, and that, technically, is a broken back. If you break your back that way, you will suffer some pain for about six weeks but there will be no serious results – no instability of your spine, no nerve damage, no degenerative change. The bone will heal by itself, and you may not even realize it was crushed.

In another situation, you can have an injury to the vertebrae when the back muscles suddenly tense up and pull off one of the "transverse processes," which are other wing-like projections on the sides of the vertebrae. Or if you get hit in the back hard enough, those little wings may crack. In either case, you have a broken back.

But, again, these are not serious injuries. Usually, the breaks heal quickly and easily, the muscles reattach themselves, and you are soon feeling fine. Nothing important will have changed – not the structure, the stability, the nerve function, or anything else. Even when a detached transverse process fails to mend itself, it remains captive within its assembly of muscles and ligaments and presents no serious problem. Mind you, it will be painful from the outset – a broken bone always is – and the pain may last for months. But hurt, as I have pointed out before, is not the same as harm.

Then you never consider performing surgery after a break of that kind?

No. In fact, most people who break their backs do not require surgery. The back has a tremendous ability for recovery and a great margin of protection. I already mentioned crushed vertebrae. You may find this hard to believe, but in a serious accident it's possible for a vertebra to be crushed – usually at the front – until it is only two-thirds of its normal height, and yet the victim will suffer only temporary pain. The body gradually adjusts to the new situation.

An older person with osteoporosis may end up with half a dozen or more crushed vertebrae over a period of years. The condition is easy to spot: the crushed vertebrae, being wedge-shaped instead of uniform height front and back, give the spine an unnatural forward curve, making the person round-shouldered.

In appearance, it's quite a pronounced abnormality and can lead to chronic backache, but it causes no nerve damage or other problems. And so, spinal fracture, per se, doesn't call for surgery.

There must be some cases when surgery *is* called for?

Yes. For example, surgery is advisable when a vertebra is not just crushed but shattered. This is what we call a burst fracture, and it is dangerous because fragments of bone can become lodged in the spinal canal, where they may interfere with the nervous system and cause partial paralysis.

Until a few years ago, this condition was hard to diagnose, because the injury cannot be seen with any certainty on conventional X-ray or even on a myelogram. Now, thanks to the computerized axial tomograph scanner – the diagnostic machine usually known simply as the CT or CAT scan – we can identify these "bursts" of the bone quite precisely. Once they have been located, a surgeon can go in and remove them. Incidentally, this is usually done from the front of the patient's body, because that route normally provides better access to the fracture fragments.

After that operation will a paralyzed person usually regain his or her normal functions?

The amount of paralysis will depend largely on the damage done to the spinal cord or to the *cauda equina* at the time of injury. But, obviously, if pressure from the bone fragments continues, removing these fragments gives the patient the best possible chance for recovery. Unfortunately, unlike so many other parts of the body, the spinal cord has very limited powers of regeneration, and once serious damage has occurred there may be little chance for a return of normal function.

My main point, however, is that while surgery is called for when there is a specific task to perform, such as restoring adequate stability or removing bone fragments from the spinal canal, most vertebral injuries can be safely left to heal by themselves. And that includes a good many broken backs.

One example is the Chance fracture, which was first described back in the 1940s by a doctor with the delightfully unlikely name of Quigley Chance.

Chance fractures are hardly ever seen any more. They were more common some years ago, when most cars had lap-type seat belts, with no shoulder restraints. When a passenger is involved in a violent, head-on collision while wearing a lap belt, the belly has no time to compress. The person's body is folded over the belt, with all the bending taking place at the front of the abdomen. This abnormal bending pattern can literally tear the spine apart. The discs in the spine are so tough and so securely attached that they are not affected, but the bone, being weaker, is torn in two. In an X-ray it looks as though someone has taken a cheese cutter and sliced the bone in half and then yanked the two pieces apart, creating a gap that may be a quarter of an inch wide.

Are you saying that people can survive such a horrible injury?

Yes – although you wouldn't think so if you could read the X-ray. And yet, usually after a few months he or she will be walking around with no serious nerve damage whatever and certainly with no paralysis. Typically, the only complaint is back pain, which gradually subsides as the gap between the two pieces of the vertebra eventually fills up with new bone growth so that the spine functions normally.

You've certainly convinced me that whiplash and broken necks and backs are not necessarily the life-shattering experiences that most people suppose.

I hope I have. I don't want to minimize the seriousness of the injuries that occur in some cases, but it's important to keep things in perspective. Otherwise, some people will worry needlessly about life-long disabilities arising out of accidents from which, in reality, they will recover nicely.

Sometimes people have anxieties about complications that can't possibly happen. For instance, I've talked to patients and their relatives who were afraid that a person who has been injured in the low back might have damaged the spinal cord. Happily, I can dispel that fear by pointing out one simple fact: in that lowest part of your spine, there *is* no spinal cord, only a bundle of more resilient nerve roots.

Surely you don't expect people to be walking around with that kind of medical information in their heads.

No, of course not. I expect people to spend their time thinking about matters of more immediate concern than how their bodies work or what certain medical and pseudo-medical terms mean. But I do hope that readers who find themselves in emergency wards, either as accident victims or as attending relatives, will be able to remember the information in this chapter and keep things in perspective.

If anyone tells you someone "has whiplash," or is suffering from "a broken neck" or "a broken back," I hope you'll realize that the situation is probably not nearly as bad as it sounds. Your best response is to ask exactly what the damage is and what the consequences are likely to be.

Ninety-nine times out of a hundred, if you ignore those ominous phrases and all the emotional baggage that goes with them, you can draw a lot of comfort from learning the facts and remembering how adept the human body is at surviving injury and healing itself.

5. ABOUT THAT PAIN IN YOUR NECK

Like many people, I'm seldom satisfied with my first attempt at anything, and I tend to worry long after it's too late to make changes. Whether it's a matter of planning an "ideal" house, or writing a first book, most of us look back on the finished product and see things we wish we'd done differently.

In the case of my first book, *The Back Doctor*, I didn't have to do the second-guessing alone; my readers offered me numerous comments that proved most helpful when the time came to plan this second volume. Many of them told me they wished I had said more about neck pain. Originally I thought I had covered the subject thoroughly enough in a book which, after all, was written primarily for people with bad backs. Even at that, the index lists sixteen references under "neck" and four others under "cervical spine."

Necks and low backs, of course, have many problems in common. They are, after all, both parts of the same biomechanical system. But many of the specific questions I was asked about the nature and treatment of neck pain were not answered in my first book.

This chapter, then, is intended to deal with the concerns I have heard expressed so often in the past half-dozen years. Certainly I have never underestimated the importance of neck pain. A full

50 percent of all the people who come to me with back problems have neck pain as well, and some 20 to 30 percent of all my patients are people with nothing *but* neck pain.

And so I dedicate this chapter to those two groups and others like them for whom neck pain is, or might become, a problem.

My doctor keeps referring to my problem as neck pain, and yet the pain really isn't in my neck. The worst of it is along the top of my shoulder and beside my shoulder blade.

If your pain runs along the inner border of your shoulder blade, it probably comes from your neck. I understand why you might think there is something wrong with your shoulder, because that's where it hurts. But often that's not where the trouble originates.

It can be quite confusing. I have a simple test I use to separate pain referred from the neck from pain arising in the shoulder itself, and it's something you can try for yourself:

Place one hand over the most painful area. Now take careful note of the location. If your hand is over the upper part of the arm, you probably have true shoulder pain. But if your hand is on top of your shoulder, it is more likely you have neck pain that is radiating into the area.

Are you saying all neck pain is felt on top of the shoulder?

By no means. Commonly, neck pain is literally, as well as figuratively, a pain in the neck. Usually you'll feel the pain most intensely in the back of your neck, and often that's because the muscles there are in spasm. Sometimes the pain radiates downward into your shoulders and back because the spasm spreads into the *trapezius*, a big kite-shaped muscle that starts with a point at the base of your skull, reaches the tips of both shoulders, and extends down over much of your back to another point on your spine above the waist.

When spasms occur, you are likely to notice little tight knots along the upper ridge of *trapezius* muscle on top of your shoulders.

This is a location where emotional tension is often felt. And if it is your neck pain that is making you tense, you get a double whammy: pain from the original cause, plus pain from the muscular tension.

Of course it's possible to have neck and shoulder pain at the same time from separate causes. In fact 10 to 20 percent of all people with neck pain have separate (though usually related) trouble in the shoulder. Your shoulders are contained in rather loose capsules that permit a wide range of movement, but if the joints are kept immobile – as they often are when neck pain spreads to the shoulder area – the folds of that capsule get stuck together. Soon you find you can't raise your arm without pain, and every attempt to move the shoulder increases the agony. The area around the joint is bound with scar tissue, and every time you move your tear it a little. This condition is aptly described as "frozen shoulder."

The same thing can happen to your shoulder if you break your wrist. Putting your wrist in a cast and your arm in a sling immobilizes the shoulder. To avoid the risk of having your shoulder seize up, you shouldn't wear the sling any longer than a couple of weeks. For the same reason, the therapy for a person recovering from a broken wrist will routinely include practicing shoulder movement.

A friend of mine told me she had pain that apparently started in her neck and went past her shoulders all the way down her arms into her hands. Is this possible?

Yes, that can certainly happen. More often, there is pain radiating into the shoulder and upper arm, about as far as the elbow, with tingling, numbing, or burning sensations down into the hand.

The fact that the symptoms are felt in areas other than the neck doesn't mean the pain is any less intense. The pain you mentioned that radiates from your neck down along your shoulder blades can be especially troublesome. In fact, it can become the dominant problem – deep-seated, sometimes causing nausea, and usually aggravated by any sort of movement or the slightest tensing of the muscles. Often, it's not even relieved by lying down and trying to relax. That pain can be excruciating, as I know from personal experience.

As you may realize, the process of pain radiating from the neck is much the same as the pain that spreads into the legs when someone has low-back trouble. In that case, the worst pain is often in the thighs, hips, or buttocks.

This similarly won't surprise you if you understand something of the structure of the human nervous system. In your neck, six nerve roots on each side combine into an elaborate arrangement called the *brachial plexus*, which sends three major nerves into your arm to perform specific functions. In your low back, you have a comparable group of nerve roots, which join together to form the more familiar sciatic nerve. It's actually a bundle of nerves that run down the leg to perform specific functions there.

As a result, if a certain nerve root leaving your spine detects a painful condition in the back, you may feel symptoms in the distant location which that nerve supplies. This spread is called referred pain and must be differentiated from pain running into the arm or leg because of actual nerve damage. One nerve commonly involved with referred pain exits between the fifth and sixth vertebrae in your neck and runs down to your thumb and forefinger. (In anatomical terms, there are seven cervical vertebrae numbered from the top. This nerve appears between cervical five and cervical six, or C_5-C_6.)

To describe the condition from the diagnostician's point of view, if you told me you felt pain or unpleasant sensations in your thumb and forefinger, I'd suspect your trouble was originating at the C_5-C_6 level, in the lower part of your neck.

You seem to be saying that pain originating in your spine is much the same whether it's in your neck or down in your low back.

Broadly speaking, that's true. The pain-producing mechanisms are similar; both your neck and your back can experience pain from wear and tear in the facet joints and discs – Type One and Type Two pain, in other words. But with Type Three pain, a pinched nerve, it's usually a different story. As we saw in Chapter 3, when a nerve in the low back is pinched, the problem is caused by either a bulging or ruptured disc or a bony entrapment. If you have neck pain from a pinched nerve, however, the culprit is likely a combination of pressure from the bone and disc.

Incidentally, one other difference worth noting here is another basic point of anatomy: as we discussed in Chapter 4, your neck is built for more mobility than your low back. That means as the years go by and your discs dry out and your spinal joints lose some of their flexibility, you'll notice the change more in your neck than in your back, simply because you expect your neck to be more flexible. You can see that difference if you watch someone back a car out of a driveway. A young adult at the wheel will simply turn the head around as far as necessary to see out the back window. But a driver who is, say, fifty or older will have to turn the whole upper body to get the necessary view.

It seems to me that many of the people I've known with stiff, painful necks also had frequent headaches. Is that also a matter of referred pain?

In some cases it is. But whether it's referred pain or muscle tension pain doesn't make a lot of immediate difference. In fact, the two are so closely associated that they are almost indistinguishable. Neck pain is usually felt through spasm in half a dozen small neck muscles that relate to head and neck movement, and these muscles are part of a larger muscle mass covering the entire skull. When the little muscles are irritated, the muscles overlying the skull become tense, and you get a headache. That kind of muscle tension is by far the commonest cause of all headaches, whether or not they are accompanied or triggered by neck pain.

Is a muscle-tension headache the same as a migraine?

Definitely not. Migraine is a term that is often misused. Many of my neck pain patients mistakenly describe their headaches as migraines. To them, the word just means severe. A true migraine is caused by alterations in the function of the cranial blood vessels. The symptoms of the common or the classic migraine can vary a great deal, but typically the pain is one-sided (although bilateral headaches are not rare) and accompanied by a loss of appetite, nausea, and sometimes vomiting. Often before the headache starts there is a period when the victim feels inappropriate mood swings or sudden cravings. In the classic migraine there is a period of visual disturbances, an "aura." A migraine attack can wake a sufferer from a sound sleep, something a muscle-tension headache won't do. One fact that surprises many of my patients is that the migraine headache doesn't always produce excruciating pain.

Muscle-tension headaches begin insidiously and disappear slowly and haltingly. The pain can last for days, far longer than the normal migraine. The associated nausea is usually caused by a misuse of pain medication.

My main point, though, is that "migraine" refers to a specific condition which can be accurately diagnosed, and should not be used to denote just any sort of severe headache, regardless of its nature or cause.

Are psychological factors important in neck pain?

They certainly are. It's no mere coincidence that a worrisome situation is often described as a pain in the neck; worry or anxiety can easily trigger neck pain by increasing muscle tension. Once the muscle spasm starts, you are in danger of falling into one of those loops where pain causes suffering, suffering causes tension, and tension completes the loop by increasing the pain.

Earlier, you described how neck pain can be carried by the nerves down into the arms and even into the fingers. Does that indicate that a nerve is damaged? Does it mean I have a pinched nerve?

To answer your second question first: nerve damage is not the same thing as a pinched nerve. A nerve may be squeezed and become painful without being damaged. And in answer to your first question: the fact that a pain sensation is being transmitted by a particular nerve – say, from a worn facet joint in the neck down to the elbow – is not necessarily an indication that the nerve itself is in trouble. Chances are the nerve is just doing its job as the messenger, carrying the pain signal without being part of the problem. This is what we mean by referred pain. Blaming the nerve would be like shooting a messenger for bringing you bad news.

Once, when I went to my doctor with neck pain, he told me it was caused by muscle strain. Does that sound plausible to you?

That's perfectly plausible, and he was probably right. Neck pain may be caused either by emotional tension or physical strain. We are vulnerable to the physical strain partly because of the way the human neck is constructed, but mainly because of the demands we make on our necks.

Just as you should if you were suffering from low-back pain, you must make the distinction between hurt and harm. Muscle spasm can be very painful, but it is usually quite harmless. Sitting in a cold draft from an air-conditioner, for example, can cause the neck muscles to tighten and cause pain. If you have simple Type One problems, that extra muscular tension may be enough to irritate the worn joints and increase the discomfort or even produce a typical attack. But unless you understand what is happening, it will seem as if the cold air blew right into your neck and froze it stiff.

The same type of muscle spasm can occur if you sleep in an uncomfortable position or with a pillow that's too thick or springy. Even turning your head suddenly may trigger a painful episode. But, as difficult as the idea may be to accept, in each case the strain and the spasm are harmless.

What can I do to reduce those strains and avoid neck pain?

There are a great many things you can do, and I'll list some of them for you. Not every suggestion will apply to everyone, of course, but I think there's something here for most people who suffer neck pain. And, for that matter, a lot of this advice also applies to people with backache.

• Make sure your body and your mind are both getting enough rest. That means reasonable intervals of relaxation during your waking day and enough sleep at night. To respect your neck's natural limitations, give it a rest every so often. Whatever you happen to be doing, don't stand or sit in the same position, hour after hour, without a change. Break away every so often, either to rest or to switch to some other activity where those tired neck muscles will have a chance to take it easy. Or, better still, if you're engaged in any activity where the choice is entirely yours, pack it up for a while at the first sign of neck pain.

We all admire achievement, but it's a fact that many people with the worst cases of neck pain are the over-achievers – people who habitually drive themselves beyond the limits of their endurance. Such people, in my view, pay an unnecessarily heavy price for what they accomplish, when a little rest and relaxation could do them so much good. I think they'd achieve just as much that way – more, actually, because they would also succeed in avoiding neck pain.

• Examine your personal relationships. Do they create anger and hostility you can't release? If so, start looking for a harmless way to work off that tension. Physical activity would help – regular workouts in a gym or chopping a little firewood.

• If you're always dashing here and there, habitually late for appointments and obliged to apologize for your tardiness, find ways to reorganize your daily routine. There are good books on time management.

• Consider the possibility that you are working longer and harder than you need to, especially if you are holding down two jobs. Many women are in that situation today, with a household to run and a family to raise as well as a full-time job outside the home. If that's what you're coping with, it may be time for a reassignment of household responsibilities and chores. It isn't easy for some people to give up that responsibility and begin to rely on others. But it may be a choice between keeping your independence or overcoming your neck pain.

• Another enemy is boredom. Spending day after day at the same monotonous routine gives you an unneeded opportunity to dwell on aches and pains not only in your neck or back but also in many other parts of the body. Without a diversion, you may even begin to feel stress from the monotony. If there is no way of adding interest to the job itself, try to find some outside interests during work breaks or after hours.

• Don't overlook the possibility that some physical or emotional injury in the past may be an underlying cause of your muscle tension and pain. Physical irritation can come from sensitive scar tissue at the muscles' attachments to the vertebrae or from an old injury to the facet joints. But, remember, pain from those sorts of problems would have recurred periodically over the years. Once a physical injury to the neck heals painlessly, it isn't likely to start up again. Emotional stress, however, can last long after all the structural problems are resolved. That second possibility is especially strong if you have had to tell yourself to "keep your chin up" – a posture that is all too symbolic of the unnecessary strain we sometimes impose on our necks. Your symptoms may include frequent feelings of sadness and discouragement and a tendency to cry easily.

• Try to avoid dozing off while seated, as so many of us do while watching TV. Napping in an upright position places a great deal of strain on your neck as you allow your head to tip forward, with your chin on your chest. If you feel the need for a nap, go and lie down.

• The way you stand and walk can make a difference. If you slouch around like a high-fashion model, you may develop too much lordosis, or swayback, in your lower spine. This posture will inevitably thrust your head and neck forward and produce unnecessary stress on the muscles and ligaments along your spine.

• Driving a car can cause a lot of neck strain unless you take special steps to avoid it. For one thing, the very act of operating a car in heavy traffic or on a crowded expressway generates a lot of tension. On top of that, as a driver you must sit in a position that strains your arms and shoulders, encourages you to thrust your head alertly forward, and forces you to remain in a fixed position for long periods. I consider myself lucky because my car has arm-rests on both sides of the driver's seat, allowing me to transfer some of the weight of my upper body to my elbows. That does a lot to reduce the stress on my shoulder muscles. An adjustable steering wheel also helps, if you can afford the car that goes with it. As for the fixed seating posture, there is no magic solution, but there are several things you can do. Avoid sitting so far back from the wheel that you must hold your arms straight out in front of you. Shift your body weight back and forth, sitting well forward now and then as a variation from your normal position. And, if you can, stop the car every hour or so to get out for a stretch and a short walk.

• A great deal of neck strain comes from reading in bed or from assuming a poor sleeping position. If you must read in bed, use some comfortable pillows to prop yourself up into a seated position. Make sure you can hold the book and see it comfortably without straining your neck, your shoulders, or your arms. Or buy a reading-stand that swings over the edge of the bed. Otherwise, do your reading in a comfortable chair before going to bed. That may not be the most convenient arrangement, but it's a small sacrifice to make for a pain-free neck.

As for sleeping in a poor position, many people have trouble if they sleep on their stomachs. For one thing, that position creates a sway back. Even worse, it forces you to twist your neck to one side, causing strain that may last all night. Another bad habit is sleeping with your head on a pillow so thick that it thrusts your head and neck forward when you lie on your back. The pillow should allow you to keep your head back between your shoulders, not jammed forward. I have found many people with neck pain have trouble with solid foam rubber pillows. I generally recommend using a pillow that will give with the weight of your head and not fight back. If you keep waking up in the morning with a painful or stiff neck, you might consider changing your pillow or even getting a special neck pillow of the type we discussed in Chapter 1. As I mentioned, it is used under the neck, not under the head, and is most effective when you lie on your back. The typical cervical pillow is firm, not spongy, and about four inches thick. Newer models, designed to allow side sleeping, require some trial and error. There are other alternatives as well: a few patients get good protection and pain relief by sleeping in soft collars or cloth ruffs.

What about using a collar to protect your neck when you are not sleeping?

Like a brace for the low back, a cervical collar acts to restrict movement and take over the normal function of the supporting muscles. Using a collar to carry the weight of your head when your neck is sore may seem like a good idea, but it leads to some difficult problems. Your neck muscles rapidly lose their strength and tone, so you become dependent on the collar. Putting a collar on is easy; getting rid of it again may require weeks of exercise and increased pain.

The neck collar is also a common source of psychological dependency. Patients with chronic neck pain frequently feel compelled to wear a single ruff fitted so loosely that it provides no support or restriction of motion. It's almost like a feeble gesture of security to mark their profound suffering.

However, a cervical support does have some value. I routinely prescribe one after neck surgery or for use in specific situations where neck pain is likely, such as riding on public transit or driving heavy equipment. If you've been advised to use a collar, try to wear it only when recommended by your doctor and for as brief a period as possible. By combining that protection with regular neck exercise to maintain muscle tone you can avoid one of the major blocks to rapid rehabilitation.

Aren't there some relaxant pills you can take to ease the muscle spasms in your neck?

There are. But, as we've seen, relaxants have limitations. The term is not wrong but, as I have said, it's misleading. I think of them as "people relaxants," because you can't say to yourself, "This muscle in my neck is tense, so I'll just relax it by taking a pill." The pill doesn't know which of your muscles you are concerned about; it will relax them all. For that reason, you shouldn't take this type of medication if you have to remain alert. Using one of those pills can be like taking a stiff drink: alcohol is the most widely used "people relaxant" of all.

However, if you are in a position to relax safely, and you need relief from pain brought on by muscular tension, the medication might be a good idea.

What about pain killers?

As I pointed out earlier, many of the so-called pain killers we use don't actually remove or block the pain but simply alter your perception of it. You still feel the pain but you don't care. The headache no longer bothers you so much – but then neither does anything else. When you combine a pain killer with a tranquilizer you certainly feel better, but you cannot expect to function normally. And that way of feeling better can be a problem in itself. It's easy to understand why some people get into the habit of handling their pain with medication instead of exercise and proper posture.

Used properly, relaxants and pain killers are just temporary remedies.

Do you recommend heat or ice packs to relieve neck pain?

As with back pain, both heat and cold can be useful. They are just two of many counter-irritants that "jam" the nervous system in much the same way as a shortwave broadcaster will jam an enemy's radio messages. When you use heat or cold or other irritants, the brain gets a strong impulse that blocks the pain signal. And so you feel heat or cold but not pain.

Sometimes even a violent counter-irritant can provide welcome relief. I have had neck pain off and on for years. One winter recently, for no apparent reason, I suffered an excruciating attack. For months it interfered with my work. The pain was predominantly along the inner border of my right shoulder blade. I could feel a muscle knot there that was extremely painful. At first I got good temporary relief from a strong back rub. Then I discovered that punching the muscle was even better, and so I would invite my teenaged son to hit my upper back as hard as he could – really pound it. The counter-irritant effect gave me some great pain-free moments. Unless you've been through it yourself, you might find it hard to believe what some of us will put up with to get even temporary relief.

Would it be fair to say that pounding on a painful knot of muscle is a form of manipulation?

No, although pounding and manipulation may both provide relief. When my son punched my knotted muscle, he was providing a counter-irritant, but he was not manipulating the spine. Manipulation refers to maneuvers that put the joints through a range of movement. For reasons no one fully understands, that sometimes relieves the spasm.

It may surprise you that when I took my problem to a physical therapist for manipulation, she ignored the back spasm and worked directly on my neck. If I'd had no medical knowledge, I would have expected her to start on that knotted muscle. But she was providing the correct treatment, gentle manual traction and manipulation. She performed this treatment by pulling up on my head with both hands while gently turning my neck to the left, away from the painful side. The action produced a faint cracking sound, but it didn't hurt.

Did the manipulation produce the results you were looking for?

After the first treatment, it was amazing. I had virtually no pain and I could move my neck any way I wanted. I hadn't realized how much I had been limiting my neck movement to avoid the pain.

Are you saying that after one session of physical therapy your neck pain was gone?

Temporarily, yes. But being a typical patient and a typical doctor, I got busy and ignored her instructions to come back within a day or two for more treatment. My pain returned, as bad as ever. After several days without treatment, I went back and had virtually the same treatment again. But this time it didn't help much. I got slight relief that lasted only a few hours. I never made it back for a third session. I simply waited it out, exercising very gently to strengthen the muscles and making the pain more bearable by assuming postures that reduced my discomfort.

So what do you think about manipulation as a remedy for neck pain?

When muscle tension is a major factor, manipulation can be very effective. As with my first treatment it can produce dramatic results. But it doesn't always work that well. Although it has been shown that manipulation can hasten recovery, it has never been proven to alter the final outcome. Manipulation provides no benefit if you are having no problems at the time it is performed. In other words, it relieves symptoms but does little or nothing to remedy the cause. That's why I tell patients there's no point in continuing to go back indefinitely for more treatments if your neck is no longer stiff or painful.

Is manipulation painful?

No, it isn't; or rather, it shouldn't be, if it is being used to relieve neck or back pain. In other areas it can hurt a great deal. We talked earlier about the way your shoulder may stiffen up with neck trouble or with an immobilized arm. This frozen shoulder can require some pretty drastic manipulation. In spite of what you may think, doctors don't usually employ a treatment that must hurt the patient in order to help him, but that's what must be done to restore mobility in a frozen shoulder.

Remember I described how the shoulder stiffens as parts of the capsule stick together? Occasionally the patient's shoulder becomes so bound up by that process that you have to put him under anesthetic and move the joint for him, literally tearing the adhesions while putting the arm through the movements the patient can't make on his own. The main shoulder movement to be restored is the motion someone makes when throwing a baseball. The manipulation is done with the patient lying on his back with his shoulder over the edge of the table. Usually you can hear the scar tissue tearing; it sounds like the crunching of footsteps in crusty snow. The patient feels nothing at the time, of course, although he wakes up with one very sore shoulder. But once the capsular folds have been separated and the range of shoulder movement restored, the patient has a chance to maintain the normal function and get rid of his pain.

Wouldn't such drastic manipulation of the shoulder aggravate the person's neck pain?

Not as a rule. Often, the neck pain which may have caused the shoulder problem in the first place has long since disappeared, and only the stiff shoulder remains to be treated. Besides, the neck is carefully protected, and this manipulation is limited to the normal range of shoulder movement.

Manipulation of the neck itself is not nearly as dramatic, but the objective is the same: to loosen stiff joints and regain normal movement. Just like the patient who has had a shoulder manipulated, you must exercise often after neck manipulation to keep your increased mobility until the discomfort disappears.

You said part of the physical therapy for your neck pain was "manual traction." What is manual traction and what does it do?

Traction for the neck means pulling on the head to stretch the muscles and ligaments around the cervical spine. In my case the traction was manual; that is, the therapist pulled only with her hands. Often, neck traction is applied mechanically, using a series of hanging weights. At professional clinics you'll find therapists using traction tables designed to apply adjustable or intermittent patterns of pull, either to the neck or to the low back. Like manipulation, traction is intended to reduce muscle spasm, to free up stiff joints, and, of course, relieve pain. Because the head only weighs about twenty pounds (9 kg), traction can slightly open the exit canals of the nerve roots between the vertebrae and put tension on the bulging outer shell of each disc. The situation is quite different here than in the much larger lumbar spine, where conventional traction produces little if any separation between the vertebrae.

For this reason, traction can be helpful in relieving Type Three (pinched nerve) pain in the neck. It also has some benefit in reducing Type Two pain from a bulging disc. In my case, the effect was mainly to relieve severe muscle spasm. Of course, the stretching action is temporary. Once the pull is released, the structures return to their normal positions.

Many people learn to use traction on their own at home. If you try it, remember that the position of your neck is important. A slight change in the amount of flexion or extension can make all the difference to the success of the treatment. If you decide to get your own traction equipment, be sure to obtain proper instruction as well.

As a victim of neck trouble yourself, what positions or movements have you found useful for pain relief?

I devised my own form of manual traction, pulling up on my head with both hands and gently turning it away from the side of pain. I found I could relieve the pain for several minutes that way, although I suspect I looked a little strange. Because I have Type Two pain, a second useful maneuver consisted of arching my neck backward. I would lie on my back with my head hanging over the edge of a bed and a small pillow under the nape of my neck. This position minimized the pressure on the discs in my cervical spine and reduced my pain.

If my symptoms had come from worn facet joints, I would likely have found comfort by hanging my head forward to relieve the load on those small joints in the back of my spine. Because there is more than one cause of neck pain there is no single position that will help everyone. It is possible to distinguish Type One from Type Two pain in the neck just as we can in the low back, but finding the right movement or posture for your own pain is a matter of careful experimentation.

What can I do to improve my posture to relieve my neck pain?

Here's a technique I recommend to most of my patients. Start by imagining that your head is being picked up like a melon on a fruit vendor's stand; now, without actually touching it with your hands, lift it up, move it back, and place it squarely between your shoulders. The maneuver takes a little practice but it's worth learning. It's a good way of counteracting the habit most of us develop of standing and sitting with the head thrust forward, a posture that produces considerable strain on the neck. If you consciously try to position your head directly over your shoulders, your muscle tension will decrease noticeably. Some people, misunderstanding the technique, tilt their heads back and look up – which is wrong. Your head should move back without tilting, and your line of vision should remain level.

That principle is especially important if you are engaged in some activity that keeps you seated for a long period. Whether you are working at a desk, watching television, reading a book, or driving your car, do whatever is necessary to avoid thrusting your neck forward. That may mean finding a different chair or a better way to sit. It may mean discarding your bifocal glasses in some situations where you would otherwise tilt your head back so as to see through the lower lenses. Many people with personal computers have this problem, and the smart ones are getting single-lens reading glasses especially for use at their video display terminals.

Whatever it takes, make proper posture one of your regular habits and you'll be doing a lot to relieve or ward off neck pain.

I gather it takes a lot of conscious effort at first.

That's right. Start by thinking, right now, about how you are holding your body, especially about the position of your neck. Keep concentrating on correcting your posture until the right habits become second nature.

Meanwhile, remember that your neck, like the rest of your body, has its limitations, and if you push it beyond those limits, you're asking for trouble.

Once you establish that awareness, you'll be surprised how often you find simple ways of changing a familiar routine to eliminate discomfort or pain. I learned that lesson when I started scuba diving. Each time I came out of the water, I had a nasty headache. At first I assumed the problem occurred because of the difference between the pressure under water and the normal atmospheric pressure at the surface. But then I noticed that if I only looked at the bottom while I was diving, my headache wouldn't be so bad. I suddenly realized my scuba apparatus was to blame. I had been wearing a type of buoyancy compensator that fits around the neck like a yoke on an ox. It pulled my neck down and forced me to strain upward whenever I wanted to see where I was going. With the next dive, I switched to a stabilization jacket – an inflatable vest that serves the same purpose but places no strain on the neck. As soon as I made that switch, my scuba-diving headaches disappeared.

What about exercise as a means of preventing neck pain? Is that a good idea?

Exercise is not just a good idea; it's a *must*. But there is an irony worth noting here, for all those who exercise to protect themselves from low-back pain. One primary objective in back exercise is to strengthen the abdominal muscles, and this is often done by practicing sit-ups.

The trouble is that when people with weak stomach muscles try to do a sit-up, they invariably raise their heads off the mat first. They use the muscles of their necks and upper back, often pulling forward with their hands behind their heads as well, to help generate the force they need to raise their upper bodies. Now if they happen to have neck problems, particularly from worn and bulging discs, the added stress from this action will produce a very sore neck.

People with low-back problems must learn to do their sit-ups properly – literally to save their necks. The correct way is to keep your head back on top of your shoulders and raise your whole upper body as a unit. That keeps the strain off the neck and places it where it belongs – on the abdominal muscles.

I want to emphasize that exercise of any kind is *not* right for someone with acute neck pain. You should treat an acute attack here as you would treat acute pain anywhere else in your spine: gently. Later, when the pain subsides, return to your exercises.

If you do them regularly, you'll quite likely find future attacks are less severe and will subside a lot faster.

It's important to remember that exercise goes hand in hand with the other measures I suggested earlier – the various habits and tricks you can adopt to achieve proper posture and avoid tension and stress. In a nutshell, these are all ways of achieving and maintaining a neck that's strong enough to handle the tasks it's called upon to perform.

My advice will disappoint anyone who is looking for magic answers or spectacular forms of treatment, but it happens to be the best advice I can provide, and it has one great thing going for it: it usually works.

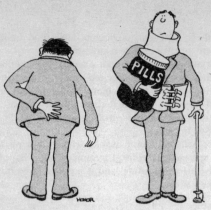

6. BACK PATIENT OR PAIN PATIENT?

Are you a *back* patient or a *pain* patient? There is a very important distinction.

If your primary problem is pain originating from a physical condition in your spine, you are a back patient. But if that *same* back pain has taken over your life, dictating your daily activities and influencing your every decision, you are no longer just a back patient but a pain patient as well.

To illustrate how you can get that way, I'll tell you about three back patients who became pain patients.

One is a woman I'll call Freda Kovacs, now forty-three. Late one afternoon about five years ago, she was offered a ride home from the factory where she worked as a sewing-machine operator. As the car waited for a red light to change, it was struck from behind by another vehicle.

Mrs. Kovacs went to hospital for X-rays and was told there was nothing wrong. The X-rays of her spine showed only the amount of wear and tear normal for her age. But within a day or two, her neck began to ache. She saw her own doctor, who eventually prescribed a full array of pills – pain killers, muscle relaxants, anti-inflammatory drugs, and tranquilizers. In spite of her repeated visits to complain of the pain, they were the only treatment she ever received.

After several weeks at home she went back to work. But even with the medication, she couldn't operate her sewing machine without suffering. She quit her job and began to withdraw from the world. First, she stopped seeing friends, then she quit doing housework. Her husband and two teenaged daughters took over her chores. Freda Kovacs had become a full-time invalid.

I met her only recently, when I was asked to examine her in connection with the lawsuit arising from the accident. In all the standard tests for diagnosing back pain, no physical cause could be discovered. Her muscle strength is normal. So are her reflexes. She has no nerve irritation. The list goes on. Everything checks out normally. There is nothing physically wrong with Freda Kovacs. And yet, no question about it, this woman is suffering genuine pain.

Why? I'm convinced it's mainly because she sees herself as a disabled person. And she got that way because she was a victim of inadequate care. Her case was regarded as a purely physical problem, and was treated with techniques that were entirely passive; no one attempted to involve Mrs. Kovacs in any part of her own recovery. She needed help with the emotional distress she suffered after the car accident. It's quite likely that with the right encouragement and reassurance, along with the proper physical training, she would have returned to her job much sooner than she did, and stuck it out until the pain subsided.

Now, I'm afraid, it's too late. Freda Kovacs, the victim of an accident that was physically inconsequential, has become permanently disabled.

In the second case, my patient was a woman who, along with her husband, had been a social acquaintance of mine for several years. She was suffering from a pinched nerve in her low back. After seven months of unsuccessful treatment, she came to me for the first time, hopeful that my professional skill and our friendship would somehow combine to produce rapid relief from her pain. After considering various alternatives, we agreed to try an injection of chymopapain, which often eliminates the pressure from a bulging disc that causes Type Three pain. But in her case the injection didn't work, and at that point she exploded with all the frustration and rage that had built up inside her through eight months of pain.

I can't remember an occasion when anyone took more trouble to enunciate a complete, unabridged list of my shortcomings as a doctor: I didn't care about her. I had callously excluded her from the process of making decisions about her treatment. I had not even asked her opinion. I was supposed to be making her well but I had done nothing to help her.... She went on and on.

I just sat there, biting my tongue and reminding myself of the things I teach my medical students about responding to pain patients. The physician is not there to win an argument; he is there to help. There are no marks for outwitting or out-shouting the patient. But how much more comfortable it is to advocate that approach in class than to follow it in practice!

And I really don't blame that woman for behaving as she did. If you'd been through months of agony and frustration with still no relief in sight, wouldn't you take it out on any doctor who failed to help you get well?

I know the feeling. I've been through emotionally destructive pain myself – not from my chronic back condition but from a form of recurrent migraine known as a cluster headache, which plagued me for years. The pain would fill my eyes with tears until I couldn't see and it would pound inside my skull until I couldn't stand still. Under those conditions, how can you possibly remain your normal, amiable self? Your whole personality changes, while you live in fear between bouts, waiting for the pain to erupt once more.

Obviously, that experience has given me a perspective on pain I never learned in medical school. I can look at someone in pain and say, "Yes, I understand what you're telling me." And understanding certainly helped me endure the tirade directed at me by that patient whose problem I had not yet solved.

Fortunately, that stormy session ended on a cheerful note. Having vented her rage, she felt better, and we knew where we stood with each other. Since then, we have moved ahead with effective treatment.

In the third case, I declined to accept the individual as my patient. My only contact with the man was a letter he wrote from another city to ask whether I would diagnose the back pain that had troubled him constantly for twelve and a half years. That time period alone told me he was far beyond the stage of simple physical back pain. It was reason enough to refer him for pain management. But there was more – significantly more. With his letter he had enclosed a loose-leaf binder containing a neatly typewritten, fifty-five-page monograph entitled "A Patient's Perspective of His Own Back Pain." It came complete with appendixes and a short bibliography. The poor man had become so obsessed with his back pain that he was making a career of analyzing it.

In response, I put him in touch with a pain clinic not far from his city, pointing out that the assessment he had asked for was the easy part; the big problem lay in controlling his chronic pain.

Although they reacted differently, all three of these patients have significant pain problems. My patient with the failed chymopapain injection had developed a strong emotional reaction that was beginning to change her personality and intensify her pain. The others had already crossed the line separating two types of pain victims: those with persistent physical pain, which is bad enough, and those who have had the greater misfortune of being entrapped by CPS – chronic pain syndrome.

In this chapter I describe the syndrome and offer practical advice which I hope will help some back patients avoid becoming pain patients.

I went to my doctor to see what could be done about my back pain but he couldn't find anything wrong with me. Now I'm wondering whether my family is right when they say I'm just imagining the pain. What do you think?

I can tell you one thing without even examining you: if you feel pain, it's real. The idea that you are imagining the whole thing is based on a common misconception about pain. Many people assume that if pain has no physical cause, you can't really be feeling anything, and your distress is somehow imaginary. But that's not true. Pain can be caused by many, many factors – physical and emotional. And they interact. The cycle usually, though not necessarily, starts with a physical cause, such as an injury. We react emotionally to the pain, and that emotion itself contributes more pain. Our reaction causes the muscles to tense, thereby introducing another physical factor – the spasm. And then we react emotionally to the spasm, and so it goes, around and around in a vicious, self-perpetuating loop.

Even after the initiating physical cause has disappeared, the pain may continue, triggered by those emotional responses.

Is that psychogenic pain?

Yes. Psychogenic pain is the technical term for pain produced by an emotional response without an accompanying physical cause; literally, pain generated by the psyche. Unfortunately the phrase is often used when the examiner doesn't believe the patient actually feels pain. And that's not correct. As I've just explained, pain originating in the mind is as real as the pain from bodily injury. Pain is pain no matter where it starts.

I wish everyone would realize that when the doctor says, "I can't find anything wrong with you" he's not necessarily accusing you of lying about your pain. What he is saying is that the cause of your trouble doesn't appear to be physical. Obviously he would allay your concerns more readily if he clarified the basis for diagnosing physical pain in one case and psychogenic pain in another. Often it's a matter of determining whether the initial cause was structural or not and whether that original cause still exists. He should help you recognize that a combination of factors may be involved – fear, anxiety, anger, depression, and various other emotions – plus muscular tension, stress, and fatigue.

Your doctor can provide a good service by exploring those additional features of the problem with you, particularly if he finds that your pain has no apparent physical origin. He will try to learn whether you have been upset about anything lately, or have been under any unusual pressure. One inevitable pressure that is often overlooked is the burden of the pain itself. Other events may intensify the problem, the way a door-slam will when you have a headache, but the very presence of the headache is enough to make you upset.

Questions in this area need to be asked in such a way that you will understand how natural and commonplace it is to feel pain that has no significant physical cause. Otherwise, the doctor's mention of emotional problems might trigger another false assumption on your part – that psychogenic pain is a symptom of mental disorders: "My god! The doctor thinks I'm losing my mind!" And, of course, that's not what's meant either.

Are you saying that people's aches and pains are *never* imaginary?

Of course there are hypochondriacs and hysterics, who react to imaginary pain. But they are rare – more rare than many people suppose – and they, too, are suffering from real diseases, forms of mental illness that can be just as disabling as the chronic pain syndrome.

But you said a person may keep on feeling pain from an injury after it heals. Isn't that the same as imaginary pain?

No, that's not the same thing. During the time the injury is there, your body develops a "memory" that may keep the pain alive after the injury has healed. If your muscles have learned how to spasm and hurt, anything that tightens those muscles in the same way – it might be fatigue, emotional tension, or even a cold draft – can trigger that pain all over again.

It's possible, too, for a person to be conditioned to feel pain merely because he or she *expects* to feel it. I actually test for this reaction whenever I examine someone with long-standing back pain. One method I use is to rotate the patient's trunk by moving his hip joints. The patient stands with both feet on the floor while I hold his arms to his sides and twist his pelvis. This movement places no stress whatever on the spine, and yet often a chronic pain sufferer will cry out with back pain. This reaction is a sign that the person expects to feel back pain (or thinks I am expecting him to feel it) and so he actually experiences the pain on cue.

One of my patients complains of numbness all down one side of his body, although he has nothing physically wrong with him. Even though there can be no purely organic cause to produce such a problem, I accept it as a genuine complaint. I do believe, however, that he exaggerates the condition, either consciously or otherwise, because he's afraid that without it I might fail to recognize the "seriousness" of his condition.

I sympathize with a patient who behaves that way. I know what chronic pain does to you, and I think it's all too easy for someone who has never had the problem to unjustly accuse the victim of exaggeration. There is simply no way to tell what some other person is actually feeling.

But that does bring up the question of malingering, which means lying about having an illness. It can be difficult to determine whether a patient is actually experiencing the pain he describes or just trying to fool the examiner for some gain, such as an increased disability settlement. Although many people exaggerate their problem, very few make the whole thing up. The factor that often decides the issue is consistency both in response to the examination and in everyday life. The patient who winces and screams with every movement in the office, and then dashes out to put another quarter in the parking meter, deserves to be viewed with suspicion.

Occasionally, a colleague of mine who runs a pain clinic in Vancouver asks a group of patients to line up along one wall of the room and then arrange themselves according to who feels the most pain – the worst in one corner and then the rest in descending order. Invariably, this request creates a small stampede. Everybody in the class tries to get into the corner reserved for those with the worst pain.

Their reaction to that test is typical of chronic pain patients everywhere, and it's not hard to see why. After all, each person has what he can truthfully describe as "100 percent of my own pain." And whatever that 100 percent amounts to, it's as much pain as its owner ever wants to have – and often as much as he thinks he can stand.

Obviously, pain is a very individual and subjective thing.

That's right. It's also very complicated. Perhaps you were taught in health class that you feel pain simply because a nerve in some part of your body sends a pain signal to your brain. That's the traditional concept. But in recent years, medical researchers have found that the process is not that simple. The signal that is sent is not necessarily the message the brain receives. The message is changed as it travels – changed in the spinal cord and changed again in the brain itself. Although we don't understand how some of these changes happen, we know there are many things that can affect the intensity of pain.

I would think that my attitude has a bearing on the way pain affects me.

You're right, it does. The amount you suffer from a bout of pain depends on a great many factors: the mood you are in, the amount of sleep you had last night, whether you and your mate are getting along well, how the "vibes" are in the office, and so on. You can be sure your chronic backache will feel a lot worse on the day your lose your wallet than it will on the day you win ten thousand dollars in a lottery.

Your perception of pain also depends partly on the efficiency of your sensory system. You have heard of people who can somehow stand a lot more pain than the rest of us – professional athletes, for instance. The quarterback who goes back into the game in spite of a broken finger is using inner resources we can't measure or even define. He may be particularly good at blocking out pain signals by concentrating on his game. Or he may simply be one of those people with a high tolerance to pain. In that case he is not any braver than the rest of us – he just suffers less because his pain transport system is less efficient or less sensitive than normal.

Is pain tolerance something that improves with practice?

No, just the opposite. Each of us has a finite ability to endure pain. The longer we are forced to cope with the problem the less reserve we have left, like a car running out of gas.

Once our tolerance is exhausted, even a minor pain produces great suffering. That's why a pain that actually remains unchanged over several months will become harder and harder to bear, and may be perceived as growing worse.

I gather you don't use the terms "pain" and "suffering" to mean the same thing.

No, doctors make a useful distinction between the two.

Pain is what results when that signal is transmitted from the hurt part of your body through your spinal cord to your brain.

Suffering describes what you, as an individual, do with that pain – how you perceive it and what effect it has on your emotional state. You may have a lot of pain and suffer very little, or you may have a small amount of pain and suffer a great deal.

People who suffer a lot from a small amount of discomfort or pain naturally become known as complainers. I've noticed that, often, when two people catch the same flu bug at the same time, one person will suffer more – or certainly complain more. But who can say the complainer is not actually feeling much worse than the other person? It's a very subjective thing, and we have no way of measuring it.

And while we're on terminology, there's a third word to mention: disability. Whereas suffering has to do with our perception of pain, disability refers to the way our behavior is altered in response to that suffering. Disability has an element of objectivity we don't find in the other two terms. It is objective because we can all see the changes in someone's pattern of activity. We may not be able to measure pain or suffering, but we can certainly count the number of days a patient stays off work.

Disability has a subjective aspect as well, since two individuals with the same problem may handle it quite differently. When two people have similar leg injuries, one person may walk with a slight limp, minimizing the difficulty as much as possible, while the other may hobble around on crutches.

That second person is in danger of acquiring a learned disability – an unfortunate phenomenon that is all too common. I once had a patient who told me with some pride that he had learned to live with his bad back and that he needed no further treatment. He no longer worked and no longer took part in any active recreation. He spent at least six hours a day in bed resting, and when he wasn't in bed he was still indoors, "caring" for his back.

Contrary to what he said, this man had not learned to control his back problem. He had learned how to be disabled. His problem was no longer his pain or his suffering. His problem was "learned helplessness," a pattern of behaving like an invalid, which he had taught himself through years of practice.

You have spoken repeatedly about chronic pain but you haven't mentioned acute pain. Does acute pain present the same kinds of problems?

Not really. Acute pain occurs quite predictably from illness or injury. If you break a leg, it's bound to be painful. The pain may last for weeks or even months, but acute pain is recognized by the patient as having a definite end point. It will disappear as the injury mends. Since we know we can eliminate acute pain by treating its cause, we don't usually treat the pain behavior, although we may provide medication to relieve the suffering.

Chronic pain, on the other hand, is pain that persists for six months or longer; a nagging backache, for instance. The patient begins to worry that the pain will never end but will persist for the rest of his life. Whether or not it ever had a physical origin, chronic pain often becomes an entity – and a problem – separate from the cause. For that reason, doctors, as well as treating the source, will often treat chronic pain independently.

One special difficulty with chronic pain arises when an acute organic cause, such as a sore joint in the spine, subsides but remains sufficiently irritable to trigger local muscle spasms and pain; or when the "memory" factor I mentioned comes into play. In either case, the actual physical problem is so minor there is nothing we can do about it. So we try to treat the pain itself. That's not impossible, but it's difficult because there are a lot of things we have yet to learn about managing pain. If we knew more, we might encounter fewer cases of people whose pain problem has progressed so far that it has become incurable.

Is there some specific point at which you can say, "This patient's pain is incurable"?

Yes, but I'm afraid with our present state of knowledge and lack of sophistication in treating chronic pain, we can't precisely identify when the transition takes place. In time, however, some patients will reach a point where, in my opinion, they are beyond help, even from the most highly skilled pain specialists. Our understanding of pain management today is comparable to our knowledge of tuberculosis half a century ago, when we treated that affliction simply with fresh air, sunshine, and rest. A great deal depends on the natural course of the disease.

A woman I'll call Hilda Carson is someone I remember well as a pain patient who was beyond help. A woman in her early fifties, she had been working as a mature model and a part-time clerk. Her problem began in the store where she worked. One day, she climbed a ladder to retrieve some stock from a high shelf, fell, and broke her left heel.

By the time I saw her she had already been through three rounds of surgery – one attempt to correct the original injury, and two others to fuse some of the damaged joints in the foot.

She hobbled into my office with a cane and told me her whole story. By now, the pain, originally confined to her heel, was surging through the entire foot and beginning to radiate into her lower leg, knee, and buttock. My examination showed that the operations had accomplished all that could be done to help her and more surgery would be of no value. Mrs. Carson was left with a chronically painful heel.

But I could see also that her pain was no longer entirely physical, since her symptoms far exceeded what you could expect from the original injury. I encouraged her to tell me more about herself and her problems. At the time of the accident, she had been happily married. But because of her heel pain, she didn't want to make love. She and her husband were soon quarreling, and eventually he left her. According to Hilda, he treated her badly in the financial settlement.

Now here she was, into her fifties, beginning to look sixty, trying hard to look forty, and unable to work as a model or a clerk. And, given her emotional state and physical problems, she was unlikely to be hired or accepted for training in any job.

As she said, "Who's going to hire a middle-aged cripple with a cane?"

And she was probably right. She had come to see herself as a totally disabled person, and for good reason. By now, her physical condition was almost incidental to the economic, social, and emotional problems it had spawned. Her broken marriage, her poverty, her inability to find work, her loneliness, her sense of despair – all these had combined to make her a classic victim of the chronic pain syndrome.

We discussed the nature of her pain, and I tried to help her understand what was happening. But she wasn't interested. If I couldn't take away her suffering with my surgery, she would find someone else. I don't often see a patient whose problems leave me feeling absolutely helpless, but that's how I felt after seeing Hilda Carson.

Is it usually fairly obvious when a person's pain problem is emotional rather than physical?

Often, but not always. Emotion, like pain itself, is not something you can measure. Sometimes it's hard to identify a patient's real emotions and then determine how much those emotions are contributing to the problem. Not long ago I saw a woman in her sixties who appeared to be coping very well with a chronic back disorder, even though it had severely limited her life. She had given up most of the things she enjoyed: bowling, gardening, ballroom dancing. She now spent much of her time looking after her invalid husband, who was confined to their home after a stroke.

Although those nursing duties aggravated her back pain, she didn't complain. In fact, she described her whole situation in a fairly calm, matter-of-fact way.

Then I began questioning her more specifically about the way her circumstances were curtailing her normal activities. At that point she broke down and cried. Abruptly, her whole manner changed. Even her choice of words was different. She was no longer speaking by rote, in the calm language she had taught herself to use when discussing her situation with friends. The extent to which she had shut the problem out of her mind became clear when she suddenly blurted out, "I only cry when I think about it."

I couldn't help feeling that a lot of her back pain came from the suppression of her emotions: the unhappiness, the anger, and the resentment she felt over the things that were happening to her. Again, here was a heavy overlay of emotion complicating a problem that was initially physical. But few, if any, of those secondary factors would be evident to anyone who engaged that woman in only casual conversation.

Is there a difference between any long-lasting pain and the chronic pain syndrome?

It is sometimes difficult to distinguish one from the other during a first consultation, but there is a crucial difference. The chronic pain syndrome – call it CPS – is a behavioral disorder. It is characterized by certain components and conditions that don't generally apply to patients who are coping with a lengthy but resolving pain problem and are able to continue functioning normally. These CPS characteristics include: pain of suspiciously long duration; pain that's out of proportion to the physical findings; the diagnosis of a soft-tissue injury; a gradually expanding array of symptoms; a preoccupation with physical complaints; "pill-popping"; "doctor-shopping"; a failure to respond to conventional treatment; a loss of sex drive; and various changes in the patient's personality and emotional makeup. These last factors usually cause marital and family problems, as they did for Hilda Carson with her broken heel.

Would you elaborate on the signs and symptoms of CPS?

All right. The first point I mentioned is, pain of suspiciously long duration. By that I mean a period of at least six months. You may have a pain that has lasted longer than you expected, but if it has been bothering you for only a week, or even a month, there's no reason to be frightened or to worry about the syndrome. Even after six months, you may have a pain that occurs only when you do a certain thing, such as putting your full weight on an ankle that was sprained and is still mending. In this kind of situation, the pain is not a result of CPS, but just the reflection of local irritation from a condition that is taking a long time to heal. With the syndrome you have pain in excess of anything indicated by the physical findings. You may even have begun to wonder whether the pain really is "all your head," as your family and friends have been saying. Most patients with CPS, however, cling stubbornly to the idea that their problem has a real and, usually, serious physical cause. In either case, the doctor can find no objective evidence of a specific impairment, such as true weakness, or loss of a reflex. The doctor detects little or nothing out of order, certainly nothing to justify the pain you are experiencing.

Again I emphasize that it's not a question of whether the pain is real; we know that if you are feeling pain, it *is* real. But by now the pain itself is not even the problem. The real problem is your *response* to that pain. With CPS, the degree and the nature of that response are excessive – that is, inappropriate – for your trouble.

Don't confuse this exaggerated response with malingering. The latter is a conscious decision, a lie, aimed at fooling someone. The chronic pain response produces real pain and real disability even though there isn't much physically wrong for the doctor to see.

Apparently there is some important point to be made as well about a soft-tissue injury as opposed to, say, a broken bone.

Yes. As I pointed out earlier, a fracture may take a long time to heal and continue causing pain for the duration. But if you suffer a soft-tissue injury, such as a pulled muscle or a bruise, you shouldn't be feeling constant pain from it after six months or so. Soft-tissue injuries heal much faster than that. Of course, there will be no sign of injury in your X-rays and, as I mentioned, no other positive indications from objective observations or tests. A patient's undue concern with simple soft-tissue injury can be the first step towards a serious chronic pain problem.

This is particularly true when we consider back pain because the element of fear is so great. A sprained spinal joint or a herniated disc will heal just as other soft-tissue injuries do, but the unnecessary worry over a "bad back" can linger on and lead to trouble.

You said the chronic pain syndrome is a disorder. Does that mean it's a disease in itself?

Yes. It *is* a disease – a behavioral disease – and it needs to be treated as such. It must also be clearly separated from mental illness. The excessive response and the development of an invalid behavior pattern can happen solely as a result of persistent pain without any other psychiatric problems. The abnormally increased awareness of pain in CPS is clearly emphasized by the next item on my list: an increasing number of symptoms. In other words, the pain tends to spread. The problem may develop in your back, but the next thing you know your whole body seems to hurt. You get frequent headaches, tingling sensations in your arms and legs, sore joints, chest pains, and many tender lumps in the muscles over the shoulders and at the back of the pelvis. To make matters worse, you now focus even more of your attention on these bodily aches and pains. The situation is especially difficult if you also happen to have a minor physical difficulty such as mild disc pain. Your whole lifestyle begins to center on these problems and you may talk or think about little else. Everything you do is weighed against the effect it will have on your pain. "I'd love to go boating tonight, but I'm afraid it might hurt my back...."

Along with this expanding array of symptoms you may experience general fatigue and probably insomnia. In fact, sleep disruption is almost an inevitable feature of the chronic pain syndrome.

You don't mean to say that if back pain keeps me awake at night I must have CPS.

Certainly not. Pain that disturbs your sleep is most likely to be just ordinary backache, and if it bothers you night after night, you may develop a pattern of sleeping poorly. Pain of this sort characteristically gets worse any time you overuse your back, and that can make getting to sleep even more difficult.

On the other hand, if there is no apparent relationship between your pain and your activity, and if pain is a major problem whenever you try to rest, your doctor will want to see whether you might have one of the rare physical causes of constant back pain, such as a bone tumor. Of course that's most unlikely.

My point is simply that insomnia, which troubles some back patients for obvious reasons, is usually a part of the chronic pain syndrome as well.

You said that victims of the syndrome are often "pill-poppers." Isn't it likely that these people tended to overuse medication even before they developed chronic pain?

I don't think so. We're not talking about an illness that affects only people with weak personalities who go through life looking for psychological crutches to lean on. While it's true that some victims are people who would probably dote on a medical problem of any kind, they are not typical. The chronic pain syndrome is something that can happen to anybody – just as a ruptured disc or sore joint can. Never underestimate the power of pain. I know what it can do to people. As the "bad guys" like to say in the torture scenes you read in spy novels, everybody has a breaking point. A lot of people have reached that breaking point before they ever set foot in my office. It doesn't surprise me that they have become pill-poppers. And it depresses me to think of how many of them got that way because a doctor prescribed medication as their only form of treatment. In many instances the patients have become completely irrational about it.

What's irrational about taking pills to relieve pain?

Nothing, if they help. But often the first words I hear are, "You've got to help me, Doctor, because I'm taking all these pills, and nothing seems to work."

"Then why do you take the pills," I ask, "if they don't work?"

"Well, I've got all this pain."

"But you just said the pills don't help. And if they don't help, why do you take them?"

"Actually, I've tried stopping, but I have to take them because of all this pain."

But isn't the person trying to tell you that without the pills the pain would be even worse?

That's a reasonable assumption, but often that's not how the chronic pain patient sees it. I ask, "On a scale of one to ten, with ten as the worst, how would you rate your pain when you use your medicine?"

"It's a ten – the worst."

"And how bad is it if you stop taking the pills?"

"Well, it's even worse!"

I sympathize with anyone in that situation, but this response only demonstrates the patient's inability to see his own problem with any sense of perspective: pain that is already "the worst" gets even worse if the pills are stopped. It has all the absurdity of those TV commercials for a washday detergent that somehow made your laundry "whiter than white."

Another thing these people fail to realize is that by taking all that medication they are getting into a vicious circle: *Why do I take the pills? Because I feel pain. Why do I feel pain? Because I'm sick. What makes me so sure I'm sick? I must be sick – look at all the pills I'm taking!*

For some CPS patients, the cycle is now complete and the treatment has become the reason for the disease which requires the treatment.

What is "doctor-shopping" and why is it part of the syndrome?

At first glance it seems obvious that patients with the chronic pain syndrome come to the doctor to get help. In a sense that's true, but typically they demand help strictly on their own terms. They don't want to hear the facts unless those facts fit their perception of their own disability. When the first doctor fails, they try a second, and then a third, and so on. They go the rounds and soon they're caught up in the system. It's all part of being sick – and of course they genuinely perceive themselves as sick people. Sick people need doctors, and so they keep finding new doctors to see. They become expert at manipulating the situation, playing one doctor off against another while remaining trapped on their own terrible treadmill.

Recently, after spending a great deal of time explaining the nature of his problem to a patient who was suffering from the chronic pain syndrome, I referred him to an excellent pain clinic. I emphasized to him that this local clinic could provide exactly the treatment he needed. After one visit to the clinic the man came back to tell me the director had found my diagnosis was completely wrong. I telephoned the clinic director, who said the patient told them I had diagnosed a serious problem of scar tissue in the spine, which would make it impossible for the clinic to help him. Both the clinic and I had come to the same conclusion about the patient. But since our opinions didn't match his own assessment, he was trying to manipulate us into a different course of action.

Just the other day, a woman came into my office for her second visit in a month. On her first, I had advised her to stop see-ing doctors, including myself, to avoid passive treatments that offered only temporary relief from pain, and to begin a regular exercise program. But she had ignored that advice and had gone to see two other doctors. One had prescribed massage. The other was an acupuncturist who stuck needles into her. Because both practitioners had, in effect, offered to take charge of her problems while allowing her to passively await the results, she liked their treatments much better than my advice. Yet here she was, back in my office, saying, "Well, your last bit of advice was no help. What are you going to do for me now?" I felt as though she had dealt me into a round of poker and was challenging me to up the ante.

Do doctors try to discourage this kind of shopping around?

Yes, we do. Obviously it's a waste of our time – and a waste of the community's medical resources.

But can't it be argued that a patient has the right to seek a second opinion?

Yes – every right. And a third opinion, too, for that matter. But when a patient goes to half a dozen doctors complaining of the same condition and then ignores each one's advice if it doesn't appeal to him – that's doctor-shopping, pure and simple. Each doctor may have a different idea of the most appropriate treatment. But that's hardly grounds for the patient to go the rounds again, telling each doctor what a failure he is compared to the others. Yet that's typical of a patient with CPS.

You said that chronic pain patients don't get better with conventional treatment.

That's right, and they often prolong their treatments to extremes. It's not unusual in these cases to see physical therapy visits for deep heat and massage extending over a year or more. And I remember one woman who was carrying so many pills that her purse rattled. In any case, it's a mistake to apply the conventional techniques of acute pain management to patients suffering from CPS. Conventional management of acute, self-limiting pain is aimed mainly at the physical problem, and that's not where the real trouble lies in CPS. More important, conventional treatment is largely passive; it doesn't require the patient to do anything or take any responsibility for getting well. Given that kind of treatment, the CPS patient is more inclined to devote all his or her energy to remaining sick.

You mentioned a loss of sex drive as one of the syndrome's components. Does that affect men more often than women?

No – the actual loss of libido seems to afflict both sexes equally. A man may feel more devastated by the experience, but if it threatens or wrecks a marriage, as it did in the case of my "middle-aged cripple with a cane," it is obviously a serious problem for victims of both sexes and their mates.

Loss of libido can be devastating whatever the cause, but associated with CPS it introduces a whole new loop: if you lose your sex drive, you become anxious. Your anxiety is reflected in increased awareness of your problem, which intensifies your pain, which then perpetuates your loss of libido. Understandably, many CPS victims see this development as a sex problem, rather than as a byproduct of their pain. Consequently, they get into sex counseling when their actual need is to learn chronic pain management. It's hard for them to realize that once they conquer their pain their anxiety will be reduced and their libido will return.

Apart from sexual problems, how big a factor is anxiety in the syndrome?

It's a big factor, and it's just one of many emotions that keep the victim off balance and unable to lead a normal life. Anxiety is almost inevitable, and so are fear, anger, resentment – plus almost any other negative emotions you can think of. And, worst of all, these emotions are not just momentary, as they usually are for the rest of us, but they become part of the person's mood, night and day, to the point where the whole personality changes.

Even if I had never encountered a CPS case professionally, I could testify personally to some of those effects – although, at the time, I didn't realize how significant they were. Early in my career, I took a year of training in Scotland. As it happened, I arrived there during a severe bout of cluster headaches, which, this time, lasted nine weeks. Every day began with four hours of excruciating pain. Although it was gone before noon, I knew it would be back the next day, and that really got to me. Months later, long after the attacks were finished, several of my new friends there told me, "You are quite a different person from what you were when you first arrived," and "We see a tremendous difference in you since we first met."

Apparently they attributed this "tremendous difference" to the bracing climate of the Highlands. In reality, I had arrived in the country fighting off that terrible migraine pain. Without realizing it, I had reacted to the pain by becoming withdrawn, humorless, uncommunicative, even rude and hostile. Then, once my headaches subsided, I returned to normal, obviously impressing my Scottish friends with my "new" personality. I demonstrated many of the characteristics I now see in the CPS victims who come to me as patients. Almost without exception they are self-centered, demanding, intolerant, and very unhappy. They are so obsessed with their pain that they have built entire new – and miserable – lives around it, allowing it to dominate every moment of their time while forcing their families and friends to cater to its tyranny.

I was fortunate; my pain didn't last long enough to take over my life to that extent. But if I hadn't gone through some of that experience I would have great difficulty realizing that most people who now come to me with CPS are normally cheerful, likable individuals – and will be again, if they manage to escape the syndrome. Treatment isn't easy but it is possible.

Suppose I suspect my problem is chronic pain syndrome – how can I go about getting the right kind of help?

Begin by finding a doctor you feel comfortable with – somebody to whom you can tell your story. If your doctor doesn't seem interested, you should look elsewhere.

If you see a specialist, make sure that it is someone who is willing to discuss aspects of your problem that lie outside his or her specialty. If you are choosing a surgeon, for example, you will be better off selecting one who will recognize and discuss your emotional problem as well, even if he or she is unable to treat it.

Don't be afraid to ask questions. Make sure you understand the nature and purpose of the tests and treatments prescribed for you. There should be no mystery about anything that's being done.

Look for thoroughness. You don't want a doctor or therapist or chiropractor giving you a hasty examination and deciding, on little or no evidence, that there's nothing wrong with you except your pain. If you do get a speedy diagnosis, you need to know that it's backed by plenty of knowledge and skill. Whatever the treatment – a special diet, manipulation, an injection, or something else – it must be tailored exactly to suit your diagnosis and your personal situation. Treatment-by-rote just isn't good enough.

Look for a doctor who encourages you to assume a positive outlook and suggests something for you to do to help yourself. You will greatly increase your chances of dealing successfully with chronic pain if you assume as much responsibility as you can and take control of the situation to the fullest extent possible.

It may seem logical to expect a doctor to provide you with medical care just the way you expect a mechanic to provide your car with service. It's perfectly reasonable to drive into a garage and say, "My brakes aren't working properly. Please see what's wrong and fix it." A mechanic who's skilled and conscientious will do as you ask, without any help from you.

But the medical treatment of chronic pain doesn't work that way. You can't expect to get well simply by handing your problem to a doctor and saying, "Here it is – please fix it." Whether you actually vocalize it or not, your approach should be, "I have this pain problem. What can you *and I* do about it?"

The patient has to take the basic responsibility?

That's right. It all comes back to the very first point I made in Chapter 1. A lot of it has to do with developing a positive attitude. If you're consciously trying to get well, you stand a far better chance of succeeding than if you just sit back and say, "Make me recover." That's true of virtually any ailment, but it's especially important when part of the problem is psychological or emotional, as it so often is with chronic pain. You will not help yourself by assuming a passive role and, by default, learning to be disabled. I can't overemphasize the value of attempting to take control, thinking of yourself as a recovering person, even if you suffer some setbacks, and working actively to succeed with the treatment your doctor prescribes.

Early in the consultation, you and your doctor should agree on a goal, such as reducing your pain or, even more important, getting you back to work.

And while setting a goal, you should get a realistic estimate of how long the treatment should take to produce the desired results. With chronic pain, you need patience. You can't expect to be rid of your problem in a matter of days; it's bound to take weeks or even months – but not forever. Whoever helps you set your goal should also help you fix a reasonable timetable for reaching it.

Finally, if your problem is definitely the chronic pain syndrome, your doctor may arrange for you to visit a pain clinic for help from a specially trained team of doctors, psychologists, physical therapists, and social workers. These specialists will try to help you by prescribing appropriate action or treatment while carefully monitoring and recording your progress. If you are afflicted by CPS, or headed in that direction, you will be encouraged to alter your pattern of living, so that you see the problem in a new light and can take charge, once again, of the decision-making process, rather than allowing your pain to dictate the decisions you make.

Does this sort of professional help work better if I'm part of a group?

Yes, often that is an important factor, just as it is for people who are struggling with alcoholism or drug addiction.

At one pain clinic, in Miami, patients are encouraged to make a contest out of breaking the medication habit. Each patient's pill consumption becomes a matter of daily record known to the whole class: "Mr. Green took seven pills today; Mrs. White took five...." Patients who manage to reduce their dosages are rewarded by a healthy sense of accomplishment and praise from their peers.

Many clinics help patients kick their drug habits by making pill-taking time-dependent, rather than pain-dependent. That is, a person isn't allowed a pill because he has pain; he's given a pill at a specified time, regardless of his pain. The patient soon learns he can't "earn" a pill by feeling pain. He has to wait until the appointed hour. The association between pain and pill-taking is thereby disrupted while the intervals between doses are gradually extended, to taper off consumption.

Do most patients who have gone through that routine learn to get along without medication?

Not as often as everyone would like. But you have to realize that apart from dependence on pills, pain itself is addictive, and giving it up can be as tough as giving up smoking, drinking, and sex – all at the same time.

You also have to allow for the fact that chronic pain clinics are bound to have a high rate of failure, because they take on the worst cases, including some incurables – people who have lived with the syndrome for too long. People like that reach a point where they don't just tolerate their pain but envelop themselves in it until it becomes virtually inescapable. Pain clinics face greater challenges than those my colleagues and I face in the classes we conduct for back patients. While our classes can often succeed by dispensing an ounce of prevention, the pain clinics have to offer a pound of cure – and, often, even a pound is not nearly enough.

As I mentioned earlier, people suffering from continual pain can become particularly self-centered and demanding, and many of them will not put up with the rigid rules and schedules that are necessary features of most pain clinics. If you check into one of these clinics, you will be told you must get up every morning at eight o'clock, pain or no pain, eat breakfast at eight-thirty, go out for a walk at nine, and so on. . . .

You aren't allowed to decide, "I won't go out for my walk today because my pain feels worse." Pain or no pain, you take that walk on schedule. The whole idea of such discipline is to reintroduce the patient to habits that bear no reference to pain. But some patients can't stick to that routine for long because it doesn't fit the pattern they have developed to suit their pain, and they soon drop out of the program.

Would such people stand a better chance with a psychiatrist?

Possibly, although the prospects are not as good as you might suppose. Some fine work has been done in this field lately by certain psychiatrists who have taken a special interest in pain. But psychiatrists on the whole have not had much success in treating the chronic pain syndrome. Without some special training or background in pain therapy, a psychiatrist may not appreciate how the patient's pain response works as part of a closed loop, with pain producing muscle tension, and muscle tension producing pain, and both factors being magnified by fear and other emotions. Often, the psychiatrist will focus on extrinsic factors such as sexual hangups, job dissatisfaction, and stress in the family – problems that are actually byproducts of the pain – without touching on the underlying cause. For this reason, many pain treatment programs use psychologists instead because of their greater emphasis on behavior modification.

Even if the psychiatrist succeeds in helping solve those extrinsic problems, the patient will still have the original minor back trouble, and, more important, the chronic pain syndrome it produced. At this point the psychiatrist, aware of the patient's back trouble, is likely to announce: "Your problem is not in your head; you need to see an orthopedic surgeon." The surgeon, finding no back condition severe enough to account for the patient's pain, and recognizing the exaggeration of symptoms during the physical examination, will probably declare: "There's nothing wrong with your back; you should see a psychiatrist."

At any rate, most pain patients are reluctant to see psychiatrists because of the implication that the pain must be a sign of mental illness. What these people need is someone who not only understands pain but also has the ability to guide them through the process of behavior modification; someone who can explain that the problem is not a mental disorder and then provide appropriate physical treatment. It matters little whether they choose a surgeon, a psychiatrist, a psychologist, or a family physician, as long as it's a professional who has had experience with the syndrome and can appreciate the difficulties of helping its sufferers re-order their habits and responses into an entirely new lifestyle.

What sort of difficulties does a person face in trying to break out of the syndrome?

We have touched on some of them already: dependence on medication, for instance. Resolving that problem will mean eliminating the use of pills completely or at least finding ways of controlling the habit, so as to avoid abuse.

Drugs, by the way, are often partly to blame for the personality changes that occur in many chronic pain victims. In retrospect, I feel that was so in my own case, during my time in Scotland. I was taking so many narcotics that I began looking forward to the pleasant floating sensation that followed every dose. Finally, I concluded I could be subconsciously nurturing my pain to justify taking the pills. I said to myself, "This is becoming a very bad loop" – and I quit the medication.

Partly because of that experience, perhaps, I am not so quick to condemn chronic pain patients who misuse their drugs.

Does the desire for medication inevitably develop into out-and-out addiction?

For some people, drug overuse for chronic pain is a route to addiction. But I know many patients who can take a high dose of pain killers day after day, without ever increasing it. While they are dependent, they do not abuse the drugs as most addicts do.

One patient of mine, after six back operations, still suffers chronic pain, for which she takes five aspirin-codeine pills a day. That means she is getting a hefty dose of both drugs. No question about it, this woman is hooked on those pills; but she doesn't abuse them. Even after a recent fall down stairs, which shook her up pretty badly, and no doubt increased her pain, she did not increase her dosage but stuck to those five pills a day.

Certainly I hope she will start decreasing her dosage. Her family doctor has threatened to cut off her prescription; he keeps telling her those pills are not good for her. He's right, of course. But should he cut off the prescription? Here we have a woman who has undergone many surgical procedures, mostly attempted fusions and refusions. By now she has enough scar tissue in her spine to give her all the pain she'll ever need. Yet, with the help of those pills, she's living with her situation. She is a successful sales representative, with one of the best records in the whole company.

I'm afraid of what will happen if her pills are suddenly cut off. She'll adopt more blatant pain behavior: she'll take to her bed, give up her job and income, and become a totally depressed individual.

I have encouraged her to cut down – even reducing her intake to four pills a day would be a real accomplishment – and I have outlined a scheme for her to follow. But meanwhile, in the choice between the two extremes, she has picked what I consider the lesser of two evils.

Is overcoming drug dependence the main problem, then, in escaping the pain syndrome?

No, there are usually several other important problems to solve. For example, some patients become dependent on their physical treatments.

How can physical treatments become habit-forming?

Many physical treatments are forms of passive therapy where the patient is not required to expend any effort or take any responsibility. Someone or something else reduces the pain and makes the patient feel better. Passive treatment from a physical therapist, chiropractor, or massage therapist can produce great temporary relief. But without a change in the patient's behavior, the pain is certain to return. So the therapy becomes the only source of hope.

But at least it gives the person some hope. On that basis, taking the physical treatment sounds perfectly logical to me.

Oh, it's logical enough. But in order to get well, you must not become heavily dependent on *any* outside help. If you do, you'll create a self-fulfilling prophecy. It's fine to believe your physical treatments can help you. But it's not healthy to believe you can't get along without them. If you are going to get well, you must believe most of all in yourself – in your ability to take charge and bring about your own recovery. Your pain may not be "all in your head" but the ability to conquer that pain *has* to be in *your* head – or it's nowhere.

When a patient asks me, "Should I go back for more physical therapy?" I have to weigh the alternatives: will more short-term management benefit this patient or merely create or reinforce an unwanted dependency?

My decision will depend partly on whether I think the patient is being positive or negative. I will approve the therapy if I believe the question means, "I want to help myself by means of more physical therapy," but not if it seems to mean, "I don't know what to do – I think I'll let someone else take away my pain."

Self-assurance is obviously the key.

It's essential, all right, but gaining self-assurance is not easy; and it may be especially difficult if legal considerations are complicating the medical and emotional situation. That can happen to accident victims who get into litigation over damages.

How does the prospect of litigation work against a pain patient?

Several ways. Early in a dispute over an injury, a lawyer will customarily obtain a doctor's report and turn a copy over to his client, the patient. We've already seen how Doctor can make an injury sound worse than it actually is, and a medical report written as part of a legal claim can make scary reading. If it supports your case, it's also likely to support your pain – and perhaps aggravate it by making you fearful that you will never recover.

Unfortunately, the legal process can drag on and on, as we all know, and as long as your lawsuit is pending, you have an unhealthy incentive to keep right on feeling pain. Especially if your lawyer calls up and says, "How's your sore back? Don't forget we go to court again tomorrow."

Just the other day, a patient made a remark to me that unfortunately is all too typical. She's a woman who suffered a neck injury in a rear-end collision about a year and a half ago. On previous visits she had told me her pain was gradually subsiding. Then, on this last occasion, she said: "I'd almost forgotten about my neck pain, but my lawyer told me to come back and see you to be re-assessed. And so I started thinking about my pain again, and it came back."

You can hardly blame the lawyer for wanting an up-to-date medical opinion of his client's condition, but there's no doubt in my mind that many accident victims would recover faster if there were no such things as legal claims and lawsuits. According to some studies, people who resort to litigation over injuries seldom get better until their lawsuits are settled.

Certainly I am convinced that for the patient's sake a case should be settled as quickly as possible. I've seen too many instances where prolonged litigation or an insurance investigation has led to the development of chronic pain problems that remained long after the back injury itself had healed.

The negative effects of litigation on a patient's recovery have been observed by specialists who have studied the problem more systematically than I have. In an article they co-wrote for an insurance journal, a lawyer and psychologist cautioned that "... plaintiff counsel should not simply push ahead with the lawsuit without regard to the effect that this has on his client. He should never be unmindful of the fact that it is just as important, if not more important, for his client to get better as ... to get compensated."*

Another pain specialist has even coined an expression, "nomogenic illness," to denote the condition brought about or contributed to by lawyers and the legal process.**

If you're embarking on a lawsuit, that's a hazard you ought to be aware of.

Does it follow, then, that patients improve dramatically as soon as their lawsuits are settled?

Unfortunately, no. Various studies on this issue have produced contradictory statistics. In one study, all but 10 percent of patients involved in litigation got better as soon as their legal cases were settled. In other studies, as many as 50 percent failed to get better even after receiving settlements.

What do you think held their recovery back at that point?

We can only speculate, but I think one reason is that money is poor compensation for what the injury has done to disrupt, if not destroy, their lives. More important, because of the duration of their symptoms, many of these people have accepted their new invalid lifestyle as permanent. Partly because of the image pre-

---

*Crawford M. MacIntyre, QC, and Dr. David T. Corey, MA, PhD, in "The Chronic Pain Syndrome," published in *Without Prejudice*, November 1983.

**Dr. Milo Tyndel, Toronto psychiatrist and neurologist, cited by MacIntyre and Corey in "The Chronic Pain Syndrome."

sented in court, they see themselves as disabled persons con-
demned to a life of pain. Any form of physical or emotional stress,
no matter how commonplace, is related in their minds to the
accident. The resultant muscle tension triggers a typical attack
of pain. They have developed a learned response that is beyond
their control.

**Can you offer a few guidelines for people with chronic pain who
want to avoid becoming trapped in the syndrome?**

Yes. The first step is to get a complete and accurate diagnosis.
That means finding a doctor who will listen to your needs, provide
moral support, and eliminate any doubts you may have about
serious physical problems. You can't hope to conquer your pain
if you keep worrying about what's "really" wrong.

Next, you have to resolve to take charge of your situation, and
not delude yourself that you are coping with the problem when
you simply avoid painful activities. It helps if you refuse to accept
the pain as part of yourself but look at it instead as an adversary
that you can struggle against – and overcome. And the truth is
that you *can* overcome the pain if you *believe* you can.

The third step is to profit from mistakes other people have
made in your situation. It's a common mistake to give in to the
pain by becoming completely inactive. The doctor tells you, "Be
careful not to over-exert yourself," and so you do nothing but
sit around and vegetate. After a week or two, you can't stand the
inactivity, and so you rush out and spend a whole day gardening
or playing golf. Next day, not surprisingly, your muscles feel sore
all over. Worse than that, you feel guilty because you didn't follow
the doctor's advice. And so you take yourself off to bed, resolving
not even to tell the doctor what you've done. That's a common
cycle for CPS patients: frustration leading to over-exertion leading
to more pain and frustration.

**What's a better course of action if you're told not to over-exert
yourself?**

Practice moderation – moderate exercise, as prescribed by your
doctor, and moderation in your daily activities. And be prepared
to tolerate some pain. Keep in mind that if you have just gone

through a period of inactivity, you should ease gradually back into your regular routine – a little each day until your muscles begin to recover their normal tone. Don't forget that simple muscular soreness is not indicative of a serious problem. And gentle exercise, even with chronic pain, won't cause any harm.

You are bound to have moments of doubt, particularly when you try slightly more strenuous activities and you find that the pain increases. You'll be inclined to wonder, "My god, what am I doing to myself?" This is a crucial point in your recovery when, with support from an understanding doctor or therapist, you need to muster all the self-confidence you can. You must appreciate that if you carry on now and put up with the pain, you will be rewarded by some real progress.

But if you give in to the pain and reduce your activity, you will fall into a destructive downward spiral. A decrease in your activity will cause your pain to subside, and you'll probably spend five or six weeks resting while telling yourself you're doing the only safe and sane thing. In fact you are not really solving the problem at all and could even be making your next attempt more difficult.

Sooner or later, possibly at your doctor's urging, you will try to get up and around again. This time, the pain will be much more immediate – much harder to take. The reason, although you may not realize it, will be both physical and psychological: after weeks of inactivity, your muscles are sure to hurt. And the moment you feel the discomfort, you will tell yourself, "There it is! I knew it would happen! My pain is back!"

Like an animal in some psychologist's experiment, you have developed a conditioned response. You have learned that activity means pain, and so you avoid activity. And each time you try and fail, you reinforce that conditioning.

Probably without realizing it, you are establishing a pattern of behavior that is carrying you to the brink of the chronic pain syndrome.

To avoid that pattern, you must recognize that if you've been inactive, muscular pain is inevitable but not intolerable. And it will not persist, once those muscles become properly conditioned again. Imagine putting your normal elbow in a cast for six weeks. When you first try to move your arm again, you'll feel a great deal of pain from simple joint stiffness and weak muscles. The proper treatment, of course, would be to start active movement in spite of the discomfort. How much more trouble would you have if you treated the pain by putting your elbow back in the cast for another six weeks?

You should realize that if you fall into the habit of saying, "Every time I do such and such, I get pain," then you certainly *will* get pain. Instead, tell yourself, "I know such and such activity won't actually harm me, and so I am going to do it whether it hurts or not."

That's an important step towards dissociating normal activity from pain. If you can do that, you will achieve what the best pain clinics try to do. Their objective, stated broadly, is to "normalize" the person's behavior by shifting his or her responses from a pain-dominated lifestyle to an activity-dominated lifestyle.

In one pain clinic, for instance, the therapists require patients to walk a specific distance every day, regardless of the pain. Each day's walk is timed and the time is recorded. On the first day, the person can take virtually all the time he wants, but he is encouraged to improve on that time during each subsequent walk. Typically, a patient will keep improving the pace without realizing it, until the records are brought out as proof. As the improvement continues, patients find themselves concentrating more on the achievement than on the pain, and gradually they come to realize that pain is not an inevitable result of walking.

If a person has felt crippled for some time, that discovery must seem like a great revelation.

It is – it's an immense source of satisfaction, not only because it shows progress but also because activity in itself is a satisfying thing. Which brings me to my final point of these guidelines: the best way to get back to normal is to start acting as though you *are* normal.

Patients say to me, "I can't go back to work – I'm still having pain." And I always say, "Don't tell anybody. Just go back to work and put up with a little pain." I point out that working regularly is far less risky than remaining idle, trying to wait out the pain and playing the role of a disabled person. I get quite frustrated and occasionally furious when a patient of mine is ready to return to work but is prevented from doing so by his company or union because he is not considered fully recovered. It's often hard to make the powers that be understand that getting back on the job is an essential part of getting better. Forcing a person to remain inactive is unnecessary and potentially destructive.

And so my advice is: *get active as soon as possible, even if it hurts a little*. How does that old expression go – "Short-term pain for long-term gain"?

Believe me, if it steers you clear of the chronic pain syndrome, it's well worth the discomfort.

7. INTERCOURSE, PREGNANCY, AND YOUR PAINFUL BACK

In my view, the impact of back pain on your sex life has to be seen in the wide context of all your living habits. Too often, when we talk about sex we speak of it as though it were entirely isolated from the rest of our experience. We forget that in sexual relations, back problems create the same cycles of fear and pain – and the same opportunities to control situations – as in other aspects of everyday living.

Sometimes, too, you may find it easier to dwell on your back pain than to work at improving your sex life. I'm not a marriage counselor, and this book can't cover all the ramifications of a sexual relationship that has a back problem as one of its ingredients. But what I have heard from a great many patients convinces me that even though back pain is real, it too often serves merely as an excuse for inadequate sexual response.

If that observation hits home, you should understand that severe back pain does not necessarily indicate a severe physical problem, that your backache can become a serious sexual problem only if you allow it to do so.

What are the hazards of having sexual intercourse if you suffer chronic back pain?

The greatest hazard lies in letting your bad back interfere with your sex life. Allowing that to happen can ruin the whole relationship.

But surely the activity involved in intercourse can be harmful in some cases.

Almost never. It may cause pain but it won't cause damage. Mind you, the fear of pain is genuine, and some people with bad backs truly believe they are going to harm themselves during the excitement of intercourse – but they won't.

You can't hurt your back that way?

No – for two reasons. First, while strenuous exertion might rarely be harmful during a brief attack of acute back pain, the danger doesn't arise, because you're not likely to feel sexy when your back is killing you.

Second, as I can't stress often enough, there's a world of difference between *hurt* and *harm*. There are a thousand things you can do to various parts of your body that will hurt temporarily without harming you. Standing on one leg for half an hour would probably hurt quite a lot but it wouldn't do you any harm. Having sex when your back is not at its best may hurt a little – it may even take the joy out of sex on that one occasion – but it's not going to harm you – or your back. On the other hand, however, great harm could come from denying yourself the opportunity for intimacy and depriving your partner of pleasure and gratification. Whenever I hear of people avoiding sex because of a bad back, I'm concerned there is something else wrong with their relationship. Without either partner being aware of it, the back pain may have become the excuse for saying no. Otherwise, the person with the back problem would say, "Let's try. Even if it hurts a little, it'll still be worth it!"

So the situation calls for a certain amount of positive thinking?

Definitely. Otherwise, it's like being a prizefighter and stepping into the ring with an opponent you know is going to beat you. If that's your attitude, you're sure to lose. If you believe your back condition will defeat you, it will. But if you take the opposite attitude, you'll come out a winner.

Obviously there's a big emotional factor at work.

No question about it. What starts out as one person's relatively simple physical problem can soon cause both partners to get bogged down in a morass of emotions – fear, inadequacy, resentment, recrimination, and guilt. And once these emotions appear, they feed on one another.

Which partner feels guilty – the one with the sore back?

Sooner or later, they both do. Usually, they feel a mixture of emotions. The backache sufferer either feels guilty for refusing to have sex or feels resentful or inadequate when they do have it. The partner feels guilty for pursuing the idea when the other person obviously doesn't want to, or feels resentful or rejected because their sex life has disappeared. Those negative emotions just keep bouncing back and forth. Pretty soon the back-pain-versus-sex issue dominates their whole relationship.

But what if one person says quite honestly, "I can't have sex because my back hurts?"

In some cases, for a short while, that may be perfectly true. But often it needn't be. It *becomes* true because of the way people respond to the idea. It's another self-fulfilling prophecy.

Picture it: two people go to bed ostensibly with a delightful purpose in mind. But they are all too aware that one of them has a back problem. Instead of saying, "Let's find a way to make love in spite of it," they just lie there asking, "But what about your [my] back?"

What chance do two people have of being happy and successful lovers when they're worrying about a worn facet joint or a ruptured disc? After a while, they're talking like people in a medical clinic instead of lovers in a bedroom. Obviously, the romantic mood is shattered. And that's the simpler scenario. It gets a lot more complicated when one partner begins using back pain as an excuse for avoiding sex.

The back sufferer's equivalent of "Not tonight, darling, I have a headache"?

Exactly. It can – and does – mask an enormous number of problems in relationships. I can think of many instances where patients of mine have gone to great lengths to point out that it wasn't the emotional side of their relationship but only the back pain that was preventing them from having intercourse. In most cases I got the feeling that these people were protesting just a little too much.

Are most back specialists conscious of this emotional factor affecting their patients' sex lives?

Oh, I'm sure they realize the potential is there. But the physical aspects of a back assessment are extensive, and it's easy for a doctor to focus on them, to the exclusion of other aspects.

Also, back examinations are seldom carried out in what you might describe as a counseling environment. For example, I see many of my patients in a clinic – a big room with cubicles where conversations are easily overheard. While my patients don't seem to mind if someone else hears them telling me about their back pains, they are not about to broach the subject of sex.

Shouldn't doctors ask patients whether their sex life is being impaired by their backache?

Many of us do – if we have any inkling there's a problem. But even when we see patients who present us with sexual problems, we haven't the time or the facilities – or for that matter the training – to provide the necessary counseling.

Then what do you do about it?

I hear the patient out and make whatever comments I think might be helpful, and then I usually refer him or her to a psychologist or other counselor. Before I recommend a referral, however, I make sure the patient understands that the problem is real and physical and that I am not suggesting for a moment that it's all in their head. I consider that important because I have found that many patients otherwise resent having a surgeon refer them to someone for psychological consultation.

Do you think many of your patients have back-related sex problems they never discuss with you?

Yes, I'm sure of it. I also suspect there are those who don't even realize that a sexual problem can originate with backache. I'm always glad when a patient confides in me, and I do what I can to provide some preliminary guidance or support.

At one of my clinics recently, I was conducting an examination on a woman who has been a patient of mine for about ten years. Still in her thirties, she had been married for the second time about six months earlier, and she brought her new husband to the clinic with her.

I had finished examining her and was giving her my assessment when she asked if she and her husband could talk to me privately. Of course I agreed, and so we found a quiet office away from the other patients and staff. As soon as the three of us were alone, I began to understand the real reason why the woman had come to the clinic that day.

She was quite frank about their situation. It seems that she and her new husband had had an excellent sexual relationship before they were married, but now they were having serious problems. Her back pain was interfering with their sex life. She couldn't lie on her back. It hurt her to place her legs in the right position. It hurt her to raise her hips up. She just couldn't perform sexually. It was all too painful. And she was really frightened that the marriage would falter because her husband wasn't able to get sexual satisfaction.

If she hadn't asked for that private conversation, I would have done the assessment and prescribed treatment – mainly exercise in her case – without realizing that the main issue was not her back pain but her sexual relationship with her husband.

What could you – or did you – do for her?

We talked about things they could do to relieve the problem, or at least get around it. Oral sex was one thing. Some people have inhibitions about oral sex, but it can be a gentle yet stimulating aid to good sexual relations. It can be especially useful in foreplay, to achieve arousal without the kind of physical exertion that so often aggravates back pain.

We also talked about various positions for intercourse that would avoid back pain or at least reduce it to a tolerable level.

Are there certain positions that are generally better for most back patients?

Yes, but it's often a matter of trial and error, and the best solution will often depend on which partner has back pain. For instance, if the woman has Type One back pain, the so-called missionary position, with the man on top, may hurt, since it requires the woman to lie on her back, causing her spine to arch. She can help the situation by keeping both knees bent, but the movements necessary for intercourse may still jar the spinal joints and produce discomfort. Instead, the couple might exchange positions, to have the woman lying on top, supporting her upper torso with her arms and resting on her knees to keep her back bent forward slightly.

Another good possibility is the spoon position, with both partners on their sides, both facing in the same direction, with their legs bent and the woman in front and slightly higher up on the bed than the man, so that he can enter from behind.

If the woman has pain originating in a disc, she may find she is comfortable on her hands and knees, so that rear entry is possible without a great deal of movement on her part.

It's possible, too, to help a woman with backache achieve sexual union even if she finds it painful to part her legs. If she lies on her back, with her legs together but with the knees slightly bent, her partner can spread his legs to straddle her. Or if she lies face down, again with her legs slightly bent, her partner will be able to gain at least a limited degree of penetration – more than you might expect. It's not an ideal way to go about it, but it can produce satisfactory results for both partners.

What about the missionary position when the man is the one with back pain?

He won't care for that position either if he has a facet problem, since it will be painful for him to arch his back. But he can improve matters by supporting his upper body with his arms and keeping his back flexed forward.

Are there any basic rules?

Not really. Try to choose a position that calls for a movement other than the one that hurts. In the missionary position, either partner may aggravate Type One pain unless he or she takes special care. In contrast, Type Two symptoms can be made worse with forward thrusting of the pelvis, a movement much like the pelvic tilt, which increases disc pressure. I know that many couples find it satisfactory for the man to lie on his back while the woman sits with her knees astride his body, using her arms or elbows to support her upper body. She may be face to face with him or facing toward his feet – whichever is preferable.

It sounds as though some couples might have to depart from their customary style.

That's right. But that can be good for any long-term relationship. In addition, a lot of people, especially after they have been together for a number of years, tend to overlook the importance of extensive foreplay. With very little foreplay, intercourse itself may involve an excessive amount of movement for both partners to reach orgasm. With prolonged foreplay, that final period of activity can probably be much shorter and less strenuous – to the benefit of the partner with backache.

Are some positions wrong for anyone with back trouble?

Yes, some positions are obviously hard on the back, and you will steer clear of them almost automatically. And if you have discovered during some other routine activity that a certain posture or stance is painful you wouldn't even consider it for intercourse.

What positions are likely to be a problem?

One obvious example, for a man with a bad back, is the standing position, where he holds his partner in his arms with her legs around his body. That's a macho stance that could strain even a healthy back.

Bending forward with the knees straight will often increase discogenic back pain – as you may have discovered in other situations – and it certainly should be avoided during lovemaking. The same can be said of any position that causes excessive arching of the back, since it can bring on pain from the spinal joints; the idea is to find a neutral or stress-free posture.

If the woman has Type One backache, she'll probably want to avoid lying, face down, over the edge of the bed, if her legs dangle free. This lack of support will require her to arch her back to maintain the position, causing stress on the small facet joints.

Similarly, if she lies on her back with her legs draped over the edge of the bed and her feet unsupported, she will automatically arch her back. She won't be able to bend her knees, and she may not have enough strength in her abdominal muscles alone to maintain a pelvic tilt and avoid the back pain. The moral, I guess, is that even if the romance of the moment has your head in the clouds, it's a good idea to keep your feet on the ground.

Incidentally, that last position is fine for a couple where the woman has no spinal problems and the man is the one with the sore back.

What would your general advice be?

The best general advice can be summed up in a word: experiment. Of course, we have to hope that the couple are able to voice their needs and desires in an open and positive way, so that nobody is fumbling around in the dark, so to speak, surprising the other person with variations that haven't been discussed and that may prove unpleasant or painful.

If you have some reservations about positions you might try, but are not confident that they will help you avoid back pain, try them out some time when you're alone. Simulate intercourse without your partner, to get a better idea whether the positions you have in mind will be comfortable.

Would it be worthwhile to get a book showing various sexual positions?

By all means. Explore the possibilities and try anything that might please you and your partner. Just remember that whatever keeps your back from hurting, and makes the rest of you feel good, is all right. There are no absolutes. Mind you, if you show up in the bedroom one night with an ironing board, a block and tackle, and a set of shoulder straps, you might not receive the response you were hoping for, no matter how good it might make your back feel.

What about sexual activity following surgery? Do you have any special rules for that?

That depends. If there are bones that need time to fuse, or stitches that might pull out, you obviously shouldn't exert yourself in any way without your doctor's approval. Other than that, the principle is the same as for other times when your back is a problem: as long as you have a gentle and considerate partner, let your inclinations be your guide.

That point is made in an old gag that some back doctors still use. The patient asks: "How soon after the operation can I have sex?" and the doctor replies, "That depends on whether you have a private or semi-private room." In other words, if you have the urge for sex, you are well enough to enjoy it – harmlessly.

Apart from potential pain during intercourse, do back problems affect people's sexual capacity in any way?

Some men with back pain find it impossible to achieve an erection, but this problem is fairly rare.

Why can't they achieve an erection?

In most cases, it's psychological. We're not talking about getting an erection during an actual attack of back pain. As I've already pointed out, hardly anybody feels sexy at a time like that.

However, even during a pain-free period, a man with chronic backache may have a psychological block that inhibits him from having an erection. He may fear that intercourse will bring on pain that can paralyze him, although that actually never happens. It's as fanciful as the time-worn story of the passionate couple who are making love when the man has a back spasm and is so paralyzed he can't withdraw. He and his lady friend, unable to separate, have to be carried away on a stretcher. In the more imaginative accounts, the whole thing happens at high noon in Times Square, while thousands of amused spectators look on. That's all sheer nonsense, of course. A spasm could interrupt a person's sexual activity but certainly not cause paralysis. The worst that happens is that a man's fear of back pain makes him impotent.

Could his failure to achieve an erection be physical rather than psychological?

Yes – although physical causes are even more rare, and of course they are not necessarily related to a back problem. One physical problem is an insufficient supply of blood, which can be due to hardening or blockage of some arteries. Another physical cause is neurological, involving nerve damage that may interfere with normal sexual function. But again, let me emphasize that compared to psychological causes, physical factors are a far less common reason for failure to achieve an erection.

Whatever the cause may be, failure to achieve an erection must be a frightening experience.

Impotence does scare a lot of men. But there is really no need to be frightened about back pain preventing an erection. It helps a man immensely to realize it's usually a temporary psychological condition that can be remedied. Otherwise, it may become self-perpetuating. If a man is afraid he can't have an erection, there's a strong chance he won't be able to. But once he knows that other men have had the same experience and have recovered easily, he can keep his back pain in perspective.

So you could almost invoke the old expression about having nothing to fear but fear itself.

As far as the actual impotence goes, that's quite true. I suspect a lot of men harbor these fears and experience impotence because, for whatever reason, they never discuss the problem with a doctor or other professional counselor.

For the same reason other sexual problems don't get discussed with doctors?

That's probably part of the answer. Not many men are likely to bring up the subject, and some doctors may see no way of broaching it without embarrassing their patients. Which is another way of saying the doctor hasn't developed his consultative techniques very well.

Or a doctor may ask questions the wrong way. "How's your sex life?" is practically an invitation for the patient to answer, "Fine." A lot of men would find it demeaning to admit otherwise. The doctor would likely get a more revealing answer if he were to say, "A lot of men with your kind of back trouble find it difficult to get an erection. It's frightening, but it can usually be corrected very easily. If you ever have a problem that way, let's talk about it." I think most men will respond frankly to that sort of approach – and a great many cases that have remained secret can be recognized and dealt with.

How does a doctor deal with impotence?

The first step, obviously, is to determine the cause – whether the problem is related to the man's back condition or to some other problem. The doctor can test for the physical reasons: that is, poor blood supply or nerve damage. If there is no physical cause, it's probably a psychological issue, and the next step is to refer the patient for counseling.

Women obviously have their own reasons to be concerned about back problems. For instance, what about menstruation as a cause of back pain?

Although some of the pain occurring during menstruation is felt in the lower back, it's different from common backache. It has to do with muscle spasms in the uterus, which occur as the result of changes in the hormone levels. Fortunately, there are now medications that can provide effective relief.

Menstruation can also cause fluid accumulation throughout the body. This leads to swelling in the tissues, including the tissues in the back. And if the woman already has sore back muscles, the added fluid – the edema – will increase their irritability and aggravate the problems that already bother her spine.

Backache is something many women fear when they consider having a baby. Is it true that pregnant women inevitably get back pain?

Not inevitably, no. And if backache is going to show up at all, it usually does so around the fourth or fifth month of the pregnancy and often disappears again by the end of the seventh month. Of course most pregnant women do feel some back pain right before delivery. I think it helps to realize that pregnancy doesn't usually initiate the problem of back pain; all it does is add temporary stress to the back.

What about a woman who has had back pain in the past? Is she certain to have back pain during pregnancy?

Not necessarily. I've seen some women with a history of back pain who went through pregnancy with no increase in their problem, or even with no back pain at all. I've seen other women whose initial attack of back pain developed as the result of a normal pregnancy. With many women, pregnancy brought them their first bout with back pain because it imposed extra strain on a back that had already become worn from normal use. Sometimes a woman will get backache for the first time while bearing her third or fourth child. It wouldn't be accurate to say her back pain was caused by that last pregnancy; all her pregnancies contributed something to the strain. My favorite analogy is the frayed rope on an old-fashioned backyard swing. Year after year, the rope encircling the tree branch becomes more and more frayed. Then, one day, some boy who's too heavy for the swing jumps on and starts pumping. Of course the rope, which is almost frayed through by now, breaks. You can't really say the rope broke because that one boy used the swing. It broke because it was worn and couldn't take the extra strain.

Then getting pregnant does entail some risk to your back?

That depends what you mean by risk. Certainly there is a possibility that back pain will develop; I suppose it's risky in that sense. But there is no danger to either mother or child from the back pain that occurs in pregnancy.

Are the causes of a pregnant woman's back pain the same as the causes of common backache?

In most cases, yes, although pregnancy may add some special stresses of its own. Even before her pregnancy is obvious to the casual observer, a woman may adopt a characteristic gait that is different from her normal walk. She leans back a little; her toes point outward, with a gait that is an unmistakable sign of her condition.

This change in her walk places unaccustomed strain on certain muscles. Her body begins releasing hormones that will relax the ligaments of her pelvis, so that it can stretch open at the time of birth. Once the ligaments have become more lax, she is more vulnerable to an attack of back pain, specifically from the joints in the back of the pelvis, at the base of the spine.

Also, in the later stages of pregnancy, the weight of the unborn baby strains the mother's back and abdominal muscles in much the same way that a fat man's pot belly puts extra strain on his spine.

All these conditions contribute to back pain. Occasionally the primary location of the pain is in the sacroiliac joint – where the spine connects with the back of the pelvis. But the distinction is rather academic since ordinary low-back pain, though starting a little further up the spine, will usually radiate into the same area. To a woman with a chronic back complaint who has lately become pregnant, it seems like the same old pain. Even her doctor will probably find it hard to decide where the pain originates. But it really doesn't make much difference. The problem is the same, simple wear and tear. For all practical purposes, if pregnancy-related back pain does occur, it should be regarded as just another episode of common backache – and treated accordingly.

Perhaps the most difficult situation arises when a pregnant woman develops Type Three back pain – that is, the uncommon variety where a nerve is actually pinched. A case of this kind can be a real challenge for any doctor to manage. Chemical injection is out of the question because of the risk it presents to the baby, and I would rule out surgery as well, except in maybe one case in a thousand where the indications for surgery were overwhelming. Fortunately, most of the cases of nerve-root pressure get better, given time, rest, and the various other remedies that assist recovery whether someone is pregnant or not.

Aren't there any specific forms of back pain that are caused by pregnancy?

Yes, there are a few that arise because of the position of the baby, and there are others related to the complications that may arise from the pregnancy. In this case, however, the back pain is always secondary to other symptoms that the family physician or obstetrician will recognize as being related directly to pregnancy. Simple back pain in the absence of any other complaints can be pretty uncomfortable, but it is harmless.

You may have heard the term "back labor." Some women in labor experience a back pain that is different from common backache. The pain is quite low, often in the flanks. It's a form of pain that is part of normal delivery – although in a slightly unusual location. While it can be very unpleasant, it is just related to the intense muscular activity of the uterus at the time of birth and does not lead to long-term problems or increase the incidence of future episodes of back pain.

Are there some women whose backs are in such bad shape that they simply should not even consider getting pregnant?

Absolutely not. I've had patients tell me they have been given that advice, and I think it's wrong. Pregnancy could increase the expectant mother's back pain, but none of the mechanical problems that affect people's backs make pregnancy dangerous or impossible.

This was not always true. At one time, the spinal condition called spondylolisthesis was a threat to some pregnant women. Spondylolisthesis is not a disease but a mechanical disorder in which one vertebra slips out of line. It was identified for the first time more than a century ago as the cause of one woman's inability to deliver normally. In her case the slippage at the lowest level of the lumbar spine was so bad that her spinal column had moved forward into her pelvis and blocked the birth canal.

But before you start worrying about that possibility, let me emphasize two points. That degree of spondylolisthesis is extremely rare, but even if it occurs it can now be identified easily on X-ray and corrected with current surgical techniques. Also, if that severe slip does occur and is still undiagnosed when the patient becomes pregnant, it can be detected early in labor, and the baby can be delivered safely by Caesarean section.

What do you recommend for women with back pain who are going to have babies?

Exercise and special habits in daily living are important – but not just for women with a history of back pain. Every woman should exercise during and after pregnancy, to reduce the unwanted effects of child-bearing and promote a speedy return to normal activity once the baby is born.

What sorts of exercises?

When she first sees her family doctor or obstetrician about her pregnancy, she will probably be told to take up certain exercises that are commonly prescribed for expectant mothers. They are intended to strengthen the muscles of the abdomen and the pelvic floor. This helps support the unborn baby and will eventually assist with the delivery. This exercise program is similar in many ways to the one I prescribe for Type One back pain but, as with any set of exercises, experimentation is important. The expectant mother should develop a program that fits her daily routine and works to minimize her discomfort.

Are there special exercises for women whose pain is originating in the sacroiliac joint?

Yes, but special sacroiliac joint exercises are rarely necessary. Most expectant mothers find that regular back exercises provide the pain relief they are looking for.

What special habits should the pregnant woman adopt for daily living?

Various tricks can spare her back from unnecessary strain:

● She probably won't need to be told to leave her high heels in the closet and get herself some flat shoes. She'll discover that high heels increase the lordosis or curve in her lower spine, pushing the mid-section further forward and increasing the mechanical strain.

● She should make use of a foot-rest while seated, whenever possible, since this will take the strain off her back by raising her legs and reducing any excessive curve in her spine. Resting with the feet in an elevated position helps support the weight of the abdomen. It's useful as well because keeping the feet up will reduce swelling in the legs and aching in the thigh muscles.

● Rest is important too, of course. A pregnant woman will find she needs plenty of sleep each night, and she should take daytime naps as well, if possible.

How soon should a new mother begin to exercise after the baby is born?

As soon as her doctor will allow. She can begin almost immediately with isometric stomach-strengthening routines, which will help her to strengthen those weakened muscles without injuring herself. After a few weeks, with her doctor's permission, she should take up most of the routine exercises I recommend for people with common backache.

Which part of the whole child-bearing experience is hardest on the back?

Surprisingly, the worst time is usually after the baby is born. Not only because of the way the birth itself stretches various muscles and ligaments and saps some of the mother's strength, but also because of what a new mother goes through in caring for her baby – all that lifting of the child and its equipment, bending over the crib, doing the laundry, and so on. But all these hazards to her back can be greatly reduced if she prepares herself for them through exercise, good postural habits, and proper rest.

From everything you've been saying, it sounds as though nobody really needs to allow a bad back to interfere with his or her sex life or prevent a couple from raising a family.

That's exactly right. No question about it. Back pain does tend to interrupt people's lives, sometimes with tragic consequences, but there is usually no medical reason why this should happen. If you understand what you're up against and know how to cope with the pain – or, better still, learn how to prevent it from happening – your back is no threat to your sex life and needn't stop you from having a baby.

8. As You Grow Older

If you are a middle-aged victim of common backache and feel trapped by the prospect of a lifetime of discomfort and misery, I have some encouraging words for you: as you grow older, your back will almost certainly get better, and if you live long enough, you'll outlive your back pain.

Most backache sufferers, of course, assume that their spines are in for the opposite experience – a lifetime of deterioration.

Happily, good old Mother Nature commonly treats us all better than that. Unless you find yourself among the small minority who suffer backache from one of the less common afflictions, you can take comfort from the statistics which show conclusively that most aching backs get better all by themselves when their owners are around seventy.

Unhappily, few physicians ever reveal this good news to their patients. Why is that? I suspect many doctors become so engrossed with the immediate situation that they never get around to discussing the patient's long-term prospects. Also, I think doctors are often wary of raising false expectations in the minds of patients who are likely to experience quite a number of painful episodes before their backs finally begin to give them less trouble.

As well, there are some afflictions associated with aging which affect a minority of the population but get so much public attention they contribute to the myth that backache is inevitable during old age. One notable example these days is osteoporosis, a widely discussed condition that is greatly feared – often needlessly. It's true that middle-aged women have special reason to be concerned about osteoporosis; it afflicts far more of them than it does middle-aged men. But it's also true that for most women and men, regardless of age, osteoporosis will never be a problem; only about 15 percent of the population suffer as a result of it, compared to the 80 percent who suffer from common backache at some time in their lives.

If I were to apportion space in this chapter to afflictions purely on the basis of the number of aging people who suffer from them, osteoporosis would rate far less space than I have given to it. But it's something that concerns many people and I believe they are entitled to be told everything they want to know about it. And so I deal fully with all the questions I am commonly asked about this condition. This discussion should reassure readers that osteoporosis is not an inevitable source of trouble or pain.

The amount of space allotted to other less common causes of backache is also out of proportion to the frequency of their occurrence, for the same reason.

I hope that, by the end of this chapter, you will have a better idea of how the aging process actually affects your back. And if only one message stays with you, let it be my opening statement: *Most people's back pain really does disappear as they grow older.*

You say backs get better with age, but I know lots of old people with stiff backs and joints, and stooped shoulders, and all sorts of aches and pains.

That's true. But most of their aches and pains come from other causes, mostly in other parts of their bodies. And don't overlook the fact that being stiff and feeling sore are not the same thing. The aging process that makes your back stiff also keeps your facet joints from moving as much, and so they cause you less pain.

Your back continues to undergo wear and tear, but you don't feel its effects nearly as much. So the stiffening of your back with age has a beneficial effect.

Also as you grow older, your whole pace of living slows down. As you place fewer demands on your body, your back gets extra rest and it's less likely to feel painful from normal use.

Of course there are exceptions to the rule. Just the other day, I met a woman of seventy-nine who had just experienced her very first attack of back pain. But she's in a real minority. It's much more common to see people who had back pain in their earlier years and got better as they grew older. This observation has been borne out repeatedly by studies all over the world.

I remember many occasions as a boy, when our family outings were cancelled at the last moment because of my father's back problems. He would simply have to take to his bed because his back was so painful. Years later, when I got into this business of telling people about back pain, I often said that backs get better with age, and of course I said so in my first book. When *The Back Doctor* came out, my father, who was then about eighty years old, called me up and said, "I don't think it's right for you to go around saying such a thing without consulting your father."

"Okay," I said, "what happened to your back pain?"

"Well," he said, "it got better."

Are you saying that someone can just ignore proper back care and still wind up eventually with a pain-free back?

In many cases, that's true. Mother Nature will always try to do her best for you, no matter how you neglect yourself. But to increase your chances of having a pain-free back in later years, and to avoid a lot of misery along the way, you should keep yourself in reasonable physical condition.

How would you define "reasonable physical condition"?

I'm talking mainly now about back and abdominal muscles. It's hardly surprising that a person reaching, say, age seventy finds it difficult to begin developing muscular strength.

People who have kept their muscles in good condition throughout their lives will find it much easier to improve their muscle tone in their older years, and that extra strength is important to protect their backs.

There are two reasons why it's difficult, late in life, to take up exercise for the first time. For one thing, you lack the habits that would help you get into an effective routine; for another, you lack the necessary muscle tissue. If you are going to exercise for the sake of your back, you need to pay special attention to your belly muscles and those ridges of muscle that run down each side of your spine – the paraspinal muscles.

Picture a seventy-year-old man with a pot belly and weak muscles around his mid-section. That extra weight out front is pulling on his spine, and he hasn't the muscles to protect his back from the strain. He's not just a candidate for back pain, he probably has some pain already.

And he could have avoided that problem by doing regular back exercises as a younger man?

To a great extent, yes, and it will be very difficult for him to start now.

What if he had started years ago and then stopped? Could he expect to start again with any success?

Certainly the more he exercised over the years the better his chances of resuming the habit. But it's one thing to keep in shape all your life and quite another thing to get back into shape once you've let yourself go. In our exercise clinic at the Canadian Back Institute we see a lot of middle-aged and older people who have delusions about their physical abilities. I call it the 65/25 Syndrome; it stands for body of 65, mind of 25. These people just don't understand, or refuse to believe, that their bodies, being older, will not respond as quickly as they once did to the resumption of exercise. Invariably they're shocked to discover they can't snap back into shape in six weeks of workouts. It takes a lot more work and a lot more time.

Is being in bad shape as much of a problem for women as it is for men?

It's a problem for both, but in overweight women, the extra pounds tend to be stored a little lower and a little further behind, which is less of a strain on the back. Of course, it's still important to be in good shape, and certainly a woman with back problems can benefit considerably from exercises that strengthen the abdomen and the paraspinal muscles.

I seem to be getting the message that there comes a time for some people when it would be pointless to exercise.

If an elderly person is able to exercise and has the desire, I wouldn't object. But others may find exercise a frustrating experience if they haven't done it before, and I would doubt their ability to keep it up. When you talk about exercise for people in their senior years, you've got to be practical and realistic.

What happens, then, to older people who have back trouble and can't or won't exercise?

Fortunately, nature is still on their side. Even without exercise, as I said earlier, the joints and discs will still stiffen up with age, making the back pain disappear. In the meantime, while the pain persists, there is a place for corsets or other forms of temporary support that will help you through a bad time. And we can all practice proper body mechanics – the right way to stand and sit, for example.

What about other causes of back pain besides wear and tear? Aren't there some to which older people are especially susceptible?

Yes, there are two that are particularly noteworthy. One is osteoporosis, which we can talk about in a moment. The other is acquired spinal stenosis, which we discussed earlier, designating it as Type Four back pain.

As you'll remember, acquired spinal stenosis is a condition where the size of the spinal canal is reduced by a chronically bulging disc, bony overgrowth, or a combination of the two. The narrowing of the passage itself doesn't necessarily cause trouble, but it may make it difficult for blood vessels to supply the nerves that control the muscles in your legs. The result is a condition called *cauda equina* claudication.

In a typical case, the backache isn't a major problem; it's the legs that are most painful. And even the legs are fine when resting. But after a few minutes' walk, they feel strange – cold, rubbery, or numb – and the person has to sit down and rest for several minutes. *Cauda equina* claudication affects the elderly more often than other age groups because their bodies have been in use long enough for bulging discs and bony growths to develop in the spinal canal.

An uncle of mine can't walk very far without his legs becoming very painful. His doctor told me the problem was a poor blood supply to the legs. Is that the problem you've just described?

No. But, because the symptoms are similar, it's often hard to tell whether the person with that complaint is suffering from poor blood supply to the nerves in the back, which is *cauda equina* claudication, or limited blood supply to the muscles of the legs themselves, which is vascular claudication.

In a physical examination, the two conditions can appear almost identical, and so we employ several tests to help with the diagnosis. Some of the tests done to confirm claudication brought on by spinal stenosis are in fact designed to rule out vascular insufficiency in the legs.

The key to the direct diagnosis of *cauda equina* claudication is the CT scan, which allows us to check the diameter of the spinal canal and detect the long-standing disc bulges or bony growths that can narrow the space. Before the CT scan was available, the only way we could get some idea of the size of the canal was to obtain a myelogram, which involves injecting radiopaque fluid into the nerve sac around the *cauda equina* and X-raying the critical area.

Apart from what we can learn through these diagnostic investigations, one of the clinical differences I have noted is that patients with trouble in the back may get the most relief when they rest in a specific position – often one that involves sitting bent forward or with one knee drawn up – whereas people with poor blood supply to the legs get relief by resting in any position.

Incidentally, the diagnosis can become particularly tricky when a patient with simple Type One or Type Two back pain also suffers from poor blood supply to his legs. The symptoms may sound like *cauda equina* claudication, when in fact the patient can have two entirely unrelated problems: simple back trouble, plus vascular claudication.

Obviously, the two types of claudication must be treated quite differently. *Cauda equina* claudication is treated surgically to enlarge the spinal canal and make more room for the nerves and their blood supply. However, as I mentioned earlier, we don't operate on a case of spinal stenosis just because the canal is narrow; we perform surgery only when that narrowing causes pressure on the nerves.

Treatment of the vascular type of claudication may require surgery directly on the blood vessels in the legs.

You also mentioned osteoporosis as an affliction that affects older people. What exactly is it?

It's a thinning of the bone, which commonly occurs with age. When you hear the term osteoporosis, don't think "disease"; it is just Doctor for a process that happens to virtually everyone who grows old. Most people are never aware it has happened to them, since only a minority of the population ever develops osteoporosis that's painful or disabling. The great majority of cases remain undiagnosed because the bone-thinning causes no problems. Technically, osteoporosis exists – quite harmlessly – in the spines of most middle-aged and older people.

Then I could have osteoporosis without feeling any pain?

That's right. The condition itself doesn't hurt. Pain occurs only when other problems develop, as we'll see later.

Does that thinning of bones take place only in the the spine?

No, it occurs in most other bones as well. For example, medical researchers have found that in people over eighty, the walls of a normal thigh bone are reduced in thickness by as much as 50 percent. The outside diameter of the bone remains the same but the thickness of the walls is reduced from the inside – just the opposite of what happens when a tree grows by adding an outside layer or "ring" of wood year after year.

If you're over forty, some of the bones in your body may already have walls that are thinner than they once were. They're thickest when you're in your late twenties or early thirties, and they begin to thin out some time after age forty. The space inside, previously occupied by bone, is filled up partly by marrow but mostly by fat. If you find this whole idea frightening, you should understand that it's just as normal for your bones to change over the years as it is for your skin to wrinkle or your hair to turn gray.

Osteoporosis is like a worn-out pair of jeans. They may get thin at the knees, but as long as they don't tear, they're still serviceable. Obviously, however, the thin material is more likely to give way under strain than when it was new, and just as you have to be careful with a worn pair of pants, you have to be careful with a back that has osteoporosis.

What causes osteoporosis?

We don't know the cause, but we do know it's related to aging and it affects some people much more than others. In many cases, it just seems to come on gradually as the person gets older. Other contributing factors are: a calcium deficiency; in women, an estrogen deficiency; smoking; heavy drinking; lack of exercise.

Specific diseases can upset the system and bring on osteoporosis. For example, your doctor might find you have hyper-thyroidism, a chronically overactive thyroid gland, which can decrease the calcium content of your bones and hasten the onset of osteoporosis. So, if a doctor finds you have osteoporosis, a complete medical examination is in order, so that any disease can be either ruled out or detected and treated.

When does osteoporosis become painful?

That will happen when the bone of a vertebra gets so thin that it cracks or crushes just from the weight it normally bears. The drum-shaped bodies of the vertebrae are made of porous bone, full of holes like a sponge. This spongy bone is not unique to the spine (your heels, for instance, are made of the same stuff) but it's quite different from, say, your shin bones or your ribs. Now, when osteoporosis sets in, the holes in those sponge-like bones grow larger. As you would expect, the more porous the bone becomes the weaker it gets. When it reaches the point where it's too weak to support the weight of the body, a vertebra can collapse.

You mean one of the bones will just suddenly give way?

That's right. The collapse can be triggered by something as innocuous as a sneeze or a cough.

A crushed vertebra sounds terribly painful.

You bet it is. It produces the kind of acute pain you get with any broken bone, and this pain usually lasts about six weeks, until healing is complete. That pain is often the first indication of a problem caused by osteoporosis.

Are there permanent effects, even after the crushed vertebra has healed?

Not usually. The healed fractures become pain free, and the function of the spine returns to normal. Sometimes the vertebral bodies are squeezed down unevenly, so that they are narrower at the front than at the back, and that part of the spine is tipped forward, creating the so-called "dowager's hump" you see in some elderly people – usually in women but sometimes in men as well.

Further collapse, or the involvement of several vertebrae, may also affect the alignment of the facet joints, which may therefore wear more rapidly and cause trouble. Also, if a disc happens to bulge against a vertebra weakened by osteoporosis, it may push right into the thin, spongy bone, and that, too, can be painful.

Is it true that women are more likely than men to be affected by osteoporosis?

Yes, they are. Most research indicates that, in proportion to body weight, a typical woman has about 30 percent less bone mass than a typical man. And so, if a man and a woman both experienced the natural thinning out of the bones at the same rate, the woman would suffer the consequences much sooner. Furthermore, women are more often afflicted by an accelerated type of osteoporosis.

For reasons we don't understand, this type afflicts Caucasian women more than those of other races. According to one recent continent-wide study, 25 percent of white women in North America over the age of sixty have one or more broken bones associated with osteoporosis.

Earlier you mentioned that smoking and heavy drinking contribute to osteoporosis. How does that happen?

We're not sure of the exact mechanism, but we think it has something to do with the body's hormonal regulating system, which controls the storage, distribution, and use of calcium. Normally, calcium is taken out of the gut, stored in the bone, and then released from there as needed for regulation of specific body functions, such as normal nerve conduction. As the blood passes through the kidneys, the calcium is routinely filtered out and some is recycled for repeated use.

This process may break down for several reasons. The kidneys may fail to recirculate the calcium. Or there may not be enough calcium getting into the system in the first place. Or, on the other hand, too much calcium may be released from the bones into the general circulation, causing an overload that is corrected through a greater than normal excretion of the mineral.

So the hormones that regulate the calcium level will fail if you drink heavily or smoke?

Not fail, exactly, but there is a strong chance they will become less effective. And this raises a point that I'm sure a lot of people don't know: the bones in your body are being renewed constantly. In fact, they are completely exchanged about every seven years. Two different kinds of cells are involved in this process. One cell, called the osteoblast, generates new bone, while another cell, the osteoclast, eats up the old bone and sends its various components off into the system. It's nature's way of replacing material that's worn down, worn out, or damaged. For instance, it's this process that enables facet joints to reshape themselves when the discs in your spine narrow, as I described earlier.

Of course there has to be a balance between the processes of tearing down and building up. If you have too much bone mass it will get in the way, and if you have too little it won't provide adequate support. Certain hormones must be present in proper quantities to regulate the cellular activity that removes, repairs, and replaces normal bone.

Throughout their early years, most people's bodies manage to maintain the proper balance between making and removing bone. But as they grow older, the process falters because of a hormonal imbalance (a common cause in women after the menopause) or for various other reasons, such as a deficiency of calcium or of additional bone-forming materials. As a result, the bone creation process slows down while the bone destruction keeps right on at its usual pace. And so the bones get thinner. That's osteoporosis.

What's the best treatment for osteoporosis?

Unfortunately, there is no fully effective treatment for osteoporosis, once it has developed. It can be arrested, and in a few patients it can be partially reversed but not fully corrected. The best strategy, then, is prevention. You can increase your chances of avoiding the problem by maintaining or increasing your calcium intake, exercising, drinking alcohol only moderately or not at all, and not smoking.

You said "maintaining or increasing your calcium intake" as though everybody were likely to develop a calcium deficiency.

The fact is that most people do have a calcium deficiency, at least in North America, where the problem has been studied extensively. To keep their bones in good shape, men and pre-menopausal women need at least 1000 mg of elemental calcium a day. Mothers who are breast-feeding and women who have gone through menopause need about 1500 mg a day. But according to most calculations, the usual intake in North America is only about 400 to 500 mg a day. In other words, most men and young women on this continent are getting only half the calcium they need and most older women are getting only a third of what they require.

Does that mean everybody ought to drink a lot more milk?

That would be one solution, but a lot of people can't or won't do it. To get enough extra calcium from milk, most adults would have to drink about two more eight-ounce glasses than they now consume; post-menopausal women and breast-feeding mothers would need about three to four glasses a day beyond what they already take as part of their regular diet. That could be especially difficult for older people, whose systems don't tolerate milk readily.

What foods besides milk contain calcium?

There is calcium in other dairy products, such as cheese and yogurt. It's also contained in leafy green vegetables, kidney beans, and canned salmon and sardines, especially in the soft bones. It is possible to get a sufficient quantity of calcium from your diet, but not many people eat enough of the proper foods regularly to get the calcium they need.

What about calcium pills?

They can help prevent osteoporosis from developing. Men and pre-menopausal women should take about 500 mg of calcium a day, to supplement the calcium they get in their normal diet. Older women and breast-feeding mothers should take twice that amount.

Is there a danger of overdosing on calcium pills?

Under normal conditions, it's not possible to harm yourself by taking too much calcium by mouth, thanks to that natural control mechanism I described. The extra mineral just passes through the system and is discarded.

Can calcium pills help people who already have osteoporosis?

Yes, but since the process is not reversible simply with calcium treatment, the pills are useful only to stop it from getting worse.

Can extra hormones be prescribed to overcome the hormonal deficiency that leads to osteoporosis?

Estrogens, which are female hormones, have been used quite

successfully to prevent the loss of bone in post-menopausal women. But there can be undesirable side effects – and estrogens don't reverse osteoporosis, either; the most they do is arrest it.

What sort of side effects does estrogen cause?

Taken by itself, estrogen increases the risk of cancer in the uterus. This risk can be eliminated if a woman is willing to take progesterone along with the estrogen. They are the two hormones in birth control pills, and when they are taken in cyclical doses they will re-establish menstruation. When menstruation returns, I recommend regular check-ups by a gynecologist.

Would that mean there is a chance of becoming pregnant?

No, there's no chance of that. But there are other considerations. You can't prevent osteoporosis simply by adding some estrogen for a month or two. It has to be a long-term commitment. If you start taking estrogen-progesterone replacement and then stop it, your bone loss will rapidly return to its normal rate, and you will be no further ahead. If you took estrogen for, say, two years after menopause and then stopped, your chance of developing osteoporosis would be the same from then on, as if you never took the hormone replacement at all.

And yet we hear a lot these days about the benefits of estrogen.

Yes, and that worries me. Drug companies have always tried to sell estrogen by persuading doctors to prescribe it for their patients. But many doctors resisted the idea, for the reasons I just mentioned. More recently, advertisements lauding estrogen have been aimed directly at the public, and many patients are asking their doctors to prescribe estrogen to help in the management of their osteoporosis.

Then what do you say to a patient who asks about estrogen?

I explain the pros and cons and I point out that it involves a decision that's not to be taken hastily or lightly.

Can't anything be done to treat people who have osteoporosis?

Curative treatment is still a doubtful proposition, but doctors have
had some success with sodium fluoride, usually augmented by
extra calcium and vitamin D. Incidentally, the amount of sodium
fluoride prescribed is much greater than the amount added to
drinking water to toughen children's teeth. The extra fluoride,
combined with the calcium and vitamin D, can actually promote
the formation of bone. However, some people respond to this
treatment while others don't.

Fluoride should be administered only by a specialist who knows
exactly what he's doing. In large doses it can cause nausea and
gastro-intestinal bleeding, and it makes the bones brittle, leaving
the patient susceptible to fractures in the hips and long bones.
It may also produce the excessive formation of bone spurs.

On the positive side, fluoride is capable of toughening up the
porous bone in the spine, preventing the rapid bone loss that
might lead to the collapse of a vertebra.

Two other substances that have shown some promise are gland
extracts called calcitonin and parathormone. But these hormones
must be given by frequent injections, and the cost is substantial –
with no assurance that the treatment will work and no convincing
evidence that they can bring about a meaningful reduction in
the number of fractures that occur.

I feel the research in this area is very promising. But at this
point, there is no simple answer to the problem of treating osteoporosis.

**You implied earlier that exercise might help. How does it relate
to osteoporosis?**

We don't know the whole answer, but it's been recognized for
almost a century that your bones respond to use by getting stronger,
in much the same way as your muscles do. And there is much
more recent medical evidence that even light exercise, if it's done
fairly regularly, can retard the loss of calcium.

Or, to be more exact, I should say studies show that people
who exercise regularly seem to lose less calcium than those who
don't exercise. Although I'm in favor of exercise, and the recent

studies are certainly promising, I have to admit that it's hard to isolate the benefit of exercise from the effects of a generally healthy lifestyle. Many people who exercise regularly are also likely to avoid unhealthy habits, such as drinking heavily or smoking. And so, to be scientific about it, you have to ask: are people better off because they exercise or because they have developed healthy habits?

Incidentally, investigations into exercise have concentrated mainly on women, because of their special need to prevent calcium loss after menopause.

Then osteoporosis is less of a threat to women who are athletic?

That's not necessarily true. There is evidence that extremely strenuous workouts can upset the hormonal balance. Doctors have found that female athletes who run much more than twenty miles (32 km) per week may develop the condition known as amenorrhea. That is, they stop menstruating. The theory is that if the amount of body fat drops below a certain critical level, the body's production of estrogen also drops. In any case, the development of amenorrhea is a pretty clear indication that the hormonal levels are askew. And without the right balance, there's a greater risk of rapid osteoporosis. Researchers have found that a woman of twenty-five who exercises excessively – and here we're talking about someone training at an Olympic level – can suffer as much bone loss as an average woman would expect at age fifty.

Then the moral of this whole exercise story is moderation?

That's exactly right. Don't become sedentary, but don't become an exercise freak, either.

The most important point to make about osteoporosis is that a certain amount of bone loss is normal with aging. You can't prevent it entirely, but you don't need to, because it's unlikely to cause a problem. Excessive bone loss, on the other hand, is preventable, and if you let it develop to the point where it allows fractures causing pain or disability, you could be in for a lot of trouble.

What about other painful back conditions that develop as a person grows older?

One is degenerative scoliosis, another type of the spinal curvature we discussed earlier. It's different from the scoliosis that occurs in children, where the curvature is the result of an abnormal spinal growth.

Do we know what causes degenerative scoliosis?

Typically it results from an uneven pattern of wear and drying out in the disc. One side of the disc flattens down more than the other, so that it becomes wedge-shaped. Consequently, the spine tilts over toward the flatter side, causing a curvature.

Is degenerative scoliosis painful? How is it treated?

This form of scoliosis often puts increased pressure on the joints, discs, or nerves, causing pain that's virtually the same as common backache. The treatment is also the same: exercise, posture training, muscle strengthening, and in some instances surgery, if the narrowing between the vertebrae is so severe that the symptoms can't be relieved in any other way.

Are there other back conditions associated with aging that people should know about?

Another condition that's uncommon but worth noting is degenerative spondylolisthesis – an ailment that is easier to understand than it is to pronounce. "Spondyl" means "relating to the bones of the spine," and "listhesis" is a slip. For reasons no one understands, this problem occurs most often at a specific level of the lumbar spine in women over the age of forty-five. The facet joints connecting the fourth and fifth lumbar vertebrae are L-shaped and positioned to lock into place. (Anatomically there are five lumbar vertebrae, numbered downward, making Lumbar 5, or L_5 as it is usually called, the last movable segment before the pelvis.) In some people, as the joints wear with age, they flatten out, and the locking effect is lost. This means the entire fourth lumbar vertebra, now held only by the L_4-L_5 disc, is free to slide forward very slowly. When that happens, you get pain.

Can anything be done about this slippage?

Treatment is not always necessary. Sometimes with further aging the area stiffens up by itself, and when the movement stops, so does the pain. If the symptoms persist, they can sometimes be controlled by exercises that strengthen the belly muscles, so that they can take some of the load off the spine. However, when there is significant slippage because the joints have completely lost their ability to lock together, surgery may be the only way to go.

Is surgery likely to succeed in a case like that?

As a rule it will. Since the problem is clearly identified and the mechanical failure is quite local, a spinal fusion is usually a successful way of stopping the slippage. In this operation we span the distance between the two vertebrae with strips of bone, and in that way we fuse the fourth and fifth lumbar vertebrae into a single, longer bone. The joints above and below the fused area remain functional, with their lock mechanisms still working normally. Of course movement at the L_4-L_5 space is gone, but that's the idea; otherwise the facet joints would remain unstable.

What about cancer of the spine as a source of back pain in older people?

Cancer can originate in the back in one of two locations. It can begin in the vertebral bone, or it can develop in the blood-forming tissue within the bone, that is the bone marrow. Either way, it's rare for cancer to originate in the spine; the occurrence rate is much less than for cancer of the lung, breast, or prostate.

What about cancer that spreads to the spine from somewhere else?

It is more common – or, I should say, less rare – to find the spine affected by a cancer that has spread from some other part of the body. But almost always, this cancer is diagnosed before it reaches the back. And, for that reason, neither the patient nor the doctor is inclined to regard the illness as a spinal problem, but rather as a cancer that is becoming a threat throughout the body.

In very rare instances, patients may complain of back pain that turns out to be caused by cancer in the spine that spread there from somewhere else even though the original source cannot be identified. To give you some idea of how rare this is: out of the more than 40,000 back patients I have examined, I've encountered only three cases of this kind.

In short, if you don't have cancer anywhere else in your body, your chances of having it in your spine are extremely remote, whatever your age.

What kinds of cancer are likely to spread to the back?

Breast cancer is one. Another is cancer of the prostate, which, as you know, is a problem for men in their older years. A third is multiple myeloma, a cancer that may originate in the spine but actually attacks the blood-forming cells of the bone marrow in many parts of the body. The incidence of these last two cancers increases as people grow older. Again, I must stress that, although the numbers go up with age, the possibility of spinal cancer is still very unlikely.

As unlikely as it may be, if I did have cancer in my back, what would the symptoms be?

Nobody should jump to that conclusion, but I will mention two symptoms. First, a pain that is constant, even at rest. By that I mean a pain that remains unchanged no matter what you do to seek relief. Bending backward, stooping forward, sitting, lying down – nothing makes any difference to the pain. Second, a pain that has been present for a relatively short time. Malignancies of this sort progress rapidly, and if you have had the same problem in your back for, say, one or two years, it is not cancer. It is probably just one of the common types of back pain. But if your back is bothering you and you don't know what's wrong, see your doctor. Chances are you'll gain peace of mind, as well as receiving advice about the appropriate remedy for whatever the problem may be.

If you suspected a patient's back pain was caused by cancer, how would you proceed?

I would order several diagnostic procedures. I'd want a series of blood tests conducted to look for the chemical changes that occur when bone is being destroyed by a malignant tumor. I would also order certain X-ray studies, such as a CT scan or perhaps a different type of bone scan in which a radioactive material is injected into the system. This material becomes incorporated briefly into the structure of the bone. On the scan, the doctor can see an increased amount of the material in any area where there is excessive bone reaction. That doesn't necessarily mean there's a tumor there, but it does indicate that the body is reacting – to something. And this can be a valuable clue in the search for what is wrong.

What advice do you have for people who are worried that cancer may be the cause of their back pain?

The first thing I want them to understand is that cancer as a cause of back pain is extremely rare. But if they have any apprehension, they should see a doctor. He may use the tests I just described, although I must point out that I don't use them routinely in my own practice, because they simply aren't necessary. I emphasize that point because I would hate to think this discussion might give anyone the idea that their doctor wasn't being thorough enough if he ruled out cancer without conducting the tests.

How would you summarize what older people should know about back problems?

We've spent quite a bit of time talking about the back pain some older people experience from causes other than wear and tear. It is important to remember that these afflictions are very uncommon. They make up only a small fraction of all backache cases. And we have effective remedies for most of them. One exception is osteoporosis. As a natural process that can become excessive, it exemplifies the adage about an ounce of prevention being worth a pound of cure.

The most important point of all, however, is one I made right at the beginning of this discussion: for nearly everybody, mechanical back pain gets better with age.

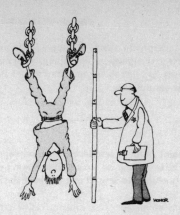

9. AEROBICS, HEEL-HANGING, AND OTHER AMUSEMENTS

Among the steady stream of people who come to me with back problems, there are always some who are looking for shortcuts to recovery.

They want my opinion, if not my approval, of devices such as gravity traction outfits or weight-lifting machines, and various "in" exercises such as yoga, as means of treating their pain or improving their backs. I'm sure some of them feel I'm being deliberately evasive when I decline either to endorse one of these alternatives without qualification or to condemn it as worthless.

My position usually lies somewhere between the two extremes. There is no such thing as *the* treatment that helps everyone. The remedy that provides dramatic relief to Patient A may prove utterly ineffective for Patient B. Knowing that, I am pragmatic enough to say, "If it doesn't hurt and it's not harmful, try it." On that basis, and if it helps the patient feel better, I'm delighted.

And of course backs do get better by themselves. Acute attacks inevitably subside, and even chronic pain recedes, in time, as a person ages and the body adjusts. And so with any treatment that is followed by apparent improvement or recovery, you have to ask: "What made the patient's back get better? Was it the therapy, or was the pain about to disappear anyway?"

Those are questions to which nobody has the answers. But I do have answers to the questions my patients most often ask about faddish exercises and therapies sometimes touted as the ultimate solutions to the painful back.

What do you think of those new devices that are supposed to relieve backache by letting you hang upside down, by your heels or in a sitting position, for several minutes each day?

They are forms of an age-old treatment called gravity traction, and the only things new about them are the upside-down position, the big price tag, and the questionable claims of success. As a concept, gravity traction is at least as old as medieval times, when a patient would be fastened, right side up, to a ladder, with weights attached to his feet, to pull down on his spine and thus relieve his back pain.

The idea of gravity traction is to provide more pull on the back than can be generated by conventional traction. In the conventional method, a patient lies on his back, wearing a waist-belt attached to weights that hang over the end of the bed and pull steadily on the spine. To keep the weights from pulling the person onto the floor, the foot of the bed is usually tipped up slightly. Even so, there's a limit to the amount of pull that can be exerted without dragging the patient off the bed, and a lot of the benefit of that pull is wasted by the friction of the apparatus and the patient against the sheets.

Does bed traction actually relieve back pain?

Sometimes it does, but probably only because it keeps the patient in bed and resting. If you put anybody with back pain in a comfortable position for a week, chances are the person will get better. I suspect the traction has very little to do with the patient's recovery. But a few doctors who believe in the value of traction decided they could overcome the friction problem and at the same time increase the traction by using the weight of the person's own body to provide the pull, suspending him in mid-air wearing a chest harness somewhat like a parachutist's gear. To give the body a chance to adjust gradually to the gravitational pull without pain or harm, the patient starts out flat on a tilting bed. Then, with each successive treatment, the slope of the bed is increased until the patient is virtually upright.

Incidentally, I tried that type of traction for my own back problem, but it didn't work out very well. For some reason, no matter how tightly I was strapped in, my body kept slipping through the harness, and I soon abandoned the whole idea.

Maybe the same harness problems gave somebody the idea of hanging by the heels instead.

Could be. That variation apparently got started in California in the 1970s. But it never really caught on until 1980, with the release of a movie called *American Gigolo*, in which the star, Richard Gere, practiced gravity traction, using boots fixed to an overhead bar. Soon, people all over the continent were suspending themselves upside down.

What happens, exactly, when gravity traction is applied – upside down or otherwise?

One of the problems is that nobody really knows. When it's used regularly, gravity traction does relieve back pain for some people. But we're not sure why. Maybe it relieves spasm in the muscles by stretching them and inducing them to relax. Or perhaps it counteracts pressure on the small joints of the spine. It's possible that if you pull with enough force on the low back, the facet joints that are sore from being jammed together will separate slightly, easing the pressure and reducing the pain. The action is the same as the one I mentioned during our discussion of neck problems. It's also possible that a strong pull on the outer fibers of a bulging lumbar disc will be enough to reduce the size of the bulge and decrease the local irritation. All these things could happen, at least while the traction is being applied.

But the evidence in favor of gravity traction isn't conclusive?

No, the possibilities I just mentioned are speculative. The problem is the size and strength of the spine in the lower back. Several studies have been done with special X-ray investigations to measure the difference, if any, in the shape of a disc's shell before and after gravity traction. According to some reports, the treatment seemed to have reduced the bulging; other reports say it had no apparent effect. Certainly the reaction is not uniform, and the weight of evidence suggests that gravity traction doesn't produce any permanent change. The most you can say for it is that it seems to help some people's backs sometimes.

But weren't the newer forms of gravity traction developed by reputable medical experts?

Many were, but that doesn't automatically make them right. Furthermore, if you find it helpful to stretch your body with gravity traction, you're not necessarily better off upside down than right side up. I've read claims that the inverted position is beneficial to the heart, lungs, and brain, but I have also seen studies indicating that hanging with your head down can produce serious side effects, such as aggravating glaucoma from the extra pressure on the eyeballs, or contributing to high blood pressure. In my view, gravity traction owes its popularity more to slick marketing than to proven statistics. The result is that people are willing to pay sometimes as much as $1,000 for an apparatus that lets them hang upside down exactly as they could, free of charge, from a jungle gym in a children's playground.

Aren't you being a little harsh, considering that some people would want to use the equipment in private, at home, and have apparently found merit in this form of treatment?

My concern here is not the potential benefits but the aggressive manner in which gravity traction is merchandized. If you read the promotional literature carefully you will see just how much hype it contains. You'll find it filled with extravagant statements that are impossible to pin down: "Many orthopedic surgeons are prescribing it"; "Nine out of ten sufferers report immediate results ... dramatic relief during their first two-minute session"; a "breakthrough [that] applies space-age technology"; "state-of-the-art"; and so on.

To me, those sound like pitches from a snake-oil salesman, updated for the 1980s.

Are you saying the manufacturers are making questionable claims?

Let's say they do a pretty thorough job of mixing fact with fancy while overlooking recognized medical knowledge. Here's an example from one pamphlet:

> Q. What about stress-related factors?
> A. Chronic pain is often associated with debilitating emotional stress, muscle tension and physical fatigue – triggering states of fear, anxiety and depression, rage, frustration. . . .

What they say up to that point is perfectly true, as we have already discussed in this book. But then the brochure goes on:

> Relaxing muscle spasm and releasing disc compression interrupts the pain cycle – while defusing stress and tension.

First, assuming for the moment that gravity traction actually does "release" your disc compression (whatever that means) there is no proof that this will interrupt the pain cycle and that stress and tension will be "defused" (which I assume is Hype for "relieved").

Second, even if these results are achieved, you have to wonder: will the traction provide more than a few minutes' relief?

And third, interrupting your pain cycle doesn't come anywhere near *altering* it. As long as it's still there, it will soon be back in full force, causing the same old agony and spasm. Yet nothing in the literature concedes that the relief is likely to be temporary.

Another statement in a brochure suggests that gravity traction can be used to treat an acute sports injury. It is saying, in effect, that if you tear a ligament in your neck, give it a good pull with gravity traction and it will get better. That's not true. Treating an acute ligament injury with traction will be painful, and it makes no more sense than pulling on a newly sprained ankle or pounding a bruise with a hammer.

The silliest claim of all is presented in some good old rough-and-tumble comparative advertising in the Coke-and-Pepsi tradition. A drawing shows two young men hanging head down. One is hanging by his heels, from a competitor's product consisting of a horizontal bar and heavy ankle straps. The other young man, using the advertiser's product, is hanging from his waist, with his thighs across the seat of what looks like an expensive version of a backyard swing. The copy reads in part:

> Medical specialists agree that the key to alleviating low-back pain is to *flatten* the lumbar curve and *stretch* the spine... [emphasis theirs]

That is startling news to *this* medical specialist, who regards a moderate lumbar curve as healthy and natural. But there's more:

> Computerized results prove that [our product] flattens the lumbar curve and stretches the spine an average of *2.7 inches more* than [the rival product] [emphasis theirs].

Never mind whether that claim is actually true, and let's not bother asking why a computer was needed to make such simple measurements. Let's consider the long-term implications for the gravity-traction industry. Will future, improved models of these devices stretch people's spines even more – an additional four, six, eight, twelve inches? Are we on the threshold of creating a whole new race of people who are totally free of back pain and stand eight feet tall? You have to wonder: where were these promoters when the Spanish Inquisition needed them?

But, all joking aside, it must be confusing for back pain sufferers who face that kind of sales pitch.

Confusing, yes, and if it diverts them from more effective long-term management of their backs, it's doing them a disservice. I'm not opposed to gravity traction in all cases, but it does have its limitations, and people should be aware of them. We do know that in nearly four cases out of five, neck traction – manual or mechanical – is effective in relieving acute muscle spasm. And it is possible that gravity traction does the same thing for the low back in spite of the greater rigidity there.

But, as I have said, it doesn't help everybody. And certainly it is not the panacea it's sometimes made out to be. Common sense will tell you that no single form of treatment is capable of relieving every kind of neck or low-back problem, regardless of its nature or cause, or what stage it has reached.

If your problem is common backache, hanging upside down isn't going to harm your spine, although it may not be good for other parts of your body. But when it is suggested to me that there are long-term benefits to be gained from a few minutes of gravity traction each day, that's when they lose me.

It seems to me that the greatest long-term benefit from gravity traction may accrue not to the people who are using the devices but to the companies that are selling them.

Would you make the same criticism of the more conventional machines people are using for exercise and body-building – cycling machines, rowing machines, weight-lifting machines, and so on?

No, I wouldn't, although I do have some reservations about them. Assuming you apply sensible training methods, warming up for each workout and practicing moderation, I see nothing wrong with using exercise machines. However, if you intend to exercise without the supervision of a competent trainer, I suggest you read up on the particular machine you intend to use, or discuss it with a qualified physical therapist or fitness specialist, so that you understand the correct procedures and safeguards.

The main hazard is that whether an exercise routine is beneficial or detrimental, an exercise machine will magnify the effect. If you do everything right, the machine will magnify the benefits you get from it; but if you do things wrong, it will magnify your pain.

I'll give you an example. Most popular exercise machines use variable weights to provide tension and resistance for muscle development. One standard routine on these machines is an exercise intended to strengthen the muscles in the backs of your thighs. You lie on your stomach with your legs straight and your calves under a padded bar. Then you bend your knees. If you do it right, this routine strengthens your hamstring muscles. But if you overload the weight on the bar, you force yourself to work too hard at bending your knees. Instinctively, you will arch your back to gain extra leverage. That extra strain on your back is likely to cause pain if your facet joints are worn and hurt every time they are squeezed together.

To avoid the unwanted effects in this case you start with a lighter load. It will take you a little longer to get the results you want, but you will avoid a great deal of unnecessary discomfort. If you are considering exercising with any sort of machine, remember: while it's bad enough to do any exercise improperly, it's worse to do one whose ill effects will be magnified.

What about aerobic exercise for people with back problems?

I see nothing basically wrong with strenuous aerobic exercise if you're already in good shape. But most of us aren't. Aerobic routines require little strength but a lot of flexibility and stamina. They won't do much to prevent or overcome common backache. In fact, the impact of jumping up and down for twenty minutes may be enough to make your back sore. And the forceful bending and twisting movements that are part of so many programs will add to your discomfort. Aerobic exercises are designed to condition your heart and lungs, but they may not suit your needs as a back-pain sufferer. There are "low impact" routines available that provide good stimulation for the heart and lungs without placing unnecessary strain on your spine.

If you get into any heavy exercises without considering their effect on your spine, you're asking for trouble. If aerobic exercises are what you want, choose some that will also help strengthen or at least protect your back – swimming or riding an exercise bike, for example.

Then you approve of aquatic exercise?

Yes, water is a good medium for exercise – you can put your muscles through their paces without the effect of gravity, keeping the load off your spine while gaining all the benefits of stretching, strengthening, and aerobic routines. Almost any kind of swimming is helpful to back patients, although the particular approach best for you will depend on the exact nature of your problem. A well-done pool program is an excellent form of therapy – a good way to augment the more specific back exercises I'll be detailing in my final chapter.

I have only two reservations when my patients tell me they have started swimming to help their backs. For one thing, I wonder if they realize that swimming will help them only if they follow a schedule of exercises. Just getting into the water to float around is not enough. Also, I wonder if they will stick with the routine. Some patients who start pool therapy in a rehabilitation department often do well until they are discharged, and then they drop their exercise program because they don't have ready access to another swimming pool. All they're doing, of course, is shirking the responsibility for their own rehabilitation. Most communities these days have pools open to the public and, in any case, you can exercise without water, or, for that matter, without equipment of any kind. You certainly don't need a swimming pool of your own to keep your back in shape.

I recall you didn't recommend jogging as an exercise for people with back problems.

Jogging provides no direct benefit to your vertebral column or to the back and stomach muscles that are important in maintaining a healthy spine. One study even suggests that joggers should have strong stomach muscles before they start running, to reduce the risk of backache. In other words, if you go jogging, you should have reasons other than wanting to control your back pain.

What do you think of yoga as a means of avoiding or overcoming back trouble?

I consider yoga interesting and useful. It is certainly not a fad. As therapy for back problems I find it a healthy combination of exercise and mental discipline. It's no panacea, but then no form of treatment is.

Yoga exercises don't do much to increase a person's strength, although they often help flexibility. On the other hand, yoga's relaxation and meditation techniques, involving deep breathing and other routines, are excellent pain-control mechanisms. In that way, they resemble some of the therapy provided by pain clinics to relieve muscle tension and diminish a patient's focus on pain.

There are, however, certain things about yoga that require caution if you are a backache victim. In performing yoga exercises, you will be putting your body, including your back, through a wide range of movements – stretching muscles in your groin and thighs as well as along your spine. These routines are good unless they overload an inflamed facet joint in the low back or put too much pressure or torque on a worn disc. Then the exercise will aggravate your back pain. For instance, the cobra, an extension maneuver, is not a wise choice for someone with Type One trouble. The shoulder stand can be a real killer if you have Type Two difficulties. Whatever your problem may be, I assume you will make the obvious distinction between a recurrence of your typical pain and the discomfort and normal aches you feel the day after any new physical routine. If an exercise causes a flare-up, strike it off your list, at least temporarily, and try it again, carefully, some time when your back is feeling better.

You should understand, too, that yoga is not designed to provide specific help for your back. Therefore, if you came to me and said, "I want something to help my back," I wouldn't likely say, "Well, go and do yoga." On the other hand, if you came and said, "I want to try yoga – do you think it's all right?" I would approve, unless I knew a particular reason why you shouldn't participate.

But, as with any new routine, the more you find out about it, the better you will be able to judge whether it has potential benefits and, if so, decide if it should become part of your individual program of back care.

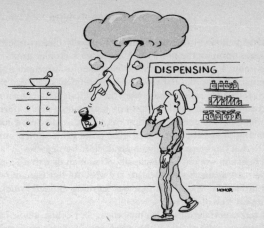

10. "MAGIC POTIONS" OR ALTERNATIVE TREATMENTS

In my practice, I keep encountering a few otherwise intelligent people who are convinced that, some day soon, someone will produce an instant cure for common backache. And I never cease to be amazed at those who believe a magic potion has already been discovered but is being suppressed by the medical establishment.

One phone call I received from a doctor in Florida was particularly disheartening. Would I mind telling him the name of the "miracle drug" I was using up in Canada? He said a former patient of mine, now living in Florida, had come asking for the same injection that I had administered to him about a year earlier. The doctor hadn't heard of any drug available in the U.S. that could cause a patient's backache to disappear instantly, leaving him pain free for an entire year. Now that the pain had returned, both doctor and patient were anxious, naturally, for a second magic dose.

When I heard the man's name, I realized part of the story was true. This patient had come to see me two or three times, complaining of low-back pain radiating to the top of his right buttock. My examination showed that the primary cause was simple

Type One facet joint pain with much of the discomfort referred
to a trigger point on the bony ridge above the sacroiliac joint.

Originally, I prescribed routine exercises to strengthen his
abdominal muscles, but the pain persisted, and so I decided that
a little temporary relief might alter the pattern and encourage
the man to continue working towards lasting recovery. Offering
the patient no greater expectation than that, I injected a local
short-acting anesthetic into the trigger point – a treatment, incidentally, that has been used by family doctors for decades.

The injection worked – dramatically. So well, in fact, that I never
saw the man again. Soon after his last visit, he left Canada and
settled in Florida, where, as I now was learning, he had evidently
spent a year free of pain.

As I recounted the history to my colleague, I could almost hear
the disappointment rising at the other end of that long-distance
line.

"Sorry," I had to say, "but I have no magic potion for backache."
The man had simply been the beneficiary of a lucky coincidence
in which the temporary relief of my injection happened to combine
with the spontaneous improvement of his back pain. The best
I could suggest was that the doctor repeat the treatment and see
what happened. Another shot of local anesthetic couldn't possibly
do the patient any harm, and, considering what the first injection
had done, it might just help again.

I never did hear how it came out, but for all I know, there
is a transplanted Canadian living in Florida today who still thinks
he was treated with a miracle drug available only in his native
land.

That wouldn't surprise me in the least. What does surprise me
is that a colleague was willing to believe I'd found a miraculous
treatment and had been quietly dispensing it to my patients here
in Canada, without sharing my marvelous discovery with the rest
of the medical community.

While I don't disparage any treatment that helps people's backs
get better without undesirable side effects, I keep stressing the
futility of their searching for that non-existent magic cure. The
search is certain to lead to disappointment and – worse still – may
distract them from the exercises and proper living habits that
offer the best long-term solution to their problem.

Many drugs, devices, and therapeutic procedures currently

touted as cures for backache would receive little further attention or acclaim if more doctors provided their patients with a thorough understanding of back pain, helping them realize that the most effective treatment usually includes their own active participation in a continuing program of management.

Physiologically, many of these alternatives have little to recommend them. But they offer new hope to the patient who emerges from the doctor's office, having received a cursory examination, a hastily scribbled prescription, and the terse instruction: "Take some of these pills and see if you feel better."

Compared to that approach, almost any other sort of treatment must seem more promising, especially if it is sold with great enthusiasm and conviction by someone claiming to have helped thousands of others with the same problem.

Unfortunately, even doctors who try to be responsive to their patients' needs will sometimes leave a mistaken impression. I've learned that from listening to the patients who come to me after seeing someone else.

"I saw my own doctor," they'll say, "but he didn't do anything."

"What do you mean? Didn't he examine you?"

"Well, yes."

"And didn't he tell you what was wrong with your back?"

"Yes, but then he didn't do anything. He just said we'd have to wait and see."

What we have here is not an uncaring doctor but a simple failure to communicate. From my own professional experience I know that "wait and see" is often exactly the right thing to do. Acute attacks subside and backs do get better by themselves. But I also know how important it is for the doctor to make it clear that waiting is not the same as doing nothing. Any time it's necessary for me to tell a patient "wait and see," I take care to avoid giving the impression that I'm not interested in the patient's problem or that I can't think of what to do next.

When I do counsel a patient to just wait, I seldom object if he or she wants to try some alternative form of treatment during that time, provided that it's not dangerous and the person has a clear and realistic idea of its purpose, its potential, and its limitations.

In this chapter I discuss a variety of alternative therapies ranging from the useful to the useless. There are many more I don't mention, but I have tried to give some idea of the kinds that offer genuine relief and those that create only false hope. The term "magic potions" refers less to the offerings of the practitioners than to the unrealistic expectations in the mind of the anxious patient.

―――――――――

I've been told that an injection of chymopapain can cure backache and eliminate the need for back surgery. Could that be the miracle cure we've all been waiting for?

Not quite. Unlike injections used for temporary relief from pain or inflammation, chymopapain can be a permanent remedy but it is useful only for Type Three back pain, when the nerve is pinched by a bulging disc. It is a chemical derived from the papaya fruit, similar to the tenderizer you might use on a tough steak. The material is injected into the disc to soften the nucleus and relieve pressure on the nerve.

Many people have the mistaken idea that chymopapain dissolves the center, or nucleus, of the disc. Actually, it denatures the protein of the nucleus, transforming a hard bulge into a soft bulge by destroying the tissue's ability to retain water. Figuratively speaking, it's like turning a walnut into a marshmallow. Usually this transformation cannot even be detected on a CT scan because the shape of the lump remains the same; only its texture is changed.

The fact that chymopapain doesn't actually remove the lump is probably one reason why it won't relieve Type Two pain, which comes from the disc itself. The bulging disc still bulges, and it continues to create a problem by stretching the outer shell. In fact, by drying out the nucleus, the injection may actually accelerate the natural aging process of the disc, and over time produce Type One or Type Two pain.

Is chymopapain safe? I heard it was banned in the United States for several years.

In the hands of a competent and experienced doctor, chymopapain is at least as safe as surgery. It was taken off the market in the

United States as a result of a large scientific study that seemed to show that it had no beneficial effect. The drug was never actually banned. It was voluntarily withdrawn by the manufacturer until further tests could be carried out. Many doctors, continuing to believe the injection was useful, pressed for its reinstatement. Meanwhile, chymopapain remained available in Canada, and thousands of Americans crossed the border to receive the drug. Eventually, further investigation reconfirmed its benefits, and chymopapain was reintroduced into the U.S.

One good thing to come out of the careful evaluation was a better understanding of how chymopapain should be used. Many of the unsatisfactory results, and almost all the complications, come from an ill-advised selection of patients (that is, people whose back problems cannot be corrected by this treatment) and from poor injection techniques.

Then is chymopapain really an alternative to surgery in certain cases?

I don't consider chymopapain an alternative to surgery; I tell my patients it's a first step that may make subsequent treatment, including surgery, unnecessary. If you have Type Three pain, and I inject chymopapain, I do so with every hope that it will clear up your problem, so that you won't need an operation. Although its success rate overall is about 70 percent, chymopapain works well in some cases and not at all in others, for reasons we don't fully understand. If the injection fails to reduce the nerve-root irritation, the only thing to do is to move on to the second step, which is surgery. Whenever I recommend chymopapain I always make it clear that the treatment doesn't always work. And so we are talking about surgery if necessary, but not necessarily surgery.

There is another way to look at the issue. Because the indications for chymopapain injection and surgery are exactly the same, if you have a condition where one of those two treatments can't help you, the other can't either. It makes no sense to consider the injection if you have already been told that surgery will not help in your case. Chymopapain isn't non-specific therapy for back pain; it is a chemical method which can provide relief of symptoms from direct nerve-root pressure.

I imagine most people would rather have chymopapain than surgery.

That's true, but chymopapain can be a painful treatment, and it has its own complications, limitations, and uncertainties. Perhaps I can illustrate what I mean if I tell you about the experience of a woman I'll call Stacey Wilson. Five years before her second episode, I had seen Mrs. Wilson for an acute attack of back pain with definite signs of pressure on a nerve root supplying part of the right leg. She recovered slowly without surgery.

The second time, her back problem was accompanied by pain running into the left leg and the loss of function in a nerve root coming from the left side of the spine. The CT scan showed two bulging discs, one pressing a nerve to the right, the cause of her previous trouble, and one pressing a nerve to the left, the source of the new pain.

I decided to use chymopapain on both discs to relieve the acute pressure to the left from the one below and reduce the chance of future trouble to the right from the disc above. Surgery at both levels was possible but would have produced more trauma to the spine and resulted in more scarring.

I gave Mrs. Wilson the injections, in both of those troublesome discs, and for three days she enjoyed complete relief. At 4:45 A.M. on the fourth day, her back and left leg pain returned with a vengeance. She endured it for almost three hours, then called me at 7:30 in the morning. I had her readmitted to the hospital. I was not alarmed by the return of her pain, since chymopapain can be initially painful and, in some cases, it will continue to produce severe back spasms for weeks. But one aspect of her problem was worrisome: Mrs. Wilson's leg pain had also returned and was worse than the pain in her back.

That symptom was significant because a routine chymopapain injection shouldn't produce increased pain in the leg. Because the injection can take several days or even several weeks to produce its full benefits, and since she was suffering so much, I kept Mrs. Wilson in hospital. When there was no improvement in her condition, I ordered another CT scan to see what was going on. I was in for a surprise. Although the X-ray appearance of the spine doesn't normally change immediately after chymopapain, in this case the scan clearly showed that a portion of the lower disc had moved further into the spinal canal.

Now it was easy to see what had happened. On the fourth day after the chymopapain injection, a fragment of the nucleus, already extruding through the shell of the disc, had torn loose. Its connection to the remaining nucleus had been broken by the chemical action of the drug. Suddenly free, the piece slid down the tunnel containing the nerve root. New pressure was causing the leg pain.

As soon as I made that discovery, I knew that surgery was the only answer. I operated, found the stray piece of nucleus, and removed it easily. From the moment she came out of the anesthetic, Stacey Wilson's leg pain was gone and her back problem disappeared. After two days' rest, she went home.

And so, that one troublesome disc required surgery after all. Like most treatments chymopapain has its benefits, but it also has its limitations.

Recently I read a newspaper feature describing how some doctors are now treating back pain with injections of steroids and morphine, and having incredible success. Is this a breakthrough?

I'm afraid not. This is one of those treatments that pop up in the news every so often, and sometimes an overenthusiastic reporter will convey the impression that it's a miraculous new cure. Usually the news reports don't make the distinction between long-term benefit and temporary pain relief, and they are vague about the kind of back problem that can be helped. In this case, the treatment is aimed only at providing temporary pain relief for patients with severe symptoms after back surgery has failed. Certainly the injection provides no cure, miraculous or otherwise.

Still, it's a fairly simple procedure. Morphine, mixed with a steroid preparation, is injected into the epidural space, the space between the bony walls of the spinal canal and the fluid-filled sac around the nerves. The relief it provides is occasionally quite dramatic, although no one knows exactly why. The morphine may have some sort of general effect on the pain mechanism, or it may react locally with the coverings of the nerves. The steroid reduces any

local inflammation and counteracts the irritation caused by the
morphine.

**The same article also mentioned other drugs that were said to be
a successful means of reducing inflammation. Are these the ones
you told me about before?**

Yes. They're commonly called NSAIDs, which stands for non-
steroidal anti-inflammatory drugs. As you know, inflammation is
the body's normal reaction to injury. It results from the rapid
collection of certain blood cells, specific enzymes, and various
chemicals needed to heal the original damage. But an inflammatory
reaction that is too strong can cause pain, so that the "cure"
becomes the cause. Anti-inflammatory drugs slow this reaction
down to a more or less normal pace and give an unnecessarily
inflamed area a chance to recover.

**That sounds like a good treatment, but from what you've said I
suppose there are side effects.**

You're right. In fact anti-inflammatories produce several side
effects. One problem is that NSAIDs don't act just on the inflammation you want to treat – the swelling and pain in a worn spinal
joint, for example; they also slow down the same reaction everywhere else in the body. In the stomach, that slowdown can cause
an ulcer or serious bleeding. To protect itself against the acids
and other digestive juices it contains, the stomach is continually
replacing its lining cells at a rapid rate. An anti-inflammatory
drug, unable to distinguish between the increased activity of
inflammation and the normally speedy turnover of stomach-lining
cells, will slow down both processes.

The NSAIDs can have other side effects. Some can cause headaches, skin rashes, or an unwanted retention of fluid. One type
has even been known to produce acute psychotic episodes. Rarely,
NSAIDs will depress the action of blood-forming tissue in the bone
marrow and elsewhere, which can lead to a serious shortage of
vital blood cells.

Most important of all, the non-steroidal anti-inflammatory drugs
don't always solve the problem. For low-back pain they are effective

only about half the time. And even when they work they must be regarded as a temporary measure to control the symptoms until natural healing can occur.

All in all, I am not enthusiastic about anti-inflammatories for low-back disorders. I prescribe them occasionally but usually as a secondary measure in the control of an acute attack already being treated with rest, counter-irritants, and gentle stretching.

A friend suggested I try acupuncture to cure my back. What do you think?

Acupuncture is a legitimate method of pain relief, but don't count on it as a sure thing, and don't think of it as a cure. According to the most reliable data I have seen, only about one-third of the people who receive acupuncture to relieve chronic back or neck pain find it effective. In some cases, the benefits seem to last a long time – for months or even for years; in other cases, the pain comes back after just a few hours or days.

Acupuncture works by somehow interfering with the normal pain-transmission system. It has no effect at all on the source or cause of the problem. The value of having tiny needles stuck in your ear, big toe, or other parts of your body to stop back pain must be weighed against the fact that sooner or later all acute attacks get better anyway and may not recur for years.

One problem with a treatment as poorly understood as acupuncture is that it breeds fads that make no scientific sense. For example, some of its practitioners have moved on to a thing called "laser acupuncture." You may know that lasers are modified beams of light that can produce enough heat to melt a brick, or be used to send signals over long distances because they travel in thin, perfectly straight lines. Neither of those properties has anything to do with acupuncture, but some people are receiving treatments with a "cold-laser probe" attached by a cord to a machine that emits an ominous hum. The whole process smacks more of Hollywood hoke than of modern medicine.

But, having stated those reservations, I'd say that if you're looking for pain relief, and conventional acupuncture appeals to you, go ahead and try it. It's harmless, and it just might help.

Is there a relationship between acupuncture and a treatment called "trigger-point therapy"?

Yes, in a way, there is. As the name implies, treatment is directed at "trigger points," small, tender lumps that sometimes mysteriously appear near the surface of the skin, usually along the tops of the shoulders or over the back of the pelvis. No one knows what causes these trigger points or even exactly what they are. They are impossible to remove surgically; they just disappear when you get under the skin. Trigger points often mark the location of pain referred from somewhere else – the neck pain you feel between your shoulder blades, for example – and these points themselves can become major sources of discomfort. But pressing on them, massaging them, or subjecting them to friction by rubbing on them rapidly, can reduce the pain they cause. Injecting them with local anesthetic is effective, and so is inserting an acupuncture needle. Many of the typical sites for these lumps correspond to the classic acupuncture points. For this reason, some practitioners believe that treating the trigger points can be beneficial to the distant site of trouble, although this two-way-street effect has never been proven to exist.

When the trigger points are widespread, with tender areas over the breast bone and at the elbows and knees as well as in the shoulders and back, the condition is often called fibrositis or tissue tension pain. Along with changes in behavior, insomnia, loss of libido, and all the other symptoms we discussed earlier, the development of numerous trigger points may accompany the chronic pain syndrome.

What about the electrical device known as a TENS unit – does it act something like acupuncture?

Sort of. TENS, or transcutaneous electrical nerve stimulation, can be an effective means of temporarily blocking unwanted pain signals. Like acupuncture, it produces a reaction that seems to liberate endorphins, naturally produced opiates that interfere with the normal transmission of pain through the upper spinal cord and the base of the brain. In the relief of some types of acute post-operative pain, TENS can reduce or even eliminate the need for other pain medication. As you might expect, the treatment has less value in chronic cases. The body can develop a resistance to the electrical stimulation, just as it can to many drugs. Consequently, a stronger and stronger input is required to produce an effect. Eventually you may reach a point where the TENS machine cannot produce an impulse sufficient to prevent the pain message from getting through. At that point the patient's symptoms will return.

On a radio phone-in show I heard a back specialist talking about thermological pain studies. Are they something new?

The term "thermological pain studies" is a fancy way of saying "thermograms," and they have been around for quite a while. Thermograms can be produced by expensive electronic techniques or, much more commonly, by latex sheets embedded with crystals that change color at various temperatures. These sheets are placed on your body and photographed to measure the temperature of your skin at various locations. That measurement, in turn, provides useful information as to the amount of blood flowing in or near the skin at that point on your body. Inflammation of the skin from any injury will produce a "hot" thermogram. So will the increased circulation in actively contracting muscles just beneath the surface.

You may have seen a thermographic study demonstrated on television. In one commercial for an aftershave lotion, viewers are shown a thermogram of a man's face right after he finishes shaving. The skin on his face records a high temperature, demonstrated by the color of the thermogram indicating an increased blood flow – which is hardly surprising, since he has just been scratching it with a razor. Then the man slaps on the aftershave and the thermogram instantly shows a remarkable change. The alcohol in the solution rapidly constricts the local blood vessels and lowers the skin temperature.

And that's all there is, really, to those "thermological pain studies" you asked about. A thermogram is a measure of local blood supply and temperature. It has some use in assessing blood flow to the limbs in vascular problems, but because it is completely non-specific a thermogram is of no diagnostic value for back complaints and it certainly does not measure pain. As a colleague of mine is fond of saying, "The most dramatic thermogram you will ever see is the picture of a blush."

I've thought of looking into a treatment called biofeedback, which is said to produce good results for backache victims. What do you think?

Biofeedback is based on your ability to exert conscious control over some of the functions of your body that are ordinarily automatic. To most people hearing about it for the first time, it sounds almost mystical. And, considering its potential for being sold as some sort of magic, I give a lot of credit to its practitioners. With rare exceptions, they are conscientious about avoiding the use of exaggerated claims or scientific doubletalk.

As a means of controlling backache, biofeedback concentrates on muscle spasm. Basically, the technique consists of recognizing that your muscles are tense, and then consciously relaxing them. During the early learning stage, you may use electrodes and meters to guide you in monitoring your responses. Once you have learned the technique, you can put the hardware aside and practice biofeedback all by yourself.

Like any other treatment, though, it has its limitations. Not everyone can master biofeedback fully, and even those who do master it cannot always apply it effectively enough to relieve a muscle spasm. Also, as you might suppose, biofeedback is a lot less useful if the chronic pain syndrome has taken hold.

In short, I offer the same advice about it as I do for acupuncture: it's harmless, and worth trying as long as your expectations are realistic. And there's a bonus in this case: if you can master it, you'll be armed with an anti-pain weapon you can use on your own, without any expense or need for medical supervision. Just remember, though, that we're talking, at most, about relieving pain – not about applying a remedy for the cause of the back problem.

Would you say the same thing about hypnosis as a means of pain relief?

That depends. If you believe hypnosis is likely to help you, it might be worth trying, provided that your doctor has assured you that your problem is primarily a matter of pain control and not something that requires direct physical treatment. I have referred patients for hypnosis on occasions when the patients themselves requested it, but I have not been impressed with the results. The idea is to change the patient's attitude, in two stages: using hypnosis first as a blocking mechanism to shut off the pain, and second as a method of motivating the patient. The pain-blocking effect works but doesn't last long, and the process of improving motivation involves functions too complex to be handled effectively by anything as simple as hypnosis. I'm prepared to believe there have been situations where hypnosis was remarkably effective, but I have never seen one.

But again, my basic rule remains the same. Alternative forms of treatment are fine if they are helpful, harmless, and unlikely to interfere with correct medical management.

A friend of mine had an operation called a "rhizolysis." Would you explain what that actually involves?

Rhizolysis or rhizotomy, as it is often called, means the deliberate destruction of the nerve supply to the small facet joints of the spine. When these joints are left without feeling, the pain from Type One problems should be eliminated.

There's nothing wrong with the theory of joint denervation, but the practice falls short. In the earliest rhizotomies the nerves were cut with a surgical scalpel, but this technique was difficult and often failed to do the job. Now rhizolysis uses a radio frequency probe that actually burns the nerves. Multiple lesions are required, since each joint may have two or even three separate nerves running to it. The problem is that it's difficult to destroy all the sensation, and even when the nerve destruction is complete, the joint can develop a new supply, allowing feeling and pain to return. Overall, for the treatment of chronic low-back pain, rhizotomy is successful in about 30 percent of patients. It is of no value in relieving Type Two, Three, or Four pain. There are risks, such as infection, related to the minor surgery. They aren't great but they must be weighed against the potential benefits of the technique.

What is your opinion of holistic medicine?

Holistic medicine is good medicine but I object to the way it is presented. Its practitioners and enthusiasts imply that no other doctors pay attention to their patients as a whole. The rest of us are accused of merely treating specific complaints as though they were isolated from the rest of the human being. This is quite untrue.

A good orthopedic surgeon, for example, will not just examine a fractured thigh bone and ignore the patient's general health. By the same token, giving that patient proper holistic treatment certainly does not mean just making him feel good and checking on his nutrition and bowel habits without paying specific attention to the broken leg. Obviously a good doctor will attend to the patient's specific problem and to his overall needs as well. Practitioners who present themselves as specialists in holistic medicine have no monopoly on good medical care.

Then you have no objection to the holistic approach?

Not when it simply represents good medicine. But I believe some of its practitioners are carrying the approach to extremes. Like many another well-meaning idea that becomes a fad, the concept of holistic medicine has been distorted by proponents who have lost the original perspective.

As a concept it took shape in reaction to increasing specialization. When the family doctor began to recede from the scene, a feeling developed that instead of going to a whole array of specialists, the patient should see one doctor who is interested in every problem. And who can argue with that? If you went to see your family doctor, I'm sure you'd want a comprehensive physical examination as well as a chance to talk not only about your head cold or your backache but also about your kids and how they're doing at school, and about your job, especially if you're having a lot of trouble at work. That's the sort of approach holistic medicine is supposed to take. The holistic practitioner is supposed to be the epitome of the good family physician.

Yet if that's all there were to holistic medicine, there would be no reason for it to exist as a separate entity, because that approach is exactly what you can expect from a competent family doctor. I think that's why holistic doctors, generally speaking, have moved away from that perfectly sensible position – so that their services will sound completely different from those of an ordinary general practitioner.

But how have they managed to sell holistic medicine as something different, if good family doctors were taking the same approach all along?

I believe a couple of other trends have helped make holistic medicine possible. One trend has been for patients to go to specialists directly, whenever they can. If you have only a bad back you probably don't want to spend time talking to your family doctor about it, because you don't believe a general practitioner knows all that much about back problems and will probably send you to someone else anyway.

As a result, people are swarming into specialists' offices with complaints that are often self-diagnosed and may or may not be accurate. Even if the complaint is not serious, most patients would rather hear that from the specialist, not from the family doctor. This trend, of course, defeats the system. The specialist sees a lot of patients who do not require his expertise, and those who do need him find it harder to get appointments.

The second trend has arisen from the first: as patients perceive that the specialist knows more about specific complaints than the general practitioner does, the family doctor comes to believe the same thing. If the doctor is told often enough that the public, as represented by his patients, is not interested in his opinion on, say, bad backs, then he stops offering his opinion. And so he abdicates the responsibility, no longer attempting to keep up to date on back care. Ironically, then, the family physician actually helps fill the system with patients referred unnecessarily to specialists.

At this point, the holistic medicine man, with the same medical training as the family doctor, enters the picture, presenting himself as a specialist. He is, so to speak, a "specialist in general practice." And whereas the family doctor may be seen as only a GP – a sort of medical jack-of-all-trades – the holistic doctor is a "specialist" specializing in everything.

Now, if he is to justify that claim, the holistic practitioner must develop special techniques. He must do things the average family physician can't do, so as to give his work a special mystique or at least an air of specialization involving knowledge beyond what you'd expect of your average doctor.

And so we find holistic medicine offering such rarefied services as hair analysis, which purports to look for trace mineral losses indicative of the body's needs. The technique has no scientific validity, and in fact a lab analysis of the same hair sample will not usually produce the same results twice. This is one reason why hair analysis is looked upon with great suspicion by all reputable scientific bodies.

That brings us to one of the great ironies of holistic medicine. Many of its practitioners provide some sort of special diagnostic technique, such as hair analysis, at the same time claiming to treat the patient as a unique organism, and then turn around and prescribe exactly the same treatment as they've prescribed for virtually all their other patients – vitamins, well-balanced diets, and proper living habits, all the common-sense things you were taught back in high school health classes.

But at least holistic medicine is harmless.

Not necessarily. Suppose you have something seriously wrong with you that hasn't been diagnosed. With the array of physical, radio-logical, and laboratory investigations currently available, it makes no sense to rely almost exclusively on a single test, particularly one so questionable as hair analysis. And yet a holistic practitioner may complete only a chemical diagnosis and then proceed to treat you with vitamin supplements and minerals, without paying much attention to the other aspects of the problem. At that point, holistic medicine, in my view, becomes dangerous, and the term "holistic" itself becomes ironically inappropriate.

What about some of the other alternative approaches – craniosacral therapy, for example?

Craniosacral therapy is based on several fascinating and totally unproven concepts. One deals with the transfer of a kind of "body electricity" from the therapist to the patient. Another describes a "natural pulse" within the central nervous system that can supposedly be felt through a periodic enlargement of the skull and an associated upward movement of the sacrum. What this theory seems to be saying is that your body behaves something like one of those instant toy poodles that entertainers construct out of balloons at children's parties: if you squeeze the air-filled poodle's mid-section his head grows bigger, and vice versa. That's more or less what the craniosacral people believe happens to your spine and head: six to twelve times a minute your spine grows shorter and your head gets larger; then your head shrinks and your spine elongates.

Proponents of craniosacral therapy also see it as a modern application of the classic yoga theory of "superphysical filaments" which, if they exist at all, have so far eluded discovery by medical science. Craniosacralists link the concept to the martial arts, therapeutic touch, and the widely publicized "Philippine psychic surgery," in which the healer appears to reach inside the sufferer's body with his bare hands and yet not leave a mark on the skin.

The scientific basis for craniosacral therapy rests on theories originally put forward by an osteopathic student in the early 1900s. Although anatomic studies showed, then as now, that the bones of the adult skull are incapable of independent movement, he felt that since joint lines were visible and since all of nature's designs have a purpose, movement must take place.

Today, craniosacral therapy exists as a manipulative technique to adjust the immovable bones in the adult cranium and to take advantage of the body's natural rhythm and the normal "direction of energy." It has never been proven to have any benefit over conventional forms of manipulation. Certainly the concept of diagnosing and treating spinal problems by perceiving and altering the expansion and contraction of the skull is well beyond the fringe of accepted medical practice.

I never dreamed that writing a book on back pain would lead me into a discussion of shrunken heads, but there you are.

What about some of the more widely accepted sources of treatment – osteopaths, for instance?

Osteopathy is a respectable and valuable profession, and I have no objection to my patients' seeing one of its practitioners, if that's what they want. Of course, I want to be sure their condition will be diagnosed properly before any treatment is undertaken.

Are osteopaths qualified to diagnose most back problems?

Yes, they are. In training and professional qualifications, an osteopath is closer to a doctor than to a chiropractor. As most people know, someone wanting to become a doctor must obtain a university degree, then attend a recognized medical school, usually in a four-year program. After that comes a year of internship, roughly equivalent to an apprenticeship. Additional training is required for a doctor to qualify as a specialist.

Generally, the educational requirements to become a doctor of osteopathy (DO), are much the same as those for becoming an MD, except, of course, that the students attend a school of osteopathy instead of a medical school. Since "osteo" means bone, you might assume that an osteopath treats only bone conditions. But in the United States, osteopaths, while concentrating particularly on manipulative therapy, are trained and licensed to perform the same services as general practitioners, and they treat such non-skeletal conditions as diabetes and high blood pressure. With extra training, they can even perform surgery.

In other countries there are differing restrictions on the services osteopaths are allowed to perform. In most Canadian provinces, osteopaths are licensed as chiropractors and are allowed to provide only chiropractic-type drugless therapy. An osteopath practicing as a chiropractor can manipulate or "adjust" your spinal joints and may administer physical treatments such as hot packs and whirlpool baths. But he is allowed to offer you only non-prescription medication such as vitamin pills.

Chiropractors have a narrower range of medical knowledge and diagnostic skills than DOs or MDs. They are trained specifically to deal with problems that can be resolved by manipulation. Typically, they are required to complete two years of university before entering a four-year course at chiropractic college, where their studies concentrate largely on spinal anatomy and manipulation of the spine. Successful students emerge with a Doctor of Chiropractic (DC) degree.

Many doctors are sharply critical of chiropractors. Where do you stand?

I have no quarrel with the treatments most chiropractors give back-pain sufferers. But I think it's important for you, as the patient, to realize that the "adjustments" a chiropractor makes to your spine have no long-term benefits. If they did, you wouldn't have to keep going for chiropractic treatments month after month or year after year. It is quite possible that a chiropractor will relieve a muscle spasm that is causing you back pain. And there's nothing wrong with that. But if you want to prevent the problem from recurring, you need to follow a long-term maintenance program that will yield long-term benefits. And that's not something you can hope to get from repeated manipulation.

Patients sometimes tell me, "I've been going to my chiropractor for the past ten [or whatever] years."

I ask: "Has he helped you to get rid of your back pain?"

"No."

"Then why do you go back to him?"

"Because he does me a lot of good."

The chiropractic profession thrives on that kind of doublethink. There aren't many patients these days who would stay with the same doctor for ten years, waiting for him to solve the original problem.

Is that why doctors often criticize chiropractors – because their treatments offer only short-term relief and have to be repeated indefinitely?

That may be one reason. But I think most doctors take exception not to what the chiropractor *does* but to what he *says* he does. Chiropractors often talk about discs and joints that have "gone out of place." Yet, as you know by now, discs don't slip and joints don't routinely "go in and out of place."

Your sore back can feel stiff and strange, but that doesn't mean the joints are out of place. And why should you assume they are? After all, when you sprain your thumb, you don't automatically assume that the joint has "gone out." So why should you think anything different about the joints in your spine? Believe me, they are encased far more securely than your thumb joints.

But I'm sure I've felt and heard my back go out – it made a cracking sound.

What you heard is essentially the same thing you hear when people crack their knuckles. The joints in your fingers and in your spine contain nitrogen dissolved under pressure in a small amount of joint fluid. If you decrease the pressure – by pulling on your fingers and enlarging the joint space, for instance – the nitrogen comes out of solution and turns into gas, going "pop" just the way a bottle of champagne pops when you uncork it. But whether the joint is in a finger or your spine, nothing has gone out of place when it "cracks." Yet some chiropractors will encourage you to believe otherwise. Just ask yourself: when was the last time you saw anyone rearrange his fingers just by cracking his knuckles?

Chiropractors have a whole lexicon of terms they love to toss around. I find that as objectionable as speaking Doctor when plain English will do. I know one woman whose chiropractor told her that her neck had lost its "motoricity." Now there's a piece of jargon for the auto-makers in Detroit to conjure with! ("Test drive the Zoomjet 88 – it's tops in motoricity!") And just in case he hadn't frightened the poor woman enough with that one, the chiropractor also told her she suffered from "multiple subluxation complexes."

But I don't think that's all just chiropractic jargon. I'm sure I've heard my own doctor use some of those words.

You're right. It's not just chiropractic jargon; it's also medical jargon. Luxation means dislocation, and subluxation therefore means "something less than a complete dislocation." Never mind the accuracy of the diagnosis; let's deal just with the jargon. Since there is no single English word that precisely means "subluxation," I give the chiropractor full marks for precision in the use of the term, even though the patient couldn't understand what he said. However, when he spoke of "multiple subluxation complexes" he was talking pretentious nonsense. "Multiple" just means many or several, and "complexes," in that context, doesn't mean anything at all. In my view, if a doctor or chiropractor tries to impress his patients with mumbo jumbo like that, he probably doesn't have much else to offer.

Some people are convinced that many doctors are jealous of chiropractors.

I wouldn't say jealous, but doctors may well envy chiropractors for developing such strong loyalty in their patients. Much as they would like to, few doctors can evoke that kind of response. One reason is that doctors, particularly specialists, usually treat patients for a limited period of time, and if the treatment is successful they don't arrange to see them again. Chiropractors, on the other hand, tend to require frequent follow-up or maintenance visits, regardless of whether the patient still has trouble. That continuing contact often creates a bond.

But there are other reasons as well. A past president of the American Chiropractic Association told me that chiropractors were kept busy treating patients with back problems partly because doctors had abdicated their responsibility. He said most MDs were not interested in treating backs and were happy to let somebody else take over. I think there is a great deal of truth in that. A doctor who shows little concern for the patients' problems can hardly expect loyalty from them.

Also, because of their broader knowledge and the caution typical of the profession, many doctors may hesitate or worry aloud over the correct diagnosis and treatment of a back problem. Their apparent indecision raises the patient's concerns that the problem is more serious, or at least more difficult, than he or she expected. Most chiropractors are far more decisive. They'll say to the patient, "I know exactly what's wrong and how to make it right. Now if you'll just lie down here on this table...."

That's what people want to hear when they're bewildered and frightened about a medical problem. It gives them hope and confidence in their ability to get better. And that's an important step towards recovery regardless of who initiates it. Once he's got that going for him, it may not even matter whether the chiropractor's physical manipulation is effective.

But every time I get treated at the chiropractor's I come out feeling good. Are you saying that manipulation isn't really helping me?

No, that's not what I'm saying. If you have pain when you go in and it's gone when you come out, you are obviously gaining some benefit. Like any other valid form of therapy, manipulation can produce desirable results if it is applied properly and in the right circumstances. But remember, it's not a cure, and if you visit your chiropractor even when you have no pain – perhaps because you made the appointment well in advance and because you know you'll feel good afterwards – you ought to ask yourself what's really going on. Is the visit simply an indulgence, on a

par with a leisurely soak in the bathtub? Are you beginning to
rely on treatments you don't really need? And, if so, to what extent
is your chiropractor actively encouraging you to become dependent
on him?

But can't I trust a professional to make the proper decisions?

This is not a matter of trust but a matter of *responsibility*. It's your
back we're talking about here, and the primary responsibility for
looking after it belongs to you, no matter what specialists you
see or how trustworthy they are. You are the one who must make
the important distinction between a treatment that really helps
your back get better and one that merely makes you "feel good."

One example of a "feel good" treatment is massage. Even from
a registered therapist, massage is just another way of gaining muscle
relaxation. It has no lasting effect. But if you are tense and suffer
from muscle tension pain, a vigorous massage can certainly make
you feel better. The problem is that patients may become dependent
on these treatments, which require no active participation and
provide only short-term comfort. The treatments become a means
of avoiding the responsibility of taking charge.

What's the difference between a chiropractic adjustment and the manipulation I might receive from a physical therapist?

Basically there is no difference. "Adjustment" is simply the chiropractor's term for manipulation. Applied to the spine, manipulation means putting your back joints through a range of movement. Whether manipulation is done quickly or slowly, forcefully
or gently, to the whole spine or part of it, and whether the range
of movement is part of, all of, or slightly more than the joint's
normal capability depends on the practitioner and the circumstances. No matter which kind of specialist performs the manipulation – a chiropractor, an osteopath, a physical therapist, or an
MD – it's essentially the same thing.

You've mentioned training for osteopaths and chiropractors. What about physical therapists?

The physical therapist graduates from a four-year university program with a bachelor degree, though many continue training in a specialty – such as orthopedics, pediatrics, cardiovascular rehabilitation, and manipulation techniques. Masters and PhD programs in physical therapy now exist in many large universities throughout North America. The four-year course also includes a clinical internship with considerable practical exposure.

In the typical situation, physical therapists are allowed to treat only at the direction of a doctor, and cannot accept unreferred patients. Unlike chiropractors, they must function as part of a medical team. Through this close association, I have come to appreciate their role in the physical treatment of back problems and have learned a great deal about the value of manipulative therapy.

From what you've learned, how does manipulation relieve pain?

We think the pain relief results from the release of muscle spasm or the return of normal movement to stiff spinal joints, but we don't know exactly why or how manipulation works. Even the experts can't determine whether the benefit of stretching comes from its effect on the joint lining or capsule, or the muscle sheath, or even the fat under the skin. All we can say for sure is that manipulation does relieve back pain for some people sometimes.

Studies have shown that manipulation has no long-term effect: those who are going to get better do so with it or without it. Its role seems to be to shorten the duration of the problem, and that's a good thing in itself. But if I were selling medical "cures," rather than dispensing advice, I could easily draw on my professional experience to "prove" that manipulation is the answer for common backache.

On one occasion I was supervising minor surgery when a nurse from another operating room came and asked whether she could have an appointment with me soon. She explained that she had a muscle spasm in her neck. Since I wasn't scrubbed for the operation I suggested we might just as well do something about her problem right there and then. I had her lie down on a spare table in the operating room and after I examined her I "adjusted" her neck. The manipulation immediately relieved her pain. She got up and left the room – pain free.

On another occasion a friend of mine and his wife were over

for a visit. When she complained of a pain in her low back, I offered to examine her. I decided manipulation might help, so I had her lie down on a table and I proceeded to manipulate her back. It was another one of those treatments that provided instant relief.

That's just the way things go, sometimes, with manipulation. Since it took only a few minutes, and neither woman was really expecting much change, if the manipulation hadn't succeeded they probably would have quickly written off the experience as just another treatment that didn't happen to work. As it was, they were delighted with the result and may well have told others about my skill.

Chiropractors thrive on that kind of selective, word-of-mouth publicity, and who can blame them? But even their successes prove nothing about the validity of chiropractic theory.

But you'd have to admit that to most patients, theory doesn't matter a lot – it's results that count.

That's usually how patients feel, and I don't blame them. Manipulation has its place, and as long as it is preceded by proper diagnosis, so there is no question about the cause of the problem and the safety of the "adjustments," I don't object to that form of therapy for anyone who wants to try it. I frequently refer patients for manipulation, usually to a specially trained physical therapist and occasionally to a chiropractor. Your chances of being helped temporarily are better than fifty-fifty, and you might turn out to be one of the lucky ones.

However, I'm thinking more generally about alternative forms of treatment when I say it's a mistake to ignore theory and simply ask whether a treatment produces results. A lot of questionable procedures have been sold to desperate people on the basis of a few good results, which may or may not be indicative of the soundness and value of the technique. In some instances, the practitioners impress prospective patients by citing testimonials from well-known doctors, medical institutions, or recognized medical journals. It all sounds very convincing and few doctors or patients ever have the time and inclination to check out the references.

Not long ago, I was asked to comment on the value of a treatment called prolotherapy, which involves injecting various fluids into the spine to "tighten up the ligaments." The whole theory is highly questionable, but that's not central to the point I'm making here. Prolotherapy, which first surfaced about thirty years ago, had recently been taken up by a local family doctor who obviously seemed to believe in it and wanted the Workers' Compensation Board to approve and pay for it. When the board refused and the doctor concerned persisted, I was asked for an opinion, and so I looked into the claims he was making.

In one of his letters, the doctor had said the value of the treatment was mentioned in a well-known orthopedic textbook. He even cited the edition and relevant page numbers. So I got a copy of the book. I found that either this doctor hadn't read the text carefully, or he'd assumed that nobody would bother to look up the reference. In fact, what the author had written about prolotherapy injections was disturbing news for the doctor and his patients.

The book cited two reports published in the *Journal of the American Medical Association*, which described two prolotherapy cases that turned out badly. One patient ended up as a spastic paraplegic and the other developed serious symptoms and then died following surgery undertaken to relieve them. The author also related first-hand experiences with patients sent to him after prolotherapy. He said he couldn't see any benefit from the injections, and that his "overall personal opinion of the technique" was "not favorable."

So much for documented references offered as "proof" that a treatment is valid. Even if the sources cited actually support the claims being made for a treatment, there may also be any number of unfavorable reports that are intentionally left unmentioned.

But what if the supportive statement has come from a highly qualified doctor whose credentials are beyond question?

You won't often find highly accredited medical specialists making declarations of that kind in support of any radically new treatment. But even if they do they can still be wrong. They may have been misled by incomplete or erroneous information, or they may be basing their statements on a sampling that was too small to be conclusive.

I realize that, as a group, doctors are regarded as arch conservatives when it comes to accepting new techniques. Some people would carry that criticism even further; they are willing to believe that superior discoveries and new treatments are continually being suppressed by the medical establishment to avoid embarrassment or the loss of income that would ensue if established procedures had to be abandoned.

That "conspiracy" theory, of course, ignores the fact that there are scores of medicines, machines, and techniques in use today that were unheard of even five or ten years ago. Certainly the establishment has no vested interest in keeping you sick – least of all if you have a bad back. Most doctors would be delighted to find a way of eliminating back pain. General practitioners don't like treating it because of the uncertainties and frustrations involved; and most orthopedic surgeons, myself included, would welcome the chance to devote more time to patients with injuries or other problems.

Meanwhile, before you try any "revolutionary cure" or "new natural therapy as seen on TV," you and your doctor should scrutinize it carefully to determine its real value and possible drawbacks. Since your own back will be the test site, would you really want to do anything less?

11. TOOLS OF THE BACK DOCTOR'S TRADE

Every so often, a patient of mine describes some feeling or observation so perfectly that I feel compelled to record it and find a place to use it in my lectures or my writing.

One of those memorable observations came from a woman who shares my enthusiasm for analogies. She told me a story that precisely described the problem of her back pain, which was defying my best efforts at diagnosis and treatment.

Her husband, an automobile mechanic, had gone to work on their own car because it was stalling frequently. He checked every possible cause, or so he thought, and replaced several parts in case they were faulty. But the stalling persisted, occurring at unpredictable intervals. Everything he did made the car run a little better but never really solved the problem.

Finally, after deducing that the trouble had to be somewhere in the gas line, he spotted a tiny thread near the end of the pipe. That was the clue he needed: a fragment of cloth, probably from a previous maintenance job, was loose in the pipe and was intermittently blocking the flow of gasoline.

And, as my patient observed, "Isn't that something like my back trouble? It comes and it goes, and there are a lot of things you are doing for me – getting me to exercise and practice good back care and lose weight – and those things are all helping a little. But you've never really gotten to the source of the problem – the real thing that makes my back hurt."

With that fitting analogy, she announced her discovery of an inevitable truth about back problems: although we have many remedies to try, they are never fully successful unless we are treating the right problem.

However, we *are* solving more and more of those diagnostic riddles, thanks to modern technology.

At a recent meeting in San Francisco, a colleague of mine declared that in his practice the CT scan has already replaced physical examination of the back. I think that's an overestimation of the machine's capabilities. It's like saying that once people can shop by closed-circuit television they will never want to enter a store again. But there are just some things a picture can't tell you about that sofa you're thinking of buying. Don't you want to bounce on the cushions and feel the texture and personally examine the workmanship?

Diagnosing back problems involves many aspects that shouldn't be left to a machine, and I don't believe that current technology can provide a substitute for the human perceptions and insights that so often make the difference in a difficult diagnosis.

And yet I certainly share my colleague's enthusiasm for the modern medical tools which have become invaluable aids to suggest and confirm the diagnoses made by traditional means. This chapter explains why.

X-rays are used routinely for back trouble. Aren't they actually quite dangerous?

Not really. Unfortunately, most people have an anxiety about X-rays that has no basis in present-day reality. Their fears may be based on stories from the early days of X-ray work when researchers had their fingers burned off because they had no idea there was any danger, or on frightening descriptions of the effects that follow an atomic explosion. There is a growing concern about the cumulative effect of low-level radiation. And, of course, there are the numerous exposés written by consumer advocates "piercing the veil of medical secrecy" and detailing "the horrors of excessive X-ray exposure."

The resulting public reaction to X-rays reminds me of an experience I had not long ago, when my colleagues and I treated an unusual illness in a recent immigrant to our country. It turned out to be a case of leprosy – not a disease you expect to find in most hospitals in the western world. Some of the other doctors were aghast at the diagnosis, and I would probably have reacted the same way if I hadn't worked for a time in the Far East, where I became accustomed to seeing perhaps three or four cases of leprosy a month. From that experience I came to appreciate that leprosy is a treatable disease with a remarkably low rate of contagion. Doctors can work among lepers for years and never contract leprosy themselves.

Everyone trained in modern medicine may know these facts intellectually, and yet there were a few of my well-educated contemporaries who reacted much the way people did in biblical times, when anyone suspected of having leprosy was not permitted to walk through a village without crying out the warning, "Unclean! Unclean!"

Many people harbor a similarly uninformed fear of X-rays. They associate them with such horrors as genetic mutations brought on by radiation poisoning. And X-ray technologists, intent on reassuring patients that no harm will come to them, take elaborate precautions to protect themselves with leaded shields and aprons, thereby unintentionally reinforcing those already exaggerated fears. No one may bother to point out that while the patient will be exposed to half a dozen X-rays that day, the technicians will have the potential for being exposed to several hundred that day and every other working day of their lives.

X-rays, in short, are not nearly as dangerous as most people believe. But there is clearly another side to the story. Some doctors and chiropractors suggest or even insist on obtaining radiographs when there is little or no indication that they will be of value. A patient of mine was seen in the emergency room of a local hospital for an acute attack of neck and shoulder pain. The record I saw later described her symptoms clearly as a typical acute attack of local muscle spasm with no nerve involvement. In spite of the simple and obvious diagnosis, no one in Emergency would treat her without seeing an X-ray. My patient really felt forced into submitting to a series of cervical spine films, which, of course, showed nothing abnormal.

Usually the X-ray's diagnostic value far outweighs the minimal risk of exposure. But charging an extra fee for unnecessary radiological tests, or getting an X-ray as a substitute for good clinical judgment, or as protection against a possible malpractice action, is unfair to the patient. The small amount of extra radiation may not be harmful, but it isn't good for you, either.

I wouldn't make such a point of discussing the balance between the proper role and the misuse of X-ray if popular misconceptions didn't interfere with the care I try to provide. I have had patients tell me they were unwilling to undergo necessary X-rays or a CT scan to assist the diagnosis of their orthopedic problem because they had already had "too much radiation" from routine chest X-rays. Such concerns are groundless. The amount of radiation you get during a routine chest film is negligible, and the amount to which you are exposed during a properly controlled CT study is not much more.

Radiologists themselves have inadvertently fed this fear by setting extremely conservative standards for exposure. When they assure people it's safe to have, say, one X-ray every six months, the implication is that it would be unsafe to have four or five X-rays a year, when in fact even at that rate, your exposure would be far below the slightest degree of danger.

I have heard people talk about EMG machines. Are they a form of X-ray?

No, EMG stands for electromyography, which is the study of how a muscle reacts when it is stimulated by its nerve. Your doctor might want to study your muscle reaction if, for instance, you have back pain and have lost the ability to lift your toes while your foot is flat on the floor. To conduct the test, the examiner will insert extremely fine needles into various muscles in your leg. The needles, which you'll find uncomfortable but not painful, are connected to an instrument that reads the electrical pattern caused by contraction of the muscle. A skilled EMG interpretation can tell the doctor whether there is muscle damage or a lack of nerve stimulus, and whether that is a new, progressing problem, an old recovering problem, or a chronic, unchanging one.

The same equipment can also study the ability of the nerve itself to conduct impulses. The needles are inserted in much the same way as for the study of muscle reaction, but in this case, the instrument is used to measure the velocity of the message or impulse traveling through the nerve from one muscle group to the next. If the impulse takes longer than normal to travel a given distance, we know there is a block within the nerve.

This test is quite useful in some parts of the body but less so near the spine, because we can't obtain measurements on both sides of the point where we suspect the nerve is being pinched. Still, the test can be used to rule out blockages at other locations along the rest of the nerve, so that we can conclude, by deduction, that the problem must be in the nerve root as it leaves the vertebral column.

Are EMGs an important diagnostic tool for back specialists?

Some doctors in my field consider EMGs very useful; others regard them as a waste of time. Generally, I've found that an EMG will not give me more information than I can get from a good clinical examination. Occasionally, though, I have made clinical judgments which changed following electromyography. For instance, I've had cases where muscle weakness was present in both legs or both arms but where one side was so much weaker than the other I concluded that only one side was involved. But when the EMG studies clearly demonstrated abnormal muscle reactions on both sides, they significantly altered my opinion. In situations like that I have learned to appreciate the value of the EMG.

Do you really need a high-tech machine like that to measure nerve function? I'm pretty sure an aunt of mine was tested simply with an anesthetic injection into the nerve.

That's not quite the same test. A nerve-root injection is done with local anesthetic to temporarily deaden the nerve the way a dentist does before he drills your teeth. In some patients it is difficult to tell which nerve root is causing pain, and freezing the roots one after another is a way to find out. When the injection stops the pain, we assume we have found the nerve carrying the message. Of course that only tells us where the trouble is, not what is causing it.

The same type of test is done by injecting the facet joints. In cases of Type One pain, anesthetizing the small spinal joints may help to localize the problem.

Both these procedures are designed to relieve back pain temporarily. In that respect they are the opposite of a discogram, which is intended to increase your pain briefly, for diagnostic purposes.

Are a myelogram and a discogram just different names for the same thing?

Not at all, but there are similarities. They are diagnostic procedures that are usually undertaken as preludes to surgery, and both are based on the same principle: the injection of a radiopaque fluid – that is, a fluid that completely blocks the penetration of the X-ray beam.

How are those injections helpful?

When the patient is X-rayed the fluid will appear white because the material completely prevents exposure of the photographic plate by the X-rays. The shape assumed by the contrast material within the body will outline structures not normally seen by X-ray – such as a bulging disc. This sort of image tells doctors more about a spinal condition than they could discover from a plain X-ray alone.

Then what's the difference between the two kinds of "grams"?

In the myelogram, the material is injected into the dural sac. This is the fluid-filled sheath that surrounds the spinal cord and the nerve roots. In the discogram, the material is injected into the disc itself.

What would make a doctor choose one instead of the other?

The myelogram gives the doctor information about the condition of the nerve sac. A tumor growing on a nerve, for instance, would block the flow of the injected material and show up as a defect on the X-ray picture. Similarly, pressure from outside the sac from a bulging disc or bony narrowing of the canal might impede the progress of the fluid and be seen on the X-ray. Determining whether the obstruction is inside or outside the dural sac requires a lot of experience in reading myelograms. And, keep in mind, the problem can be seen only if it directly affects the dura – the membrane sleeve around the nerves – and alters the flow of the fluid.

The discogram outlines the center of the disc itself and can detect abnormalities even when there is no nerve pressure. Discograms are sometimes used to localize the site of disc pain or determine whether a disc adjacent to the one selected for surgery is normal.

Discograms can give information only about the specific level that is injected. Myelograms can screen an entire section of the spine.

Incidentally, there are two more "grams" I should mention. One is an epidural venogram. In this test the radiopaque fluid is injected into the veins that run inside the spinal canal. The idea is to observe a blockage in the normal venous flow outlining a bulging disc. The other procedure is an epidurogram, in which the fluid is injected around the dural sac, rather than inside it as in a myelogram. The test was developed to avoid possible toxic effects from the older types of contrast medium on the nerves inside the sac. The epidurogram has the same basic purpose – that is to enable the doctor to detect and study a bulging disc – but since it produces a picture that's very difficult to interpret and since the new radiopaque materials are much safer, this procedure isn't used much any more.

What do they do when they give me a myelogram?

You are asked to lie down on a tilting table. The radiologist uses a long needle to inject the fluid into your dural sac, and has the table tilted in a gentle, see-saw motion. The tilting causes the fluid to flow slowly up and down your spine, filling the space around each nerve. As this is going on, X-rays are taken from various positions. All this takes about fifteen to twenty-five minutes, depending on which kind of fluid is used. The older type is an oil-based liquid that must be removed by means of a second needle when the test is finished. That extra step adds a little time to the procedure and accounts for certain post-myelogram problems. The newer type of material is a water-soluble liquid, which rapidly disappears from the spinal fluid by itself and is eventually excreted from the body.

Is a myelogram painful?

Sometimes, but not always. Some people find it painless with only mildly uncomfortable after-effects. One patient of mine, a young woman, said she "didn't feel a thing." Another patient, a middle-aged man who considered himself "a pretty tough guy," said later that the myelogram aggravated his sore back, produced terrible neck pain, and left him with a raging headache.

Is that why you hear such horrible stories about myelograms?

Could be. But a lot of those stories are greatly exaggerated. If you believe them, you may arrive at the hospital expecting the worst and be much more likely to have an unpleasant time. The headache that sometimes follows a myelogram is usually due to a lowering of the spinal fluid pressure within the dural sac, which also surrounds the brain. Most of the liquid removed is taken out when the oil-based contrast material is extracted at the end of the procedure. The body rapidly replaces the missing fluid, and the headache disappears. Obviously, with the water-based compound this is less of a problem. Other reactions may occur because of the patient's sensitivity to the material itself or because of irritation at the site of an obstruction. But in many cases, a lot of the trouble arises from tension. Everything seems to hurt more when you are tense. If you manage to walk in relaxed and unafraid, you could be pleasantly surprised at how routine and painless the procedure can be.

How can I avoid being nervous?

A lot depends on how much you understand beforehand. Ideally, your physician will give you a good briefing in advance. But some doctors don't communicate as well as they might, and if you're already upset or anxious about the prospect of surgery, you might not be taking everything in.

The radiologist, or whoever is actually administering the test, is usually responsible for making sure you understand what the myelogram is all about. While helping you overcome any fears you may have, the radiologist should also make you understand that a myelogram is more than a quick needle and a couple of X-rays. Most radiologists I know clearly outline the procedure, discuss the possible after-effects, and mention the risks involved.

Are you saying it's a risky procedure?

Only in the sense that there's some risk involved in any invasive procedure, whether it's having your tonsils out or getting a tetanus shot. There's always a possibility, however slim, that you may develop an infection, encounter unexpected bleeding, or react in an unusual way to the injected material. But to put it in perspective: having a myelogram is far less risky than driving on a busy highway.

Does it take long to recover from a myelogram? What about the after-effects?

The after-effects vary a lot from one person to the next. If your experience is average, you will have a mild headache for a day or two. A lot depends on how carefully you obey the doctor's instructions. The usual prescribed post-myelogram routine is bed rest in the hospital for eighteen to twenty-four hours. The more you raise your head the more likely you are to feel the effects of the pressure-drop I mentioned earlier. Again, this is more of a problem with the older oil-based medium. If you've had that material injected, some doctors won't let you sit up at all, not even to take nourishment. When you want to eat or drink, all you can do is stay horizontal and roll sideways.

The routine is similar if you had the water-soluble injection, except that you don't have to lie down for as long – eight to twelve hours is average. And in this case you are instructed to lie with your head slightly raised, on two pillows, for instance. The headache after this type of myelogram comes directly from irritation by the injected material. Raising your head helps keep it out of the fluid around your brain. For many of the reasons I've mentioned, this material is rapidly replacing the older oil-based type.

Some people go home from a myelogram thinking they can

cheat on the doctor's orders. Usually they pay a price, with more severe headaches, nausea, and vomiting. Fortunately, although they may be very uncomfortable, they aren't doing themselves any lasting harm.

What happens during and after a discogram?

With the usual technique, you lie on your side while the radiologist inserts a stout needle with a removable core into your back. He views the insertion on a fluoroscope screen to make sure the position is right and then slips the core out. Now the needle serves as a guiding sleeve into which the radiologist slips a slimmer, longer needle. Once this second needle is positioned in the center of the disc he injects the radiopaque fluid.

The doctors will study two things – the behavior of the contrast material in the disc, as shown on the X-ray plates, and the change in your pain. If the X-ray shows a white blob remaining in the middle of the disc, the outer shell is probably intact. If the injected fluid can be seen leaking out, there has been a tear and the disc is considered abnormal.

More important than the X-ray appearance, however, is the pain produced by the test. As the material is injected, you are asked to report whether the pain you feel is identical (or almost identical) to the typical pain you have been having. If it is, the radiologist knows that he has found the offending disc.

That sounds like a pretty uncomfortable test.

I've never met anyone who enjoyed a discogram, but there are some consoling aspects. For one thing, the painful period is quite brief – only a couple of minutes. Also, the after-effects are generally less than those of the myelogram. It's not unusual for a patient to get up after a discogram, with no need for a recovery period.

Earlier you called myelograms and discograms "preludes to surgery."

Yes, and a colleague of mine calls them "road maps for surgery," and that is about right. These tests shouldn't be used to tell the surgeon *whether* to operate – that decision should be based on sound clinical judgment – but they can certainly find the trouble and show *where* to operate. Determining exactly which disc is causing pain, or just where the nerve root is being squeezed, leads to precise and successful surgery. Some of the newer techniques, such as the CT scan, are beginning to take the place of the "grams," but for now these contrast studies remain the standard against which other tests are measured.

You have mentioned the CT scan several times, and of course I have heard of it before, but I'm still not sure exactly what it is.

CT, or CAT, is short for computerized axial tomography. It is the image produced by an extremely sophisticated computerized X-ray machine. Tomography has been around for quite a while. The name means X-rays taken at various depths of focus. The effect is sort of like a loaf of sliced bread: one tomograph gives you a view of one slice. From these X-ray "slices" the CT scanner integrates and constructs views of the body that could never be obtained in any other way. The machine also enhances minor differences in density that the human eye alone could not detect on an X-ray plate. In other words, the CT does for the X-ray what computerized photographs have done for pictures of the planets. You have probably seen photos taken during space exploration, where computers have interpreted and enhanced what the camera saw. In the same way the CT scan allows us to see things such as nerve roots and disc bulges that are invisible on plain X-rays or conventional tomograms.

In the course of a few years the CT scan has become an invaluable tool for diagnosing certain problems in the human spine. Nowhere is this more apparent than in the assessment of spinal stenosis. The CT scan provides the surgeon with cross-sectional X-ray views of the spinal canal, showing exactly where the nerve roots are in relation to the bony sidewalls or a bulging disc. This one machine has changed our understanding of spinal stenosis and how it causes nerve-root compression. Personally, I won't operate on a patient with *cauda equina* claudication from a narrow spinal canal unless I have seen a CT scan.

Another area where the CT scan has produced dramatic results is in cases of severe spinal trauma. For the first time we are able to see the pattern of the vertebral fractures and identify fragments of bone or disc that may have burst into the canal. With this information, the surgeon can operate to decompress the spinal cord or nerve roots and may be able to reduce or prevent paralysis.

In many situations, the CT scan is obviously superior to the myelogram; but the myelogram is still used extensively, either because a CT scan is unavailable, or because the doctor has encountered a case where the CT image doesn't provide enough information. However, as this technology improves and the machine becomes more widely available, we are steadily moving closer to the day when the CT will completely supplant the myelogram as a diagnostic tool.

I value the CT scan the way people prize their personal computers: once you have come to rely on the machine you wonder how you ever got along without it. Certainly that was true in the case of a policeman who came to me with an unusual complaint – and an unhappy history of injuries. While he was working as a traffic officer, a car collided with his motorcycle and he was thrown onto his back. A few years later, as a mounted policeman, he suffered a second episode of back pain while mucking out the police stables.

Three weeks before he came to me, he suffered another low-back attack accompanied for the first time by pain in his left leg. After two days' rest, the pain subsided from both locations, but he noticed his foot was slapping on the ground as he walked. He had no power to lift the foot normally.

I knew that the weakness of ankle movement indicated nerve damage. But my examination produced some confusing findings. The policeman could perform sit-ups easily and without pain (which ruled out acute disc trouble) and his straight-leg raising caused no discomfort (which ruled out nerve irritation). But arching the spine backwards was painful, a finding which usually indicates facet joint pain. However, facet pain and damaged nerves don't commonly go together. And so I had a riddle on my hands: if the patient had only facet trouble, what was he doing with a slapping foot caused by nerve damage?

It seemed to me there was only one possible answer. The policeman's third attack had begun with an L_4-L_5 disc rupture. A piece of the nucleus had blown out through the shell and completely left the disc. It hit the L_5 nerve root hard enough to stop the nerve from working. That would cause the foot drop, and the sudden pressure without local inflammation wouldn't cause the typical signs of nerve-root irritation. After the fragment broke free, the shell of the disc closed up and repaired itself, which accounted for the lack of acute disc symptoms. That piece of nucleus was left in the spinal canal to continue pressing on the nerve. And so when the patient arched backwards he not only brought the facet joints more tightly together – the usual cause of Type One pain – but he also narrowed the nerve's exit tunnel, increasing pressure from the loose chunk of disc.

That was my hypothesis, based on my examination of the policeman's back. It fitted the history and the findings exactly – but how could I be sure I was right? A few years earlier, I would have had nowhere to turn for confirmation. A routine myelogram rarely fills the nerve sleeve far enough into the root canal to show the defect caused by a fragment stuck in that location. Now I simply ordered a CT scan and, sure enough, it showed the piece of disc lodged at the L_4-L_5 level and pressing on the L_5 nerve root. A difficult riddle had been translated into a clear indication for a straightforward surgical procedure. I operated to remove the fragment. There was no need to work on the disc, which had already decompressed and healed itself.

Is there any relationship between the CT scan and the new brain-monitoring process known as SEP?

Only in the sense that SEP also aids spinal surgery. SEP (or SSEP) stands for somatosensory evoked potentials. It's an exciting new tool but it is enormously expensive, highly experimental, and still of limited use. SEP is an electrical signal picked up from the cortex of the brain by a series of monitors placed on the patient's head. They measure the way the brain responds to nerve stimulation, usually as it is applied to the limbs.

During some types of spinal surgery, typically during surgery to correct spinal deformity, it is necessary to monitor the functions of the spinal cord. The conventional way of making sure the patient's nervous system is still all right during surgery is to wake him up part way through the operation – not enough to make him fully conscious but enough to get him to respond to commands, such as wiggling his toes.

Now, that practice becomes unnecessary when there is access to a SEP machine. While the spine is manipulated, technicians can monitor the cord's function by stimulating a nerve in the arm or leg and observing a change in the electrical reading from the brain. Any minor alteration in that function will be noted on the instrument, and the surgeon can respond accordingly.

SEP monitoring requires a highly trained team. At the moment, its use is limited to major centers that do a large volume of surgery for spinal deformities, fractures, or tumors. As experience with the equipment grows, however, the machine may well pass from its current experimental phase and become one of the tools of our trade.

Some of the newest work involves measuring the reaction in a single nerve root. SEP can be used in the diagnosis of spinal stenosis to tell exactly which nerve is being squeezed and causing the problem. And it even seems possible to use the equipment during surgery to tell the surgeon just how much bone he must remove to completely decompress the affected root. SEP can't guarantee a good operative result but it certainly can give the doctor a great deal of help along the way.

It sounds like an amazing piece of equipment. Do you see any other use for SEP?

I am excited by its potential for providing a real assessment of pain. We spoke earlier about the difficulty the doctor has in determining the intensity of pain that a patient feels, or in fact whether the patient feels any pain at all. Pain perception is completely subjective, and at the present time we have no way of measuring it. A person may report that he or she has severe pain in an arm or leg, but we have no method of gauging the real strength of that sensation.

Now SEP may provide a means of recording the brain's response to nerve stimulation and therefore to pain. When SEP technology is developed further, we might be able to test and analyze the electrical impulses from a patient's brain to the point where, for the first time, we will actually measure and describe pain objectively.

I read recently about a machine that scans the body by using a magnetic field instead of X-rays. Is this a significant development?

It certainly is. The machine you are referring to performs a technique called magnetic resonance imaging, or MRI. The process is also known as nuclear magnetic resonance or NMR. The MRI equipment operates by subjecting your body to an extremely strong magnet – generating 3,000 to 28,000 times the strength of the earth's magnetic field. This causes the molecules within the body's tissues to align themselves along the magnetic lines of force. You are then bombarded by radio frequency pulses that knock the atomic particles out of alignment. As the nuclei return to their former positions within the magnetic field they give off radio signals of their own. The effect has been likened to lightly tapping a spinning top: it wobbles and then returns to its original upright position. In the nuclei of the atoms, that "wobble" creates a characteristic electrical discharge. A computer records the signals produced specifically by the nuclei of the hydrogen atoms and creates a visual representation of all the hydrogen-containing tissues. Incidentally, hydrogen was selected because so many living tissues contain this element, usually in the form of water, and because no other element responds with a stronger signal than hydrogen does.

Is "visual representation" just Doctor for "picture"?

No, I'm not speaking Doctor here. MRI images are not pictures but finely detailed representations – reconstructions, if you like – of information the computer has gathered and processed. The result is something like the digital recording that is taking over from conventional methods of reproducing sound. As you probably know, when you hear a digital record, you are not hearing a reproduction of the music itself but a numerical reassembly of the notes played by the musicians and recorded on a computer disc. Digital recordings are remarkably "clean" to listen to because they contain no extraneous sounds – only the music that has been translated into numbers and then converted back into sound by the computer.

In an MRI image, you get a visual recreation of what the machine "saw" in the patient's body, but you can understand now why it's incorrect to regard it as an actual picture.

Does an MRI produce a better image than an X-ray or a CT scan?

It's not so much a better image as a different one. X-rays and

CT scans are really shadow-pictures of the body. The image from
the MRI computer never existed anywhere else. Compared to an
X-ray, the MRI has one big advantage: whereas an X-ray shows
only bone and not soft tissue, the MRI shows both and provides
much clearer differentiations between them. The difference is
less apparent when MRI is compared to a CT scan, but the MRI
image is still impressive.

The appearance is certainly different. Because of their low
hydrogen content, bones appear black on the MRI, whereas on
the X-ray and CT scan they appear white because they block off
most of the X-ray beam. The MRI can actually show the difference
between a healthy disc and a worn one, by indicating the amount
of water they contain. Not only can the MRI show the structure;
it can also reveal what it is made of. That's something an X-ray
or scan could never do as well. But because the MRI is a representation rather than a direct visual image, it needs a great deal
of human interpretation. The surgeon who is used to reading
X-rays needs some practice before he can decipher an MRI.

Is that a skill most back doctors have acquired by now?

Not yet. I am enthusiastic about MRI, but the machines are expensive and scarce. The process is just coming into its own for the
diagnosis of back problems, but it's bound to have a major impact
on the decision-making process in surgical procedures.

Is the high cost of MRI machines responsible for the time lag?

It's one reason; but MRI is still in its early stage of development.
At the moment, it can't quite do everything a CT scan can do.
For example, from a CT scan I can get a much clearer picture
of the vertebrae with slices as thin as 1.5 mm – less than 6/100ths
of an inch. The MRI, at the present time, hasn't reached that
degree of precision.

Is the patient in any danger from the magnetic field of an MRI?

No one can answer that question with absolute certainty, but by
all indications so far, there is no danger. Thousands of patients
have had MRI images taken and have been monitored carefully,

with no evidence of side effects of any kind. In assessing the risks from the radio frequency impulses, some authorities have estimated that the present strength could be 100 times more powerful before there was any cause for concern.

There are special exceptions, however. Patients who have cardiac pacemakers or metal implants of any kind must avoid MRI. The extreme magnetism would knock the pacemaker out of commission and cause a harmful reaction from any other metallic implant.

So far, MRI machines have presented only one minor drawback for patients: people who are troubled by claustrophobia find it difficult to climb into the MRI chamber and remain there for the necessary twenty to thirty minutes.

I see the MRI as the wave of the future for diagnostic work, partly because it is non-invasive and it completely avoids the concern some patients have about exposure to radiation. The MRI computer can even color the images and produce a stunning display of living anatomy as it has never been seen before.

My doctor was talking about another computerized instrument, a densometer. What is that?

It's not as dramatic as the MRI, but in some ways it's just as exciting. The dual photon densometer promises to revolutionize the diagnosis of osteoporosis. As you will recall, osteoporosis is a condition in which there is a reduction in normal bone mass below the level needed to maintain skeletal support. This is normal with aging, and it is not painful in itself, but it makes the bones susceptible to fracture, which can lead to problems that are both painful and disabling.

Until now, the onset of osteoporosis has often been hard to detect because we have not had an accurate method of measuring bone density. Conventional X-rays are not up to this task. Thirty to 50 percent of the bone mass can disappear before routine X-rays are able to detect any difference.

A more direct method of assessing osteoporosis is the bone biopsy – that is, removing a small sample of bone for laboratory study and analysis. But that's an operation, a painful process that still produces results which can be unreliable, since it is impossible to be sure that the sample taken is typical of the other bones.

Now they have come up with a computerized measuring technique which, even in its early stages of development, is capable of analyzing bone density with amazing precision. A specific radioisotope is injected into the patient's bloodstream. As in a conventional bone scan, the material is taken up by the bones, where it remains for a short while. But unlike the isotope normally used, the new compound emits radiation on two distinct frequencies. A computer records both levels and performs some complex calculations on the two pieces of information. Then it conveniently prints out the percentage of bone loss, comparing it with the average for a person of the same age and sex, and in some cases even estimating the probability of a fracture.

Both dual photon densometry and magnetic resonance imaging are two excellent examples of the new medical tools that will soon enable us to diagnose and treat back problems with unprecedented accuracy and effectiveness.

12. ANYONE FOR SURGERY?

In a medical world seemingly divided between "cutting doctors" and "talking doctors" I feel comfortable in both camps. Although I spend almost half my working days in the operating room, the patients I treat there represent only a small fraction of the backache victims I see. For the others, the appropriate treatments involve less dramatic action – physical therapy, exercise, good posture, and healthy living habits – all constructive ways of working with nature to encourage the healing process.

Because I put so much effort into counseling my patients in back care, many people conclude, quite erroneously, that I disapprove of surgery, or at least that I am reluctant to operate on any back patient except as a last resort.

.This isn't true. My low ratio of surgery cases is based on a perfectly sound principle: to be remedied by the scalpel, a back problem must be structural, localized, and specific – an unstable joint or pressure on a nerve root. There is no practical surgical procedure for repairing generalized wear and tear down the length of the spine, and I have yet to acquire forceps capable of reaching into a patient's back and simply plucking out the pain. Even when the trouble is localized to a specific structure, surgery isn't usually the answer.

Most back problems, in other words, are inoperable. Which is not to say that they are hopeless but only that they call for non-surgical treatment. An operation is not a last resort but a particular remedy suitable for selected cases. Whenever these cases are referred to me, I recommend surgery with an alacrity that would surprise those who consider me an "anti-surgery surgeon."

On the other hand, I flatly refuse to operate when I'm convinced surgery is the wrong way to solve the problem and is unlikely to succeed. Not long ago, a woman walked into my office and announced: "I need a back operation." After reading my first book, she had diagnosed herself as the victim of Type Three back trouble (a pinched nerve) and had decided surgery was the remedy. When I examined her I found she was wrong on both counts. I explained this to her, declined to operate – and lost her as a patient. I have no doubt she has since been making the rounds in search of a "cutting doctor" who will do as she asks.

In contrast, I remember a genuine Type Three patient who should have had surgery. The man had been lifting some files out of the back seat of his car when he lost his balance and twisted his body. Three months later, he came to me, and the CT scan I ordered showed he had a large disc herniation in his low back. The affected disc was pressing on a nerve root, causing severe pain and a progressive weakness of muscles in one buttock and the calf of one leg. I recommended surgery and predicted that he had a 90 percent chance of making a complete recovery. Naturally I also discussed the possible complications of the operation, such as infection or local nerve injury, and I stressed the need for continuing back care when the post-operative period was over.

Unfortunately, my warnings must have scared him off. He declined the operation and has been suffering ever since – from inactivity, unemployment, financial problems, his weak leg, and the back pain itself. The choice was his, of course, but clearly he would have been far better off having the operation.

I would feel much happier about both those patients if I had managed to provide them with a clearer perspective of spinal surgery, to help them make better-informed decisions. I hope this chapter will provide that perspective for many back patients facing comparable situations.

Just the idea of having a back operation frightens me. Do many of your patients feel the same way?

Many are frightened by the very word "surgery" and everything they associate with it – from the intimidating atmosphere of the operating room to the possibility of never regaining consciousness after a general anesthetic. Some of them believe the spine is such a complex and mysterious part of the body that the very prospect of having it invaded or disturbed is terrifying.

And that's with *elective* surgery. Imagine an accident victim who is lying in Emergency when a surgeon – a total stranger – walks in and says, "How do you do. I am going to operate on you in about an hour." No wonder patients are frightened. Not just at the thought of surgery but because someone they have never even seen before has just announced he is going to do something drastic to them. Feeling that absolute loss of control, and the need to depend so completely on someone they don't know, must be terrible. In that situation I always take a little extra time to get acquainted with the patient and the family and explain what the surgery is all about.

On the other hand, I have patients who are so convinced they need surgery that they won't follow my advice about doing anything else to help themselves. They just keep waiting for me to agree to operate on them and assume full responsibility for their recovery. They view the operation as an easy way out, often expecting it to alleviate not only their back problem but many of their non-medical complaints as well. Some patients seem to believe back surgery will improve everything from their short temper to their falling hair.

It must be important to know what your surgeon plans to do and how he believes it will help.

Certainly the more you know the more comfortable you will feel. Listen carefully to what you're told, first by your family doctor, and then by the surgeon, who has a responsibility to help you understand your operation. With my patients I spend a lot of time explaining what I'm going to do. I know they have certain expectations, and I know the operation is capable of correcting certain things. It's in everyone's best interest to make sure those two elements match up. If your expectations are unrealistic, you are not likely to be satisfied with the results.

Often, it's a simple matter of clear communication. Although the onus lies primarily on the surgeon, for your own sake as a patient you should do everything you can to make sure the message you're hearing is the message that's intended. If the surgeon says, "You'll be fine in a week," and fails to elaborate, the two of you may have wildly different notions of what that means. You may think being "fine" means suddenly becoming twenty years younger and able to leap tall buildings in a single bound, while he probably means you'll be well enough to get out of hospital, perhaps with a little help.

The only way to overcome such gaps in understanding is to talk. Ask questions. Get an explanation of any point you're unsure about. Clear up any discrepancies between the things you have heard elsewhere and the things your doctor is telling you. You're a rare patient indeed if you don't have at least one or two misconceptions about back surgery. No matter how hard I try to present my patients with a clear picture of the procedure, I'm sure some of them remain convinced, for instance, that I plan to completely remove one or two discs from their spines. That operation, commonly referred to as a "disc removal," actually entails something far less drastic; only the *nucleus* of the disc is removed – and only a part of the nucleus at that.

What *is* back surgery all about? There must be many different kinds of operations or procedures.

Surprisingly there are just two basic types of surgery for common backache, although, as you might suppose, wide variations are practiced within each type.

One is decompression, involving the removal of pressure being exerted on the nerves within the spine. That pressure can come from several sources – a disc bulging into the spinal canal and pressing against a single nerve root or against the dural sac containing the *cauda equina* or, higher up, the spinal cord; a bit of nucleus that has escaped from a disc and lodged somewhere in the canal; a bony growth from a facet joint or the wall of the canal that is reducing the size of the tunnel. If you remember what we said earlier about the four types of backache, you will realize that all the conditions I just mentioned are forms of Type

Three pain (the pinched nerve) or Type Four pain (spinal stenosis). Decompression, broadly speaking, involves removal of whatever is pressing on the nerve.

The other basic operation is stabilization, or fusion, as it is commonly called, which is a remedy for Type One and Type Two pain. It involves fusing two or more vertebrae together to eliminate any painful movement. The problem may be either worn facet joints rubbing together, or a bulging disc that is no longer serving as the firm cushion it was intended to be. To join two vertebrae, the surgeon bridges the joints and disc space between them with pieces of bone that are permanently incorporated into both vertebrae. The joints are immobilized, the disc is replaced by solid bone, and the two vertebrae become fused into one structure.

Do some back patients need both types of operations – decompression *and* fusion?

Yes, in some patients with Type Three or Type Four pain, decompression may be combined with fusion. For instance, after a decompression that clears up the problem of a pinched nerve, the surgeon might find that removing the required amount of material has produced a mechanical instability requiring a fusion.

Are the two types of operation performed at the same time?

Sometimes. If a stenosis patient needed several facet joints removed for decompression, the surgeon could anticipate a degree of instability that would need stabilizing, and he might very well perform both procedures during the one session.

Are most back operations successful?

If by successful you mean that the operation gets rid of your symptoms, the answer is yes, they are. Your pain is gone and you can function normally. Realistically, you can't expect surgery to transform a worn old back into a brand new one; that kind of success will always elude us.

Success depends on two important conditions. First, the operation must be done for the right reason: you must have a condition that can be remedied by the proposed surgical procedure. And second, the operation must be done properly. If these basic conditions are met, the chances of success are excellent. As you might expect, however, the prospects are better for some types of back surgery than for others.

The back operation with the best success rate is one of the decompression operations, the simple discotomy. In this procedure, the surgeon cuts out a small portion of the bony plate on the back of the vertebrae (the plate is called the *lamina* and this part of the operation is called a laminectomy). Through that little hole into the spinal canal the surgeon can reach the disc and remove the bulge that is pressing on the nerve. Nine out of ten patients who undergo a routine laminectomy and discotomy get rid of their symptoms and return to normal living. The success rate for the simple discotomy is high because it is a straightforward operation for which the indications are very clear.

For the benefit of those who like to pick up a little Doctor language now and then, I should explain that the suffix "otomy" means "to put a hole in," and so the first part of the operation really ought to be called a laminotomy. The suffix "ectomy" means "to remove," and so the second phase of the operation should actually be called a "partial discectomy." But in common surgical jargon these "pure" terms have been slightly corrupted, and the procedure is known instead as a "laminectomy-discotomy."

Do all the people who need simple discotomies have the same problems?

Yes, with minor variations. The symptoms include a predominance of leg pain and other leg complaints, such as loss of power in certain muscle groups, decreased sensation, or the disappearance of a reflex. The exact pattern depends on the specific nerve root involved and that depends on the precise location of the disc rupture. The patient's complaints either fail to get better with well-controlled bed rest and physical therapy, or they actually grow worse. When the indications are that clear, surgery is likely to be done at the right time, and the chances of success are consequently very good.

Other forms of decompression surgery may be carried out for problems that are hard to determine so precisely, such as an area of spinal stenosis causing *cauda equina* claudication, and accordingly their success rate is somewhat lower. Even at that, surgical enlargement of a short length of the spinal canal to reduce nerve pressure has a success rate well over 85 percent.

The reason for that lack of precision isn't hard to understand. The surgeon may correctly diagnose the problem as one involving pressure from bony overgrowth in the canal without being able to tell exactly how much bone needs to come out. Consequently he may go in and remove some bone without taking quite as much as he should, thus failing to relieve all the pressure on the nerve. Or the surgeon may err in the opposite direction, overdoing the bone removal. Destroying too much of the roof and sides of the tunnel can allow an excessive growth of scar tissue, which can choke the nerve as much as the original stenosis did. And eliminating the entire posterior joint structure will lead to segmental instability.

Instability caused by decompression surgery is not nearly so common today as it was in the sixties, when we knew less than we know now about spinal stenosis and its remedies. In those days it was not unusual for surgeons to remove the posterior elements of four or five vertebrae. Although the early results were satisfactory, over half the patients had their back problems return within two years. Some had spines that were so unstable that the vertebrae actually began to move out of alignment. The only remedy was fusion, which was a pretty "iffy" proposition with so many levels of the spine involved.

What about the success rate for fusion operations generally?

If you have a condition where you need a fusion at just one level – that is, where only two vertebrae are to be joined into a single unit – the chances of success are good, approaching 90 percent. The percentage is slightly lower for a fusion at two levels, and lower still for three levels, which is pretty well the surgical limit in cases of ordinary Type One or Type Two back pain.

Instability is a subtle and complicated condition that's hard to assess. Although one level of your spine might show definite signs of wear with abnormal movement, the neighboring levels may also be involved to a lesser but significant degree. By stabilizing that one level, I will be shifting the load to the other levels, which may consequently become unstable. Because of these inherent uncertainties, I never recommend or perform a fusion unless I am convinced that the person is seriously disabled, with pain that cannot be controlled by a rigorous exercise and training program. And when I make the decision to operate, I have to take into account the fact that fusion will set up new conditions that can cause new trouble.

Fusion is generally a larger operation than decompression. Because more muscle is stripped away from the bone to gain access, it causes more scar tissue to form. Scar tissue is tender stuff and can cause considerable local discomfort for a year or more. Usually the bone used in the fusion is obtained from the patient's pelvis, and this "donor site" becomes a second source of pain during the convalescence.

All in all, it's a process so complicated that no one can say with certainty that a fusion operation will get rid of all the pain, even if the bones unite to provide a solid bridge between the adjacent vertebrae.

To make matters a little more confusing, a few patients will have good results from their fusions with excellent pain relief and return of function, while their X-rays clearly show the operation has failed to produce a bony connection between the vertebrae. In other words, although the surgery was a technical failure it was a clinical success.

Perhaps the one exception to the uncertainty about low-back fusions is the operation for spondylolithesis at L_5. This is a condition where a defect in the normally solid bridge between the upper and lower joints of the last mobile vertebra allows the body of the bone to slip forward. Fusing to restore normal stability is one case where a technically successful operation almost always solves the problem.

You must walk a tightrope, trying to help a patient understand what the chances and risks are, and yet not discourage or frighten off the person who would probably benefit greatly from surgery.

That's exactly right. Like most other surgeons, I try to achieve what has become known as "informed consent." That means asking the patient to accept treatment with a full understanding of both the positive and negative results that could ensue.

Is this idea of "informed consent" a new concept for surgeons?

Yes – in the deliberate and expanded manner that is customary today. The traditional routine of signing the consent form merely gave your permission, whether you understood or not. The evolution of informed consent as a concept was pointed up to me recently by a friend who described an experience he had about thirty-five years ago. As a young man, my friend needed minor surgery for the removal of a couple of sebaceous cysts in his scalp. A few days before the operation, the surgeon told him that while the operation was pretty routine, there was always the chance that the cysts would not come out completely; some portion might remain to cause trouble in the future. When my friend mentioned this caution to his uncle, a retired doctor, the uncle laughed and said: "He's just making up excuses in advance, in case he botches the operation."

The uncle's response shows how most doctors viewed such cautions in earlier times. Today, with the public more aware of surgical risks and with doctors feeling more vulnerable to malpractice suits, the surgeon, for ethical and legal reasons, must forewarn the patient by spelling out the potential risks entailed in any procedure. If he fails to do that, he could be accused of operating without the patient's informed consent.

I fully approve of informed consent. As you suggested, however, it's sometimes a hard principle to apply. Where do I draw the line between informing my patient as fully as necessary and scaring him out of his wits? It's easy to describe what I think I am going to achieve and how well I hope it will go. It's much more difficult to dwell on all the possible causes of failure and still maintain the patient's confidence in my ability as a surgeon.

And my approach won't be the same for all my patients. Each of them is a unique individual with his or her own intelligence, emotional makeup, and expectations based on a mixture of real experience, valid information, vivid imagination, and folklore.

For most operations, we know the percentages of successes and failures, but these don't really tell the whole story. As a patient, you are a person, not a statistic. There is not much consolation in having known beforehand that the general success rate is 90 percent if it turns out that the success of your own surgery is zero. So I attempt to explain where the problems may come from and what can be done about them should they arise. Most of all I want the patient to realize why in his or her particular case the operation is worth the potential risks.

This concept of informed consent is something to keep in mind, against the day when you may have to listen to the pros and cons involved in having your own back surgery. If your doctor seems to be telling you more than you want to hear about the risks, remember: if you are to share in the decision intelligently, you must have a thorough understanding of what you're getting into.

If I have an operation on my back, is it possible I will need surgery later on for the same problem?

The majority of people who have one operation never have or need to have a second one. If the results of your surgery have been good for at least a year after the recovery period, you can be reasonably sure that it was a technical success and you won't need an encore, at least not for the same problem. On the other hand, if your original trouble returns within six months, a second operation to try to make things better usually fails. Unless a new problem can be demonstrated clearly, more surgery is not often the answer.

I have been presented with all too many sad examples of second surgery. On one occasion I was asked to provide a consultation on another surgeon's patient who had serious problems. The woman (I'll call her Mrs. Wallace) had been through three back operations, all of them fusions. All three operations had failed, and she still had disabling back pain.

Mrs. Wallace had just had another myelogram, and I could see that while the attempts at fusion had partially stabilized several of the worn areas, her spine was a long way from normal. At every level of her low back there was one problem or another – here some narrowing of the spinal canal, there a bulging disc, here an arthritic joint, somewhere else a failed fusion. Through a combination of normal aging, natural wear and tear, and three operations, the poor woman had a spine that was beyond salvaging.

And, as I suspected, I had been invited there with more than simple consultation in mind. Mrs. Wallace wanted me to operate on her. She had read my first book and made up her mind that my surgical skill was the answer to her problem. I know she was disappointed when I said there was no operation I could perform that would help her. But it was true. There was not even anything new to be found that would justify any drastic change in her treatment. Every problem I spotted in her myelogram was already known to her own surgeon, who had performed those three failed operations. I offered her a program of chronic pain management and exercise, but Mrs. Wallace clearly wasn't interested. I left the case with the distinct impression that her surgeon would soon give in and take her into surgery for a fourth round. I wish them both well but I don't give them much chance of success.

I gather you don't hold much hope for a third or fourth spinal operation.

That's putting it mildly. I often say to patients, "Your first chance is your best chance, and your second chance is your last chance." Unless, as rarely happens, the back surgery is for a completely different condition.

I first made that observation many years ago, and it was borne out later by a study done in co-operation with the Ontario Workers' Compensation Board. We reviewed cases where patients had undergone two or more unsuccessful back operations, looking for reasons why the surgery failed. We found that the most common reason for the failure of a second operation was the same as the reason for the failure of the first: most of these patients shouldn't have had surgery at all. Typically, the indications for the original surgery were unconvincing or confused. The patients had few if any clinical findings that suggested the need for any operation. Some patients had normal myelograms; others had myelograms that did not match up with their clinical findings. Almost all the other tests that were done revealed nothing significant.

It was hardly surprising, then, that those first operations had less than six months of apparent success, followed by a recurrence of the same old trouble. Having undergone the original surgery for inappropriate reasons, these people went through the same process all over again, with the same poor result.

Of course there were other cases, too, where surgery failed the first time around, even though it had been the proper course to follow.

Why would surgery fail if it was done for the right reason?

Perhaps it wasn't performed properly or thoroughly enough, or maybe the patient didn't follow the doctor's instructions about post-operative care. Or there could have been a complication or a second problem that wasn't diagnosed at the outset.

However, in cases where the need for surgery was clear from the beginning, the second round of surgery undertaken to salvage those first-time failures had a high rate of success. When it came to a third operation, no matter how valid the indications had been for the first two, the chances of improvement fell dramatically. Which is why I say that when it comes to back surgery, your second chance is your last chance.

Are you saying, then, that it's futile for anyone to have more than two back operations?

Generally speaking, yes, it is, particularly if the successive operations are all intended to remedy the same disorder. It's a different matter if new back problems develop after successful surgery. One patient of mine has gone through three operations for herniated discs – twice at the same level and the third at the level below. The operations took place a year apart, each time near Christmas. The timing and regularity of her surgery became a bit of an unhappy joke between us. But every operation was justified and all of them succeeded. In each instance she had fully recovered and remained symptom-free for longer than six months, the critical period for gauging the potential success for "second try" surgery. She simply had the rare misfortune of developing three separate disc herniations (one at the site of previous surgery) on three separate occasions.

That patient was lucky: her last surgery, many Christmases ago, left her with a functional, pain-free back. Another patient of mine wasn't as fortunate. He had had a series of operations, each of which solved an immediate problem but left his spine less stable. His original problem was a routine case of stenosis; several nerves were being squeezed in an abnormally narrow part of the spinal

canal. I corrected that problem with a decompression operation.
Three years later the man was struck by a car, injuring his spine.
Our findings indicated the need for another decompression, and
when I operated I found a distinct ridge of scar tissue right across
the area we had opened up earlier. The impact of the accident
had either added more scar or disrupted a comfortable balance
between the scar left from my first surgery and the local nerve
roots. I removed the excessive fibrous tissue, enlarged the canal
a little more, and my patient got better.

Then, a full year later, his back pain recurred, and I decided
he needed a third decompression. This time he had developed
a large ingrowth of scar at the upper end of the previous
decompression. Scarring, as you probably know, is one of the body's
natural responses to injury, including surgery. It produces many
benefits but it has its drawbacks; scar tissue can choke off a nerve
and cause severe pain. In this man's case, I felt there was little
choice but to remove that ingrowth of scar along with some more
of the bone on the back of his spine and hope for the best.
Unfortunately, that additional bone loss deprived his spine of still
more of its natural stability. The only possible remedy for his
fourth recurrence of disabling back pain was yet another round
of surgery – this time a fusion, which, I am happy to say, was
the last operation the man needed. He still has chronic back pain,
but he can control it well enough to lead a normal life.

It's worth noting that while every one of those operations was
a success in itself, the earlier surgery made the subsequent
operations necessary. While it's true that the final outcome in this
case was satisfactory, it was far from perfect. If you are facing
the prospect of surgery, don't limit your discussion with the doctor
to the immediate problem. Consider the long-term effects of the
operation on the function of your spine, the chance of increased
trouble in other areas of your back, or even the chance of a
recurrence of the original difficulty. Be sure you understand your
role in the rehabilitation process and whether there will be any
need for a permanent adjustment of your activities.

**What about neck surgery? How is it different from operations on
the lower back?**

There are a few significant differences. The canal in the cervical spine contains the spinal cord rather than the separate nerve roots found in the low back. The cord is very sensitive to pressure, and for this reason the operations are designed to avoid any pulling or pushing on it. And, of course, damage to the spinal cord would have far more serious consequences than injury to a single nerve root lower down.

But the indications and techniques of surgery are otherwise much the same. The most common reasons for an operation are: painful wear in a disc (Type Two); or pressure on a nerve root as it leaves the spine (Type Three). This pressure produces pain or loss of function in the arm or hand. Most neck problems can be managed with non-surgical treatment, however, and of all the patients I see with neck pain, only about 1 percent require an operation.

Decompression operations can be done through the back of the neck in the same way we perform decompressions in the lumbar spine. But because of concerns about moving the spinal cord aside to reach the disc, many surgeons make their approach from the front. A small incision is made on one side of the neck and then deepened through the muscles before passing between the carotid artery (a major artery to the brain) on one side and the trachea (the windpipe) on the other.

The front of the spine can be seen at the bottom of the wound, and most of the nucleus of the troublesome disc is easily removed through a hole cut in its outer shell. It is possible to work all the way to the back of the disc to eliminate bulges pressing on the nerves in the spinal canal.

Because the neck is more flexible than the low back and because the frontal approach removes a large amount of the nucleus of the disc, this technique usually produces a degree of instability. For that reason, decompression is almost always combined with a fusion. A small block of bone taken from the pelvis is fitted into the disc space between the vertebral bodies.

In other cases, such as when treating a major injury to the facet joints of the neck, a fusion can be done from behind, in much the same way as we usually fuse the low back.

After surgery the patient wears a rigid collar but is usually able to be up within a day or two. Until the bone graft forms a solid union, which takes about three months, the neck must be protected. During convalescence, the donor site on the pelvis often hurts more than the fusion in the neck.

Are neck operations generally safe and successful?

Yes. Although most people don't need an operation to solve their neck problems, when surgery is required the success rate is high. The same complications that sometimes result from low-back surgery can occur after neck surgery, but they rarely do. Special care is taken in handling the major vessels to the head, in protecting the spinal cord, and in making sure nothing is done to disturb the nerves that control the vocal cords.

What circumstances would prompt you to recommend back surgery for me?

Since the symptoms and the treatment wouldn't be the same for every type of back problem, I'll describe my approach to a typical situation involving the commonest form of back surgery, the discotomy (which really ought to be called a partial discectomy, since only some of the center, or nucleus, of the disc is removed).

By the time we considered a discotomy, you would probably have seen me several times, for pain that is in your back but much worse in your lower leg and foot. Under my direction, you would have gone through several weeks of conservative management consisting primarily of bed rest and gentle extension exercises.

My decision to consider an operation would be prompted by your signs and symptoms either failing to improve or growing worse. And that raises a very important point: I would not suggest an operation simply because you have pain. I would have to be convinced you are suffering from a loss of nerve function that could not be restored through rest and non-surgical treatment.

How could you tell if there is a loss of normal function in a nerve?

Earlier, when we discussed the causes of common backache, we talked about the tests for irritation of a nerve root. We also discussed the ways to tell whether a certain nerve is failing to conduct impulses properly. These examinations would help me make my decision.

Nerve irritation, the source of most of your leg pain, can be measured by the straight-leg-raising test. I'd have you lie flat on your back with your knee extended while I raised your leg. If you felt pain in the back of your thigh, calf, or foot with an elevation of less than sixty degrees, I would know you had nerve irritation. Other tests could indicate the same problem. For instance, if pressure applied behind your knee caused pain to spread up or down your leg, there would be abnormal irritation somewhere in the sciatic nerve.

If you had a loss of sensation in a specific area of the leg, an absent reflex at the knee or ankle, or, most important of all, decreased power in certain groups of muscles, I would know that one of the nerves coming from the lumbar spine was unable to carry its normal signals. The failure of these functions and their lack of recovery over a period of time are factors in determining the need for surgery.

Even at this point, however, I might bring you into hospital for several days to see whether complete bed rest would improve your condition. At home there are just too many temptations to get up and join the family for dinner or help with the chores. Once you were in that hospital bed you'd stay there. You could get up to use the toilet or take a daily shower, but that's all. Otherwise, you'd be lying down, even while eating your meals or watching TV. The physical therapists would keep a close eye on your resting positions and direct a program of gentle exercise. No sitting back against plumped-up pillows all day. As I said earlier, sitting is hard on your back, and in this situation it could defeat the purpose of your time in hospital.

You'd be surprised at how many of my patients begin to get well during that short stay. Often, those few days of bed rest under close supervision are enough to start them on the road to recovery. They can go home without surgery, get some more rest, and then start on a long-term program to get their backs in shape.

What would happen if I didn't respond well to hospital rest? Would you automatically schedule me for the discotomy?

Not automatically. The next items on your agenda would be a few diagnostic tests. Special studies would be carried out, along with some ordinary X-rays of your low back, routine blood work, and a general physical assessment. You might be given a myelogram or a CT scan or both, to determine the exact location of your bulging disc. If the results of your tests confirmed my diagnosis and located the problem, you would be scheduled for surgery.

What do you do, exactly, when you perform the discotomy?

It's a straightforward matter of going in and removing the nucleus of the disc that's bulging out against the nerve.

I begin by making a one- to two-inch-long incision in your back, at the appropriate spot, as determined by your myelogram or CT scan. On the way to my destination, I carefully strip away the muscles that block my entry and temporarily retract them to one side. Next, I remove a small portion of the roof of the spinal canal (a section of the bony plate, or *lamina*, and the yellow ligament, or *ligamentum flavum*, that spans the space between the bones).

Once inside the canal I gently push the nerve sac and root aside to reach the disc located on the floor of the tunnel. The bulge is usually quite easy to see; the inflammation makes it look like a large pimple. Curled up in the middle of that bump is the material that escaped from the center of the disc. After extracting the loose fragment I may or may not attempt to clean out the remainder of the nucleus still contained within the disc's outer shell. I know it's impossible to remove all of it, but I can probably take out about 75 percent. I don't remove the thick walls that bind the disc to the vertebrae on either side. Nor do I worry about the hollow that I've left in the center of the disc, since this will fill harmlessly with scar tissue stronger and more resilient than the part of the nucleus I removed.

Whether or not I proceed to remove those portions of the nucleus remaining within the disc will depend on how I judge the situation. Usually the surgeon scrapes out all the nucleus he can get, to ensure that another loose piece isn't lurking inside the disc waiting to cause more trouble. But if I find that the *anulus* – the outer shell of the disc – has healed so well that no more nucleus can get out, I'd be foolish to disturb what nature has already mended.

Once I have removed the necessary amount of material, it's just a matter of withdrawing from the site, covering the exposed dura (nerve sac) with a thin layer of fat to reduce future scarring, moving back the muscles that were pushed aside, and closing up the incision. The whole operation is briefer than the average movie – sixty to ninety minutes – and a lot less bloody than some.

How am I likely to feel right after a discotomy? Will my old pain be gone?

Yes. The first thing you are likely to notice when you wake up is that your leg pain has disappeared, although the incision in your back will be sore. You will be told that if you need to get up in the night to use the toilet, you are free to do so, and you will be encouraged to start walking the next day as much as you can. You won't even need a corset.

On the second day, your leg will still be pain free, but you will begin to realize your back is hurting more and more. I always warn my patients about this in advance. I tell them what other patients have told me: after a discotomy you feel as though you've been kicked by a horse in the small of the back. The pain is the result of muscle bruising, which occurred when I pushed those muscles aside to get at the disc. Muscles don't like being pushed around. They gradually become swollen and sore, and they complain accordingly.

Your back pain, however, will be quite different from the pain you had before your operation. The new pain will be easier to endure, like a tender bruise that's sensitive to the touch. Something about the quality of the pain makes most patients realize that it is temporary and will be gone in a few days. I remember one patient who had his discotomy on Friday morning and was out enjoying dinner in a restaurant on Sunday afternoon.

Even during those uncomfortable first days, you can be up and around, although you'll be moving cautiously. You'll learn to roll onto one side and then push yourself up to a sitting position to avoid stressing the area of your surgery. Walking is good because it stimulates the circulation in your legs, and that helps prevent blood clots from forming in the veins there. It keeps your lungs working well. And it's a morale booster. You'll find yourself thinking, "Hey – I'm getting better already!" The current emphasis on early activity is quite a change from the old days when patients were kept in bed for a week or more after simple disc surgery.

For the first week or two you can do anything you want, but you should avoid sitting for extended periods, since that puts quite a load on the area of the surgery. You are encouraged to stand, lie down, or perch somewhere, leaning with your backside against a counter or window-ledge.

How long will I have to stay in the hospital?

After simple disc surgery, you can usually expect to go home in less than three or four days. Some surgeons keep their patients in hospital for a week; others pride themselves on sending people home after forty-eight hours or less. The general trend these days is to get patients up and out as quickly as possible.

What are the chances of a complication following a discotomy?

The risks are small. But there are potential complications from the anesthetic, the chance of damaging a nerve root during surgery, and the possibility of a wound infection later on. You must also be aware that for a few vulnerable patients, typically those well along in years or with previous medical problems, the stress of an operation and the period of convalescence which follows can precipitate a heart attack or a stroke, or a blood clot in the lungs. I often remind my patients that having back surgery is not like having a haircut; there are a number of potentially serious complications. I hasten to add that the chance of trouble is small, less than two in a hundred for all complications combined. And the surgical team is highly skilled in avoiding or minimizing these problems.

One minor complication that can cause you a good deal of pain is an attack of muscle spasms in your back. I'm not referring to the bit of backache that results from bruising the muscles during surgery; I'm talking about really bad muscle cramps quite unlike anything you felt before the operation. If these occur, they will likely start soon after surgery, while you are still in hospital.

How long do spasms like that usually last?

That's unpredictable. They might last just a few days, or they could drag on for several weeks. The only consolation is that they eventually end. I have never seen any, or heard of any, that didn't.

What can be done to stop the muscles from cramping?

Unfortunately, not much. Unlike other kinds of spasms, which may respond to even a single treatment of massage, manipulation, heat, or medication, these post-operative cramps seldom yield readily. The important thing is to avoid panic, which will only make them worse.

From all I have just said you may be vowing never to undergo a discotomy no matter what your doctor advises. But you must not lose sight of the fact that the removal of a disc fragment is an excellent decompression procedure with an extremely high rate of success and an extremely low risk of complication.

Would my chance of success be better if I had a microdiscotomy?

Microdiscotomy means that the surgeon uses an operating microscope while performing the surgery. The actual operation is much the same as the one I just described. Increased magnification may make it easier to avoid damage to a nerve root, but for a competent surgeon this is not necessarily a difficult feat even without a microscope. Microdiscotomy also means the use of specially designed surgical instruments, smaller and more delicate than those normally employed. And viewing the wound through the microscope may make the surgeon more aware of minor problems and the need to maintain a meticulous operative technique.

But the microscope has its disadvantages as well. The apparatus is large, awkward, and very expensive. Positioning it above the operative field is time-consuming and may contaminate the sterile area. So the operation usually takes longer, and there have been cases where significant pathology was missed because it lay outside the surgeon's necessarily restricted field of view.

The indications are the same no matter which style of discotomy is selected, as are the chances of success or complications. I have no objection to microdiscotomy so long as it isn't regarded as a guaranteed method or used as a gimmick to attract business and raise the cost of surgery.

What about other kinds of decompression operations?

The discotomy is the commonest type. As I mentioned earlier, getting to the disc usually means removing a portion of the *lamina*, the bone that forms part of the roof of the spinal canal. Occasionally, removal of this bone alone is done to eliminate nerve pressure, and the procedure is labeled a decompressive laminectomy. As far as the patient's perception goes, there is virtually no difference between a discotomy and a laminectomy.

Another fairly common but slightly different form of decompression is the type performed for spinal stenosis – removal of bony growths that are narrowing the spinal canal and interfering with nerve function. This is usually a more difficult operation than a simple discotomy, because it's harder to remove bone than it is to remove loose fragments of disc. For this reason, the operation takes longer and often means pushing aside more muscle, since the bone removal may be required from both sides of the tunnel. In addition to the decompressive laminectomy, the surgery may entail partial removal of the walls of the canal and the overhanging facet joints. Compared to the discotomy, decompression for stenosis leaves a lot more scar tissue and requires a longer period for full recovery.

During recovery, you may need to wear some sort of back brace or support, which is unnecessary after a simple discotomy; otherwise, the post-op situation is much the same. Often, you will wake up with your pre-operative back pain and your leg symptoms gone, although you won't know that for sure until you are up and around again.

Can you judge beforehand whether decompression is needed on one or both sides?

Yes, I'm usually able to tell from the CT scan and my assessment of your signs and symptoms. Once in a while, there is a disparity between what I see on the X-rays and the clinical examination. My physical findings may suggest that significant compression exists only on one side, while the CT scan shows bilateral narrowing. In that situation there may be a case to be made for decompressing both sides: the potential trouble is real enough to justify preventive surgery. I generally adhere to the old adage, "If it ain't broke, don't fix it," but I don't allow it to overrule my judgment in a specific situation.

I gather that, compared to a discotomy, decompression for stenosis is a more difficult operation for the patient to get through.

That's true. The stenotic patient doesn't always get the immediate relief felt by the discotomy patient. If you have extensive surgery for stenosis you will probably be required to stay in bed a little longer afterwards, and you'll likely take two or three months to get back to your normal routine instead of the few weeks needed by most discotomy patients. But even though your progress may be a little slower, you will likely enjoy some early improvement, and within the first few days, your doctor should be able to predict a good outcome for you.

What complications may follow decompression for stenosis?

The complications, if any, are about the same as for a discotomy. If the decompression has required a great deal of bone removal, there may also be problems with instability. It's possible to remove so much of the posterior part of the spine that the joints begin to slip out of place. That doesn't commonly occur, but it can happen, and if it does, you may need stabilization. Because of this potential problem, surgeons sometimes decide to perform a fusion during the same operation.

Now, tell me about fusion. Is there a single, standard procedure for it, or are there several different types?

Spinal fusion can take many forms. Basically, any time you join one vertebra to another with a bridge of bone, that's a spinal fusion. You can fuse one level, two levels, or multiple levels. Multiple-level fusions are not usually practical for common backache, but they are used to correct a deformity such as the abnormal, side-to-side curvature found in scoliosis patients. When it is severe, the curvature can be partially straightened and then held in the corrected position with a fusion.

It's possible to fuse segments of the spine using only bone (routinely taken from the patient's pelvis). To fuse several adjacent levels of the spine into one unit, we often secure the vertebrae with plates, rods, or wires to prevent movement while the bone graft heals. You can fuse from the back, from the front, or from the sides of the spinal column. As you can imagine, each of these techniques and approaches has its advantages, and each poses its own set of problems.

What are the usual reasons for fusing in cases of common backache?

The reason is always instability, which in most cases will have developed as a result of normal wear and tear in the discs and facet joints. The worn or damaged areas are believed to produce pain when they move, and since fusion stops movement it should eliminate the pain. Occasionally, the spine may become unstable as a result of previous remedial surgery, and a fusion will be needed to maintain normal alignment.

Please describe a typical fusion.

The routine fusion is done without metal, usually involves just one or two levels, and is approached from the back. The surgery takes more time than a simple disc removal. It usually lasts from one and a half to three hours.

To perform the operation, I make an incision about three inches long at the appropriate location. By pushing aside muscles, ligaments, and fat, much as I do for a discotomy, I arrive at the vertebrae which are to be fused together. I enlarge the exposure so that I can see not only the *laminae* but the full extent of the facet joints and outsides of the vertebrae down to the transverse processes, those little bony "wings" that serve as muscle attachments. Now I use a chisel-like instrument to rough up the surface of the bones and destroy the slippery linings within the joints where the grafting is to take place. This deliberate damage causes the body to activate its healing processes, without which the fusion could not take place.

With the fusion site open and ready, I make a second incision, this time along the back of your pelvis. When I get down to the bone, I slice off several strips of the outer bone to reveal the spongy bone inside. I use a gouge to remove this spongy bone in the form of thick little ribbons.

Next I return to the first incision and pack those little ribbons and strips into the facet joints and onto the damaged surfaces I prepared along each side of the vertebrae. These pieces bridge the adjacent segments. As the body reacts to this situation, it treats that bone graft as fragments that have broken away from the spine. With normal healing the graft is gradually incorporated until the new bone and the two vertebrae are fused into a single, solid unit.

That, essentially, is what fusion surgery is all about, although variations are always being introduced in efforts to improve the results. For instance, I often approach the spine through two incisions on either side of the mid-line, splitting the spinal muscles rather than pushing them aside. This gives me a better view of the bed where I want to lay my graft.

An aunt of mine had a fusion operation some years ago and had to spend several weeks on a special bed – some kind of rotating frame. Is that standard post-operative treatment?

Not any longer. There was a time when fusion patients routinely remained for several weeks on a turning frame so that they could be rolled over without any movement of the back until healing of the fusion was well along. Such treatment, however, is generally passé now, thanks to improvements in our surgical techniques.

What improvements in surgical techniques have made the turning frame unnecessary?

In the earlier techniques, strips of bone graft were placed behind the vertebrae directly on the *laminae* or wired to the large posterior projections located under the surface of the skin. In that position, the grafts were quite vulnerable; even a slight amount of movement could prevent them from adhering to the spine.

In the newer techniques, we locate the fusion towards the front of the vertebrae near the point known as the axis of rotation. To understand the principle involved, think of the last time you rode on a merry-go-round. You probably noticed that the closer you were positioned to the outer edge, the faster the ride and the more ground you covered. If you wanted to reduce the amount of movement, you picked a horse near the middle. Similarly, in the newer types of fusion we place the graft as close as possible to the center of rotation, where movement is minimal. Since there is less danger of disturbing the fusion, the patient doesn't need to remain immobile on a turning frame.

The more extensive fusions undertaken to correct major structural damage or significant deformities such as scoliosis now routinely use some form of internal fixation. Excellent techniques have been developed to insert screws through the walls of the spinal canal into the large vertebral body in front. Those screws can be used to secure plates, rods, or heavy cables. In other methods, the devices are held in place by wires that loop around the bones in the roof of the canal. To correct a scoliotic curve, the surgeon may use hooks that slip under the *laminae* and are pushed apart or pulled together along thick metal rods. But no matter what implant is selected, its primary purpose is to provide temporary stability while the bone graft slowly converts the multiple mobile segments into a single, rigid piece of bone.

Even after a multiple-level fusion with solid internal fixation, the patient is often able to get up within a week, wearing a carefully fitted brace. A body cast can be made and then used to mold a plastic shell to cover the entire back. The patient will wear this shell day and night for months until the fusion is solid.

With all these advances, it has become unnecessary for a patient with a spinal fusion to use the turning frame or even to undergo prolonged bed rest. Such progress has also opened the way for surgical treatment of previously unsolved spinal disorders.

I've heard that some hospitals have bone banks. Are these sometimes used to provide bone for fusions?

Yes, occasionally they are, when too much bone is required to take it all from the patient himself. As long as enough can be obtained from a suitable donor site, however, the patient's own bone is preferred, since it is never rejected by the body and is thought to have the potential to stimulate new bone growth. Bone bank bone, on the other hand, has no such potential but merely serves as a scaffold that allows the body's own bone-forming cells to grow in and bridge adjacent vertebrae.

How long does it take to recover from a typical fusion?

Depending on the extent of the fusion I will recommend you stay in your hospital bed for a few days to a week or more, and to keep you immobile I will fit you with a corset or brace. For a day or two you may not be able to get up without help from the nurses and physical therapists. Once you get over your weakness and soreness and can walk comfortably, I will let you go home.

I won't pretend that you'll have an easy time of it for those first few days. Besides the pain and soreness from the fusion, you will have the added discomfort of the incision in the pelvis where the bone was taken out. In fact the donor site may go on being sore long after the fusion has healed.

Once you get home, you should spend at least three to four months avoiding movements that could endanger the fusion – no prolonged sitting, no heavy lifting, no vigorous bending, no violent twisting. You need that period of limited activity to give the graft a chance to become fully incorporated. It may take up to six months for you to feel the full benefit of the fusion – that is, to recover completely from your original symptoms and your post-operative discomfort.

Is there some certain way of knowing when a fusion has completely taken?

Not easily. Plain X-ray can give a very misleading impression, and even the CT may be difficult to interpret. X-rays taken with the spine bent forward and backward may be helpful, but usually the success or failure of the fusion is judged according to the patient's clinical response. However, some surgeons have gone as far as to suggest that if severe, disabling symptoms persist, the only way to tell whether a fusion is solid is to open up the back and look at it.

You may find yourself among the group who get almost immediate pain relief. This is a puzzling phenomenon, and no one understands fully how such a rapid response can take place. After all, the surgeon has not actually grafted one bone to another; he has merely created the conditions under which nature will gradually produce a fusion. Yet many patients will feel a change in their symptoms right after surgery. The old intolerable pain has been replaced by a new discomfort that seems certain to disappear.

How do you think those speedy recoveries can be explained?

I can only speculate, but I believe the most important factor is the temporary reduction in movement that comes from wedging bone between the vertebral bodies and into the facet joints, or from linking the bones together with metal plates. After all, reduced mobility of the affected segment is the ultimate goal of fusion. Another factor is how severely the patient's activities are restricted. If you just put on a brace and stay in bed, your back has a good chance of becoming pain free as long as you remain that way. I have noticed, too, that with some patients, extensive surgery destroys the nerve supply to the muscles of the back. For several months, those muscles are incapable of going into spasm. At least temporarily, the patient will have some relief from muscular pain. There's also an emotional factor: having been through a big operation, the patient probably tends, subconsciously or otherwise, to minimize any residual pain. Of course, that emotional factor can work in just the opposite way; a sudden back spasm or twinge of leg pain may produce acute anxiety.

But the short-term effects are different from the permanent pain relief you hope the fusion will achieve?

Yes. In a successful fusion, you'll get lasting pain relief because a solid bar of bone guarantees there is no movement.

Can spinal fusion lead to specific complications?

Yes, it can. Loss of movement at one level puts extra stress on the discs and joints above and below. With time, a few patients will develop new trouble at a different location and start the cycle all over again.

In rare instances, fusion outside the spinal canal will cause the bone inside to produce new growth that narrows the tunnel. This leads to spinal stenosis and nerve-root compression that may require further surgery.

More often, the complications are not so serious or long-lasting. For example, a fusion patient may become too dependent on his back brace, and the doctor will have difficulty weaning him away from it. To do so, the doctor will prescribe a rigid schedule: go without the brace for one hour a day for one week, then two hours a day the second week, and so on. The patient is instructed to put the brace back on after the prescribed time, whether or not he feels the need for it. Knowing he'll soon be wearing the brace again, he's unlikely to panic without it. Meanwhile, the act of wearing the brace becomes dissociated from the sense of need, and the patient begins to feel confident that his back is regaining its normal stability.

What about the recovery period at home? Do you have a standard list of do's and don'ts for patients recuperating from decompression or fusion surgery?

As you know by now, I am not generally inclined to write hard and fast rules for my patients, but there are some necessary cautions and a few complications I always mention, on the principle that forewarned is forearmed.

The most important points cover daily living habits. For the first few weeks, be conscious of your body movements and posture. Sit, lift, turn, and bend with moderation. After the fourth day, you can wash the area of the incision, as long as you pat the wound dry, but because tub bathing requires sitting in a poor position, you're better off under a shower.

I have found an early return to regular exercise remarkably helpful. With proper supervision some patients can begin to work out within two weeks of surgery. Everyone should be given an exercise routine before the end of the second month. Surgeons sometimes neglect this aspect of post-operative management because they expect the physical therapist to set it up. The physical therapist, on the other hand, is often reluctant to start such a program without the surgeon's approval. As the person with the most to gain, the patient mustn't be afraid to ask how soon exercise can be started.

Is convalescence likely to be a painful period?

Not as a rule, but a few unpleasant things can happen to make you fear the surgery has failed and your old trouble is still with you. The post-operative pain is more likely to arise from other causes, and you'll be better off knowing about them because unexpected pain produces fear, which greatly aggravates the problem. You may develop a cramp or troublesome tingling feelings in your leg where the pain used to be, because the involved nerve is still irritable and inclined to reproduce the old symptoms. The amount of discomfort will vary according to several factors, including the amount of pressure there was on the nerve before surgery, how long that pressure had existed, how much inflammation was present, and how much force the surgeon had to use to retract the nerve to get at the location of the trouble. Remember, your symptoms are only "leftovers," and now that the irritation has been removed the nerve will begin to recover.

Another possible complication, which is less likely and usually less serious than you may suppose, is a vascular condition called phlebitis. Lying on a special frame or in a "knee-chest" position during surgery may interfere with the flow of blood in the veins of the legs. The problem can be aggravated if you are required to remain in bed after surgery. Although the term phlebitis means inflammation of the veins, the real problem is the small blood clots that form at the sites of inflammation. These small clots may lead to the formation of larger clots that can break loose and travel up the vein. One of these mobile clots, now known as an embolus, may lodge in the lung, causing a condition called pulmonary embolism. This, in turn, can put the affected area of the lung out of commission, although even that is not a serious matter if the area is small.

If phlebitis does occur, what can you do about it?

The leg pain from the local inflammation can be treated with elastic support stockings, rest, and elevation of the affected leg. Some doctors use anti-inflammatory medication, and anti-coagulants which will stop the clots from forming. In fact, for certain types of back surgery, it has become routine to use anti-embolic elastic stockings during the operation and to administer an anti-coagulant, as preventive measures. The incidence of phlebitis, a rare complication to begin with, has been further reduced by these precautions.

Because they may have been told about phlebitis by their doctors, or heard about it from friends, many patients worry about this problem. Fortunately, most people who fear they have developed phlebitis after surgery are in fact suffering temporarily from conditions that need cause no concern. For instance, if you had surgery for disc pressure on the nerve that supplies your calf muscles, cramps may recur during the healing period, causing temporary soreness. Or if you lie in bed for several days – and this is true whether you've had surgery or not – you'll find your leg muscles will complain when you try to get up. Both these conditions can be mistaken for phlebitis. The correct diagnosis should be made after careful physical examination, and in some cases after specific blood flow and isotope studies.

Are there other problems likely to occur during convalescence?

You may have a difficult time getting back to normal living, both for physical and psychological reasons. It can take you a while before you feel like eating normally. Right after the operation you may have no appetite at all. Major spinal surgery often shuts down the gastro-intestinal tract for a few days. If you eat during that period the food doesn't go far; it just lies there and gives you stomach cramps. Even when you're home again you may take some time to get your old appetite back.

But while accepting the limitations mentioned so far, you should be trying to return to your customary living habits as soon as you can. Don't be shy, for instance, about asking your doctor when you can resume sexual intercourse. Your doctor has heard that question before and will be quite prepared to give you specific advice. As a general rule, the answer is: "The sooner the better."

Recovering from surgery is really quite an art – but an art most people can master with ease. Apart from a few basics, there are no techniques that suit everybody, and there's plenty of room for individual style and judgment. I well remember one patient of mine, the owner of a clothing store, who came out of hospital after disc surgery late in November. Two weeks later, I dropped by his store, and there he was, standing cheerfully behind the counter with one foot up on a block of wood. Perhaps he should have been resting at home, but he couldn't bear being away from the business during the Christmas rush.

I wish I could have pointed him out to another man I operated on for the same problem. This patient was obviously brought up in a family that doted on high drama. Two days after he came out of the operating room, I visited him at the hospital, and there he lay, hands folded over his chest in funereal repose, while a dozen ashen-faced relatives sat around the room, whispering solemnly to one another. If Central Casting had been looking for a convincing corpse, I could have steered them to a prime candidate. Of course, he didn't die but went home instead, with the entourage of mourners in tow, and spent at least three months playing out his role as the family's critically disabled convalescent.

If you want to get off to a good start at home, resolve not to play invalid or load your spouse and family with guilt if they decline to cater to your every whim. Certainly you want them to be aware of what you're going through and what you are up against, but it won't help anyone, least of all yourself, to overstate your difficulties or limitations.

It would be a mistake to underestimate the influence that interpersonal relations can have on your physical well-being. I had one woman patient whose symptoms during her time in hospital were clearly aggravated by her husband. Whenever he was around, she lost her ability to walk and suffered excruciating pain. The moment he went away, she returned to normal.

By all means, follow the basic rules of good physical care throughout the early weeks of convalescence. But never ignore the psychological side. Nothing can help you recover more swiftly or more completely than a positive attitude on your part and a readiness on the part of those around you to help you return to your normal style of living.

What about the long-term results of neck and back surgery?

Once you get a good result it tends to stay good. There is some natural wear and tear, of course, and both the site of the surgery and the adjacent levels remain slightly more vulnerable. But in a recent study of the long-term results of spine surgery, over 95 percent of the patients felt satisfied with the outcome, and only 15 to 20 percent showed signs of new trouble that might require further treatment.

What do you see in the future for patients needing a back operation?

There are some amazing possibilities, and the technology for most of them already exists. Outpatients might be sent through a CT scan and a magnetic resonance imaging (MRI) machine that could locate, analyze, and diagnose the surgical problem. Under local anesthesia the patient could undergo an automated discotomy with

X-ray control using a power cutting tool introduced through a large needle in the back. Somatosensory evoked potentials (SEP) would tell the operator when enough nucleus had been removed to relieve the nerve pressure. Through the same needle the hollow disc center could then be filled with a mixture of bone and biological glue to create an immediate solid fusion. The whole experience might eventually become as routine and brief as a visit to the dentist.

I'm sure doctors of the future will marvel at how we ever managed to produce *any* satisfactory results with our primitive twentieth-century equipment.

13. IF YOU'RE THINKING OF GOING TO COURT . . .

Like many other specialists, I devote a certain amount of my professional time to legal cases, examining accident victims whose injuries fall within the range of my work as an orthopedic surgeon.

Most of these patients come to me on referral from lawyers, either their own or those on the opposing side. A few come from insurance companies who also want to determine the effects of the accident and the extent of disability.

While such evaluations are necessary, I am disturbed by the way they and the other steps in litigation often hamper accident victims in their recovery. Unavoidably, the extensive legal preparation and the trial itself force patients to relive a bad experience, perhaps reviving dormant pain and prolonging the present condition. Even worse, the situation compels them to focus constantly on remaining symptoms and other negative aspects of their condition.

That increased awareness of pain and disability is, of course, exactly opposite to the attitude a person should adopt if he wants to recover swiftly from injury and return to normal living. Clearly, a preoccupation with the problem is one important step in the development of the chronic pain syndrome which, as we have seen, is a behavioral disease from which some people never recover.

The motives for going to court are understandable. We all like to see justice done – to see the guilty called to account and their victims compensated for all losses and suffering. And, of course, with the increasing size of awards handed down by our courts these days, the prospects of a successful lawsuit are becoming more and more attractive.

After years of direct experience with thousands of accident victims, however, I have concluded that the financial rewards of personal injury litigation are seldom worth the price. This is a message many patients would rather not hear – especially those who are already committed to legal action – but I believe it needs to be said.

I have included in this chapter not only some practical tips for accident victims who decide to sue, but also – and more important, I think – some observations on the destructive side effects of litigation. I hope readers will consider my arguments and form realistic opinions before they have reason to become embroiled in a personal injury lawsuit, exposing themselves to the emotional stress and family pressure that so often propel an accident victim into court.

Suppose I'm to have a medical examination for a lawsuit. Do you have any advice?

There are two basic points. First, try to answer the doctor's questions as factually and concisely as you can. Since the information you provide will go into a report to be read by many other people, and may also be presented in court as verbal evidence that is subject to cross-examination, you should take special care to make yourself clearly understood. Keep in mind that the doctor is interested primarily in your mental and physical condition. This will include the mechanism of your injury but it has nothing to do with the potential liability. For example, it's important for you to describe the direction of impact in a motor vehicle collision, but it doesn't matter to the doctor who had the right of way or whether the other driver had been drinking.

Second, try to describe your condition accurately in words that are not overly dramatic or emotionally charged. For example, it's not helpful to say, "Whenever I try to move, an excruciating pain shoots all over my body." Instead, be as specific as you can: "Usually, the pain is worse when I try to walk, and it seems to be mostly down my right leg."

It might be useful to make some notes about your symptoms and how they have changed since the accident. But keep the descriptions brief; jot things down in point form.

It's not always that easy to describe your own back pain, especially in a few words.

You're right – it isn't. But the doctor is trained to help you by asking specific questions that are easy to answer. Is the pain steady or throbbing? Does it feel sharp or dull? Is the pain associated with burning or tingling sensations? These are the types of standard questions doctors use in helping patients describe their symptoms. Which reminds me of a conversation I overhead when I was a medical student. One of my teachers had just come back from a vacation abroad, and another doctor wanted to hear about it. But he didn't just ask, "How was your trip?" He asked, "Was the weather hot or cold? Was it wet or dry? Was the tour interesting or disappointing?" And so on. And in response to each question, my clinician was solemnly choosing the appropriate answer. I'm sure they never realized that, out of force of habit, one doctor was conducting a professional inquiry into the other doctor's vacation.

In a medical examination, this style of questioning helps you avoid offering descriptions that are unrealistic and therefore unhelpful. In their sincere attempt to convey the full magnitude and intensity of the problem, some patients will tell me, "It feels exactly like I've been stabbed with a red-hot spear" or "It feels just like I've been kicked by an elephant." I sympathize with anyone suffering that amount of pain, but those sorts of descriptions don't help me define the problem, since I've never been stabbed with a red-hot spear or kicked by an elephant. It isn't that I don't understand the meaning of the comparisons but they give me nothing I can write down and use in my report.

It must be difficult to prepare a report when you believe the patient is deliberately exaggerating for effect.

It is. And it's even worse when the patient, consciously or otherwise, seems to be hiding the truth. For instance, I remember one case where four people, injured while riding in the back seat of a car, insisted they had all been wearing seat belts, which are compulsory in Ontario. Their story was difficult to believe, since the back seat of the car was equipped with only three belts. Someone had to be wrong.

In reporting a case like that, I would write, "The patient says he was wearing a seat belt," not just "the patient was wearing a seat belt." In other words, I would record the patient's claim in a non-judgmental phrase, without accepting his statement as fact.

I can understand why the victim's own lawyer wants your report. Are you ever asked to examine a patient sent by a lawyer representing the opposing side?

Yes, it happens frequently. A personal injury victim involved in litigation is legally obliged to submit to an examination by a doctor selected by the other side. This is generally referred to as an IME, "independent medical examination." Obviously the patient can feel threatened by this situation and in rare instances may even refuse to answer the doctor's questions during the assessment.

What do you do if someone refuses to tell you anything?

First I try to explain that my role is not to judge the case but only to determine the patient's medical condition. In most instances my report should be virtually the same as the one prepared by the patient's own doctor. If you asked me whether you should co-operate in that situation, I'd say yes, definitely. I think you'd be foolish to do otherwise, because your refusal could suggest you have something to hide. Besides, the IME is really just a second opinion on your problem from a designated expert in the field. That specialist might even find something significant that your own doctor missed. You will get a useful opinion only if you participate willingly in the examination.

When a patient absolutely refuses, I simply report that I conducted the examination but could not elicit all the information I wanted because the person declined to co-operate. I don't imagine it helps their case if this fact is brought out in court, but that's not my concern.

If you had examined me for litigation, would you be willing to tell me what you intend to say in your report?

As a rule, I'm very open about my opinion. I believe you should know as much about your problem as you can. And I don't think it matters whether you hear it from your own doctor or the one who examines you for the other side. Besides, once the reports are prepared and filed with the court, they become public record and anyone can read them.

Do you have any special advice about the way I should handle myself in court?

Your lawyer will give you a more thorough briefing, but I can tell you a few things I've learned from my experience as an expert witness. The most important thing is also the simplest: tell the truth. Don't try to improve your case by coloring your answers or holding back relevant facts. If you are trying to establish that you have a serious injury, nobody will expect you to minimize your suffering; but if you present the facts in a balanced way, the court is more likely to believe you. For instance, if you have been able to do certain physical things in spite of your pain, I suggest you say so right from the start. Don't leave it for the other side to introduce the evidence in a way that will cause embarrassment for you or your doctor.

I was once embarrassed in the witness box when I learned for the first time that my patient, whose disability I had just described in considerable detail, was in fact well enough to be working seven days a week. He was putting in five days a week as a taxi driver and making a long trip out of town every weekend to work as a ski instructor. The man had carefully avoided telling me this, and so had his lawyer. Of course when the defendant's lawyer presented these facts and asked me whether they would

alter my assessment of the man's disability, I naturally admitted
they would. I wasn't surprised or, I admit, disappointed when the
plaintiff lost his case.

I have also learned that if you are asked a question you don't
fully understand, you shouldn't be afraid to get clarification before
answering. No one should object if you ask the lawyer to repeat
the question. To avoid confusion you might rephrase it in your
own words before you respond.

Don't pretend to know things that are outside your knowledge
or experience, such as the speed of the approaching car you
glimpsed for only a second. That last bit of advice is something
I heed myself, as an expert witness. Sometimes on the stand I
am asked to give an opinion about something I just don't know.
For example, I might be asked to compare the victim's pain before
and after a second accident that aggravated his original injuries.
Since pain is a totally subjective experience that defies direct
measurement, there is no way to answer that question with any
degree of accuracy. In such a situation I would explain my reasons
and decline to speculate.

**Do you think many patients deliberately lie about their disability
for personal gain?**

True malingering is rare. Very few people invent all their symptoms
just to collect money in court. Most patients accused of malingering
are probably not lying as much as exaggerating. They're afraid
that if they aren't blatant enough about their pain the examiner
won't fully appreciate that there is something wrong. I think we're
all inclined to cope with the same injury in different ways, depending on the situation. Suppose you were a member of a wedding
party and you twisted your ankle on the way into the church.
Wouldn't you do your best to disguise your pain and injury
throughout the ceremony? But if that same twisted ankle needed
examining in the course of a lawsuit, surely you would limp into
the doctor's office. Yet it would hardly be fair to say you were
faking your injury to increase your chances in court.

Of course, there are exceptions. As a surgical resident I examined
a man with back pain who I was sure had no real problem and
was trying to fool me. But after I discharged him from the
emergency room I had second thoughts, and so I slipped out

a side entrance to follow him up the street. I must have been quite a sight in my white suit hiding behind parked cars and peering around the corners of buildings. However, he never saw me, and after two or three blocks, sure enough, his limp disappeared and he began to walk normally.

Besides following someone out of your office, how can you tell if a patient isn't being honest with you about his condition?

Like all experienced back examiners, I have developed physical tests that are designed to weed out people who are consciously exaggerating their symptoms. The results tell me whether the person is reporting honestly.

Even if someone takes the trouble to discover these techniques, many of my tests require movements that simply can't be faked. Here's one example. Suppose you describe weakness of your ankle that causes you to walk with a limp. I will ask you to sit in a chair with both feet flat on the floor. Next I will have you raise your forefoot on the affected side while keeping the heel of that foot on the floor. Now I squat in front of you, place one hand over the instep of your foot, and ask you to maintain your position against the downward pressure of my hand. If you have a true muscular weakness, your foot will yield smoothly until it's flat on the floor. But if your power is normal and you are trying to fool me, the forefoot won't sink smoothly; instead, it will descend unevenly in little "cogwheel" steps that tell me you're faking. The interesting thing is that even with practice, you can never develop the smooth muscular release that denotes true weakness, and so the test works even if you know all about it.

I'm careful not to rely on just one or two such examinations. I use several, and they all have to produce consistent results. Also, I often test the same condition in three or four different ways, without the patient's realizing it. For instance, if a patient complains of neck pain and exhibits a greatly reduced range of movement, I sometimes stand behind him and start talking. It's remarkable to watch someone who can't move his neck at all during the examination turn his head around quite comfortably to look at me when I speak. People whose complaints are genuine won't react that way.

**Have you found that accident victims involved in litigation
exaggerate their pain more than other patients?**

In many cases they do. And that exaggeration can become a
problem in itself. I think the extent of the behavior depends on
what patients expect from the doctor and what they believe they
have to do to get him to meet those expectations.

Most of us are skeptical about those who go to court seeking
large awards for their pain and suffering. It's easy to assume that
accident victims merely suffer until their cases are settled satis-
factorily, and that once they collect a big award, their health
suddenly improves.

Certainly most lawyers and doctors can recall one or two victims
who had a "miraculous" improvement once they received a large
financial settlement. But if you consider the thousands of personal
injury actions initiated each year, you will find that such "miracles"
are exceptions rather than the rule.

When a person decides whether or not to enter into a lawsuit
over his injuries, he may well be deciding, without realizing it,
whether to set out on the road to recovery or to assume the role
of a suffering litigant for years to come.

**Are you saying that all accident victims who take legal action will
be trapped in the role of an injured person?**

No, not always, but it does happen far too often. To achieve what
he sees as a just settlement, the accident victim may concentrate
on his disability until it becomes an obsession. He will tend to
focus on his symptoms and magnify or at least sustain the pain
in order to further his case. Soon, he is thinking and talking
about little else. He becomes a "professional victim" whose
disability affects every aspect of his life, destroying his ability to
work and straining his relationships with family and friends.

Often a marriage suffers badly. Like patients with the chronic
pain syndrome, people emotionally involved in injury litigation
can experience sexual problems brought on by the psychological
strain and the preoccupation with their health. It's difficult for
a worried mind to become sexually aroused. As a "professional
victim," a man may be impotent or a woman unresponsive for
reasons that do not stem directly from the disability or any physical
impairment of sexual function.

When you consider what these changes in personality can mean to the way the person will live, you have to ask whether any amount of money awarded in court can be worth the price. Those problems will not happen to everyone, but you should be aware of the possibility when you choose to sue over a personal injury.

As you realize by now, the psychology of prolonged litigation disability is much the same as that of the chronic pain syndrome, and in fact some accident victims make the unfortunate transition into CPS. Partly because of the way the legal process holds their recovery in abeyance during the usually lengthy process, these people maintain the expected pattern of behavior to the point where it becomes permanent.

It strikes me there is something wrong with a system that allows such a thing to happen.

It's easy for some professionals to criticize "the system." But we are very much part of that system and have to take responsibility for the way it works. There are many advantages to the adversarial approach in law, and I am not suggesting we change the method. But every lawyer and doctor involved on either side of a personal injury action has an ethical obligation to settle the matter as fairly and as rapidly as possible to help the patient get on with his or her life. Yet it would be naive to suggest that there are no incentives for us to prolong an accident victim's recovery. If a case is settled quickly and inexpensively, there are no substantial legal fees. And there are fewer charges for conducting medical examinations and writing depositions. Many delays are unavoidable; the courts are overburdened. But prolonging the litigation also has significant financial benefits for the law firm or medical practice.

In some instances a doctor may unwittingly retard the process for fear of being wrong and jeopardizing the case. He may say, "I can't be sure yet – let me see the patient again in a year's time." A request like that means nobody is going to settle for at least a year, and meanwhile the patient must keep on feeling pain. Yet, medically, there's no basis for it. Without the pressure of providing a medical-legal opinion, no competent doctor would wait twelve months before deciding on a course of treatment or giving the patient some idea of what to expect.

And I suppose that if the patient has already decided to stay home from work to avoid jeopardizing his case, that postponement will reinforce his decision.

That's right – and it's an extremely important point. Usually, the best way to recover swiftly from an accident is to return to work and resume all other normal activities as soon as possible.

But suppose, as the accident victim, I'm still in pain?

My advice may, at first, sound cold and uncaring, but I would still say: get back on the job, pain and all, and do your best to stop behaving like a disabled person. How you see yourself, or more precisely how the legal action *forces* you to see yourself, is critical. The more you think you can achieve the more you will be able to do. Of course, the speed of your return to work will depend in part on the nature of your job. You may have to wait longer before getting back to heavy construction work than to an office job. But resuming your regular employment is great for your self-image, and there is no medical basis for arguing that an early return to work will harm you. It may increase your pain temporarily, but it will not physically damage you or prevent your ultimate recovery.

Consider whether you'd rather put up with a little extra backache on the job while you get better or face the prospect of months or even years of suffering and disability that must be endured before the litigation is settled. Until recently the seriousness of that enforced delay in recovery wasn't fully appreciated. But new studies are changing our understanding. In one study of ninety-nine people who filed suits over injuries they suffered in industrial or car accidents, thirty-three were found to have returned to work before their cases were settled. Of the other sixty-six, only nine were found to have returned to work within sixteen months after settlement.

Isn't it likely that many of the remaining fifty-seven patients just needed more time to recover and would return to work later?

No, I'm afraid that's not likely. As we have found from other studies and experience, if you don't return to your job within two years after your back injury, chances are you never will. You may work at something light and inconsequential, perhaps part time, but you are most unlikely to return permanently to your regular employment. On the other hand, it was found that when a group of accident victims got the help they needed to physically overcome their injuries and develop a healthy pattern of behavior, 70 percent of them returned to work before their litigation was settled. In other words, litigation doesn't necessarily deter most people from going back to work if they are properly treated, if they want to go back, and if there is a job waiting for them.

Does the prospect of a large settlement have any influence on the person's inclination to sue or file a claim for disability?

Yes, it appears to. One study has shown that in jurisdictions where the average compensation award amounts to more than 55 percent of the pre-injury net income, the number of claims increases drastically. Some people even take this opportunity to leave the work force permanently. It's bad enough to be a disabled person, without becoming a prematurely retired disabled person. Retirement can be a happy state if it is planned and carried out willingly, with a sense of purpose. But under these circumstances, it's a dismal and wasteful way to spend the rest of your life.

What about the accident victim who says, "Sure, I'll go back to work later, but I'd be a sucker to make any move until I get the big settlement I deserve"?

Unfortunately, a few people do concentrate on the money. I had one patient who had been injured in two accidents. Right after the second one, she declared she had made a serious mistake settling her first claim too soon – and by that she meant too cheaply. Now she was determined to collect enough from the second injury to make up for that earlier deficiency. There was very little logic in her approach, and I knew with that attitude she had no chance of making another rapid recovery. But the amount of her previous award would have no bearing on the size of her second settlement (if she won her case). The new award, if any, would be based entirely on the minor injuries caused by the more recent accident. After the legal fees and disbursements were deducted, her potential financial gain would be modest. More important, no financial award of any size would compensate for the way her spiteful approach was distorting her personality and lifestyle.

Fortunately, that woman was not typical of the injured people I normally see. In my experience, few are that calculating. Initially, at least, most accident victims just want to return to work and get on with their lives. But if they embark on litigation, they take on a commitment they feel they must keep. Later, as the action drags on and on, their physical condition deteriorates and they lose their job skills, their self-discipline, their work habits, and their motivation. They feel like strangers to their old colleagues or workmates. By then it's too late to get back on the job.

A friend of mine who went to court over an injury in a car accident was encouraged to keep a daily record of how she felt. Is that helpful to the doctor or lawyer?

I would rather you asked whether it's helpful to the patient. Then my answer would be: that depends on why the person is keeping the "pain journal," as it's commonly called. That daily log is useful if it is kept as part of a treatment program designed to help the patient recover from the injury and conquer the disability. The person will find it encouraging to look back and see how function is being restored while the discomfort and pain are receding.

It's quite a different thing, however, to keep a pain journal for legal purposes. Some lawyers recommend it to their clients, but medically I consider it a harmful practice when there is no accompanying therapy. The diary becomes nothing more than a daily record of misery that encourages the victim to focus his attention on his pain. That approach may help win court cases but it certainly doesn't help people get well.

It can be difficult to write a journal that satisfies both your doctor and your lawyer. While your doctor will be hoping to see a record of steady recovery, for the sake of the litigation your lawyer will want it to show a pattern of continuing disability. I recommend you use the pain journal as an aid to getting well, not to staying sick. Keep the litigation secondary in your mind and concentrate on recovering. Everyone's goal should be a rapid and complete return to a normal lifestyle and the prompt settlement of the lawsuit.

Have you found that a family's support can help the patient keep those priorities straight?

Some families provide positive encouragement that helps hasten the patient's return to normal life. But others unconsciously reinforce the harmful reactions that delay recovery.

If there are grounds for a lawsuit, a family may rally around the victim – "Mother's been hurt, and we will see to it that the person responsible pays for her injury." Although everyone's intentions are the best, the last thing Mother may need, for her own good, is the added stress of becoming a litigant. But there are no pressures stronger than those imposed by a person's own family. After all, the family has already done so much. They have arranged the medical care, visited Mother in the hospital, and begun tending her at home. In a situation like this, the family members have developed their own expectations, and everyone – Mother included – tends to react accordingly. Now they've hired a lawyer to see that justice is done. Mother can hardly turn around at this point and say, "Never mind, I don't want to sue anyone. I'm going to be fine."

Declining to go along with the family could be the smartest thing Mother ever did – but how many of us could do it?

And so, unwittingly, the family creates and reinforces the patient's new self-image as a disabled person, smothering the victim with over-protection and receiving, in response, the sad compliment of child-like dependence.

To cope with the new stress of a protracted legal action and the accompanying lengthy period of disability, the family not only provides increased support but also restructures itself, forming new relationships that are ostensibly benign, temporary, and helpful. In truth, they will change the lives of all those involved. The formerly passive spouse suddenly takes charge, and the once-dominant mate, as victim, meekly complies. Or Big Sister, once eager to further her career by handling a full-time job and a heavy course at night school, abruptly quits both to stay home and look after Poor Mother. What loving family could do less, especially now that the Disabled One is facing the strange and frightening obstacles of litigation?

The problem becomes even more complex when two or more family members are injured in the same accident. I once examined a mother, father, and three children, all involved in a lawsuit over a rear-end collision. No one had been seriously hurt, physically, but the ensuing legal battle had a devastating effect on the structure of the family. The suit became their principal family business. Unconsciously, everyone was reluctant to let the team down by getting better. And no one did.

With the inception of personal injury litigation we may begin a self-perpetuating situation that can alter the lives of all who buy into it. As one litigant's spouse said with rare insight, "It would take a miracle for us to be like we used to be."

Is there something the injured person, or the family, can do from the outset to avoid that trap?

Yes. With sound legal advice and medical support, the accident victim and the family should agree from the start to share just one objective: getting everyone back to normal living as soon as possible. And if that means putting up with some temporary pain, or passing up the "opportunity" to pursue a supposedly rewarding lawsuit, so be it.

14. A NEW APPROACH TO HELPFUL EXERCISE

People often ask me, "What's new in back care?" And, just as often, I surprise them by answering, "Exercise!"

Of course, I don't mean I have just discovered that proper exercise is useful in preventing back pain. I've been spreading that message for years. But we are now beginning to understand that exercise can also help to relieve the pain of a subsiding attack and so can assist in short-term recovery. Meanwhile, doctors and physical therapists who specialize in back care are achieving significant discoveries and developments to make back exercises more effective than ever.

For my part, in the seven years since I wrote *The Back Doctor*, I have been continually reassessing and refining the exercise routines I recommend to my patients and to classes at the Canadian Back Institute (formerly the Canadian Back Education Units). While I have found nothing to suggest that those earlier workouts were anything but helpful, I have devised ways of improving the program by modifying some exercises and emphasizing the importance of others.

I have come to appreciate more fully the value of combining two complementary types of exercise – flexion (forward bending) and extension (backward bending) – and I have learned from clinical experience that for most patients the best program consists of a comfortable balance between the two. This evolution in my thinking means, among other things, that although I included extension exercises in *The Back Doctor*, I now place greater emphasis on them. I also focus more attention on exercises that stretch the back muscles and put the small joints through a range of movement.

Readers familiar with the exercises contained in *The Back Doctor* will see both similarities and differences in the routines presented here. Perhaps the first new thing they will notice is the way the presentation makes clear distinctions between flexion and extension and between stretching and strengthening. While such valuable old standbys as the sit-up are inevitably included, they are presented in a fresh context that reflects my new approach.

Since my philosophy of back care remains unchanged, people who are comfortable with the exercises I favored in my earlier book should feel equally at ease with those they find here. My view that each person must bear the ultimate responsibility for the care of his or her own back applies especially to exercise. It's up to each of us to find, and practice, the routines that suit our individual situations. After all, we come in various shapes and sizes, with individual muscular strengths and weaknesses, differing attitudes towards exercise, and unique personal habits and lifestyles.

No arbitrary set of exercises could possibly fill the bill for everyone who reads this book. What I offer here, then, is not a prescription but a list of recommendations, an assortment of routines from which you, as a backache sufferer, can choose in creating your own custom-made exercise program, subject only to certain limitations I mention along the way. If you are using exercises from *The Back Doctor* and they're working, I suggest you continue them and perhaps try a few I've presented here.

On the other hand, if the idea of back exercise is new to you, you will want to look over the possibilities and experiment with several routines that apply to your situation before you create your permanent repertoire. You can make a more intelligent choice if you understand which form of back pain you have – Type One, Two, Three, or Four – but, even then, you may have to continue your search for exercises to accommodate the special needs of your situation. Think of yourself as a watchman, new on the job, equipped with a huge ring of keys. Several are necessary to unlock the doors along the passages where you want to go; but only by trial and error will you find the right assortment.

The choices shouldn't be hard to make on your own, but if you are already seeing a doctor or physical therapist, you might like to take this book along and ask for comments and suggestions about the program that would suit you best.

While the exercises you find here bear my stamp of approval and that of the Canadian Back Institute, they are not my inventions, and I make no claim about their being original, much less uniquely mine. But whether you think of them as Dr. Hamilton Hall's exercises or not, I suggest you make some of them your own. I think you will find them helpful, and you can be sure that if you do them as directed, they won't harm your back or any other part of your body.

My advice, then, is to move carefully but confidently. It's quite likely that within these next pages you can find a lasting solution to your back problem.

I'm anxious to get started on an exercise program to get rid of my back pain, but I'd like to know how long I'll have to keep at it.

There's no time limit. As long as you want the benefit to continue, you'll have to keep on with your exercises. Otherwise, you'll be making the mistake often made by people who want to lose weight. They attend special classes and go on special diets until they've shed the pounds they want to get rid of. Then they go right back to their old eating habits. And we all know what happens to their waistlines after that.

But you're suggesting a lifelong commitment! Do you really mean I have to do my exercises every day for the rest of my life?

Why not? You put your clothes on every day, don't you? And brush your teeth and comb your hair? What's the difference? We're talking about an additional allotment of ten or twelve minutes a day – probably less time than you spend showering and toweling yourself dry. You're quite accustomed to performing those other simple tasks of personal care, and if you think of your exercises as just one extra item, no more difficult or complicated than the rest, you won't find it hard to fit them into your life. It is the main reason I keep the exercise program short and simple. The truth is, that if people find their daily exercises don't take long, they are more likely to continue with them. On the other hand, if you look upon your exercises as something to be dreaded, you'll eventually give up on them and lose a lot of the gains you've made.

Are you saying that once I get started, I'll be in trouble if I quit?

You won't be worse off than you were before you started exercising, but many people who have begun a back exercise program and then neglected it have told me their pain returned when they stopped. And the cause-and-effect relationship seems evident, since they also say that once they started their exercises again, the pain subsided. Part of the problem in recognizing the value of exercises is the length of time they require to produce results and the gradual way in which they improve the situation in terms of reduced severity of pain and accelerated rate of recovery. You won't feel any change immediately, and no patient ever says, "I remember that after I had been exercising for exactly six months, I got up one wonderful Thursday morning and my back pain had disappeared." If you're tempted to quit, you might remind yourself of how much more fun you have when your back is in good shape and you can enjoy your favorite activities.

I'm interested in getting into an exercise class for general fitness. Should I do that if my doctor has told me to take care of my back?

Yes, you can safely take part in almost any general exercise program if you carefully pick and choose the exercises you do. Talk it over with the instructor beforehand and discuss any exercises you might want to avoid. Your decision of course depends mainly on the type of back or neck pain you have. For example, if you have discogenic pain, which I call Type Two, you may find that sit-ups are painful, and you will want to avoid them and work out some substitutes.

If you have neck pain referred between your shoulder blades, a program specifically designed to strengthen the shoulder muscles, using free weights or an exercise machine, may provide you with the only source of lasting relief.

You may want to postpone your enrollment in a class until you have developed your own back or neck exercise routine. By then you'll have a better understanding of which exercises are painful for you and which are all right.

You said earlier there are certain aerobic routines that aren't good for your back. What substitutes do you suggest?

Among the exercises that have caused the most trouble for back patients are the "high-bounce" aerobics – that is, those where you jump up and down violently. It's possible to give your heart and lungs the equivalent workout by performing a shuffling movement that is rapid but not as violent. Standing in one spot, quickly slide your feet forward and backward alternately, letting the soles of your feet graze the floor with each stride.

Or, to use another example, you can stimulate your heart and lungs with the familiar arm-raising exercise – standing with your arms at your sides and rapidly raising them to shoulder height, then dropping them back again – without the stride-jumping that is usually part of that routine.

Are there any exercises you never recommend because they irritate muscles or joints without providing much benefit?

Yes, I can think of two or three that everybody ought to avoid. One consists of rolling your head around and around in a circle from shoulder to shoulder. People do this imagining they are relaxing their neck muscles, but all they are doing in reality is making themselves feel dizzy, while the backward part of the roll compresses their neck joints. If you want to exercise your neck properly, I suggest you try the routines I will describe later.

Deep knee bends are another item on my forbidden list. They don't stretch or strengthen your leg or back muscles any better than half knee bends do, and they are far too hard on your knee joints. In the half knee bend, you should lower your body to the point where your thighs are parallel to the floor, as if you were seated in a chair. The half knee bend and its variation, an exercise called The Imaginary Chair, both appear on my list.

A third exercise to avoid – and the silliest one I can think of offhand – consists of lying on your back and forcefully flexing your spine so that your pelvis is above your head and your feet are kicking the ground over your shoulders. It was part of those old macho athletic training routines abandoned years ago by more enlightened instructors. The action offers no useful benefits and creates needless strain on the neck, back, and thighs. There was a time when training exercises in sports were based mostly on tradition. Coaches simply perpetuated the routines they had learned as players, many of them based on the premise that "if it hurts it's good for you." Today, trainers and coaches know otherwise. They have access to a large body of research in ergonomics – the study of human movement – and to various computerized and photographic devices that enable them to measure the benefits and effects of each specific exercise.

At the CBI we have rejected several traditional exercises, and reached new conclusions about several others. We have found, for instance, that one familiar routine, toe touching, has notable limitations. Traditionally, it was done with the legs straight and the feet together – a position that imposes considerable strain on your back but does nothing to strengthen your paraspinal muscles. Toe touching can be useful as a stretching exercise, but it should be done with care. Start with your feet comfortably apart and your arms at your sides. As you bend your trunk, let your arms swing loose. As long as your upper body drops down enough to stretch the muscles of your legs and hips, it doesn't really matter whether your hands actually reach far enough to touch your toes. Remember, you're supposed to be *exercising* your body, not torturing it.

Never begin this exercise by stretching your arms over your head and swinging them down to your feet in a giant arc. That's known as a "ballistic" movement – one that's sudden and violent and uses gravity and momentum rather than muscle activity to produce the result. It's far too vigorous for most people, especially those with low-back pain, and it adds nothing extra to stretch or strengthen the muscles.

Before I try to make my personal choices from your list of recommended exercises, can you give me some basic advice as to what I should be looking for?

In order to pick the back exercises that will be the most helpful for you, make sure you know what type of back trouble you have, what the exercises are supposed to do, and then make sure you are performing them properly. I'll be including that basic information along with my descriptions of the exercises themselves.

It's unfortunate how some fitness buffs waste their energy on misguided exercise. I talked to one patient who told me he was doing forty sit-ups a day to develop his belly muscles. I decided to test him. When I had him lie on his back with his knees bent and his feet unsupported, he was amazed that he could do only three sit-ups. Normally he hooked his feet under a couch, never realizing that the exercise, as he was doing it, was strengthening his thighs but doing virtually nothing for his stomach muscles. Experiences like that have taught me to be a little skeptical whenever a patient assures me that he or she is doing back exercises regularly. Usually I check with the supervising physical therapist or, as I did in this case, ask for a little demonstration. "Regularly" and "correctly" are not the same thing.

How do you decide which exercises to recommend for a particular patient?

The easiest way to understand the principles I apply is to think of your spine as not just one column but three: a front column consisting of discs alternating with the bone of the vertebral bodies; a back column consisting of a series of interlocking facet joints; and a middle column that is the canal containing the spinal cord and nerves. This is a handy concept because it enables us to identify the source of pain – that is, whether the symptoms originate mainly in the front column, the back column, or the middle column. Although the underlying cause (usually the ordinary wear and tear of normal aging) routinely involves more than one column, you will probably be feeling most of your pain in only one location. You should begin with the exercises designed to cope with the pain you feel.

Can you be more specific about the relationship between types of pain and the exercises that help control them?

Type One pain originates in the back or posterior column. There-fore, exercises are designed to open up that column and reduce the load on the small joints. For that reason, this condition calls primarily for flexion (forward bending) exercises.

Type Two pain is found in the anterior or forward column. And so the remedy calls for extension (backward bending) exercises that reduce pressure at the front.

However, since both Type One and Type Two problems can lead to a general stiffness, once the severe pain has subsided, everyone should do both flexion and extension exercises to limber up. Before choosing your routine, you should pay as much attention to the stage of your recovery as you do to the source of your pain.

Type Three pain originates in the middle column. In this case the problem is nerve pressure, which is not so readily relieved by exercise. Although Type Three pain comes from the nerve that is being pinched in the middle column, the culprit is usually a disc bulging backward from the front column. Flexion, which increases pressure within the disc, is not likely to be of any help at all, but often you can relieve the pain somewhat by extension (arching backward). According to physical therapist Robin McKenzie's theory, extension exercises shift the water content of the disc's nucleus forward to take pressure away from the nerve.

Type Four, spinal stenosis, is a narrowing of that middle column. Its pain can sometimes be relieved by altering the position of your back to increase the space available to the compressed nerves. This effect may be achieved through a series of flexion-stretching exercises. (Strengthening exercises are not particularly useful because the area is already rigid, so the increased stability produced by stronger muscles has no effect.) Bending forward tends to open up the posterior column where the exits for the nerves are located. If you manage to enlarge these exit holes, you may reduce the squeezing. Not all Type Four cases respond to exercise, however, especially if the affected passages are extremely narrow. And for reasons no one understands, the occasional Type Four pain will respond to extension-stretching exercises.

You keep distinguishing between stretching and strengthening exercises. How important is that difference?

Very important. Stretching exercises are designed to loosen tight joints or ligaments and allow a free range of movement. Without that normal range, back pain will persist just as pain may persist in any joint that has not been allowed to move for some time.

Strengthening provides muscle support for that increased movement which the joint might otherwise be unable to tolerate. Without this stability, the newly acquired mobility could cause pain by overstretching the adjacent soft tissues.

It becomes obvious that both stretching and strengthening are necessary. In a proper exercise routine, the joints are stretched so that the range of movement can develop and then the muscles are strengthened to protect that range. Stretching without strengthening can lead to unnecessary pain as a result of poor support, whereas strengthening exercises alone seldom produce pain relief in stiff joints.

What exercises do you recommend for people with osteoporosis?

Exercise in general helps maintain bone calcium levels. Bone grows stronger in response to the load applied to it, and therefore exercise is an excellent way of stimulating your bones and maintaining their bulk. However, if you have, or suspect you have, bone that is already thin, you should be careful not to engage in too-vigorous exercise, particularly when it involves extreme flexion or extension that could cause fractures. If you are in your late middle age and you are embarking on a strenuous exercise program for the first time, you'd be wise to check with your doctor first.

The choice between flexion and extension exercises should still depend on the origin of your back pain. If you have no pain, a combination of both seems reasonable. Where osteoporosis is present, strengthening is more important than stretching.

I'd like to know more about the pelvic tilt. Is it still among the exercises you recommend?

I never considered the pelvic tilt an exercise, even though, for convenient reference, I listed it as such in *The Back Doctor*. The pelvic tilt is really a starting position for many of the flexion exercises and should be maintained during some of them to protect the discs from excessive load. It's possible, of course, to tilt the lower part of your pelvis forward while standing (ask any belly dancer), but for our exercises, the pelvic tilt is performed as you lie on your back with your knees bent and your feet flat on the floor. Without holding your breath, you tighten your abdominal muscles and flatten the small of your back against the floor by rolling your hips forward and contracting the muscles in your buttocks. You can raise your buttocks slightly but do not push with your feet. This may sound complicated, but it's really a very simple and gentle movement – one of those maneuvers that is (if I may twist a phrase) easier done than said.

Before the roles of stretching and extension exercises were emphasized, the pelvic tilt was considered the basic element in maintaining proper low-back posture. Although its role is now more specifically defined in relation to flexion-strengthening exercises, its general value has not been diminished.

*   *   *

So we come to my list of recommended exercises. Before we get into them, I have a few comments. The routine that will be right for you can come only from experimentation; there is no single pattern that will work for everyone or even for the same individual at all times. Consider both the source of your pain and the state of your recovery.

Keep your exercise period short (ten to fifteen minutes) so that it fits your day. Some people find that two daily sessions are helpful. The number of different exercises you do doesn't matter. There is no benefit in rushing through a dozen in fifteen minutes. Work steadily but perform each one carefully and with control. When the allotted time is up, save the rest of the routine for tomorrow. Varying your program day to day adds interest.

For those with neck problems, I've supplied several neck exercises. For those who wish to help lighten the burden on their backs, I've included some leg-strengthening exercises. These extra routines may be done alone or combined with the back exercises.

I encourage you to read the next section completely before making your decisions. Don't focus on just one or two items that sound useful; give yourself as much information as possible before you start.

For handy reference, I've also assembled the back exercises I outline into two easy-to-read charts. These are designed to provide at a glance suggested programs for all four types of back pain, both in the early stages of recovery and for long-term maintenance. They cover flexion and extension exercises, encompassing both stretching and strengthening routines.

EXERCISES FOR YOUR NECK, LEGS, AND BACK

Although the precise number of times you repeat a given exercise during each session may not make much difference in the long run, most of the exercises I describe here are intended for eight to ten repetitions each, unless my comments suggest otherwise.

Whatever number of repetitions you choose, take your time with them. You aren't in a race, and going slowly is not a matter of pampering yourself. In fact, it's more difficult, and therefore more beneficial, to do your exercises slowly than to repeat them as rapidly as you can, because speed can create that undesirable ballistic effect I mentioned earlier. The idea is *to provide gentle, controlled stretching and gradual strengthening while avoiding stress that may provoke pain*.

Most back patients who start to exercise worry about causing pain and wonder how much pain can be safely accepted. They should realize, however, that the pain caused by their original problem is not the same pain that comes from unaccustomed activity – that's a different sensation. Therapists at the Canadian Back Institute call it "sweet pain." It's a sensation I find impossible to define, but once you experience it I think you will agree "sweet" describes exactly the feeling of pain you know you can accept.

Neck Exercises

Strengthening the neck is just as important as strengthening the low back. In one respect, exercises for the neck are even more critical, because there are fewer passive ways you can protect your cervical spine. We have already discussed some easy ways to relieve stress on the lumbar area, such as standing with one foot raised on a rail or stool, or sitting with a pillow tucked into the small of your back – but there are no equivalent tricks you can use for your neck. Whether or not it remains free of pain depends almost entirely on the posture of your upper body and on the strength of the neck and shoulder muscles that support your head. That's a fact worth remembering when you are deciding whether to begin doing neck exercises regularly.

Ironically, one of the commonest causes of neck pain during exercise is the improper performance of low-back routines. When doing any flexion exercise for the low back, you should bring your neck and shoulders forward as a unit, keeping your chin tucked in. Straining with the neck to help lift the upper body puts unnecessary stress on the cervical spine and can lead to pain. It's been my experience that about two out of every ten patients who exercise for the low back report an increase of pain in their necks. It's almost always due to exercising improperly.

Stretching Exercises for the Neck and Shoulders

Neck Exercise 1: THE SHRUG

To start: Sit or stand in a relaxed manner.
The action: Raise your shoulders as high as you can. Hold that position to a slow count of eight. Then relax and pause before repeating.

Neck Exercise 2: BACKWARD THRUSTING

To start: Stand up or sit erect on a hard chair with your shoulders well clear of the chair back.
The action: With your arms loosely at your sides, thrust your shoulders as far back as they will go. Hold that position for a slow count of eight, then relax and pause before repeating.

Neck Exercise 3: **FORWARD THRUSTING**

To start: Stand up or sit erect on a hard chair with your shoulders well clear of the chair back.
The action: Thrust your shoulders forward as far as they will go. Hold that position for a slow count of eight, then relax before repeating.

Neck Exercise 4: **NECK ROTATION AND TILT**

To start: Stand or sit erect.
The action: Turn your head slowly to the left side and bring your chin down towards your shoulder as far as it will go. Return your head to the forward position. Now tip your head gently to the left as far as it will comfortably go, as if trying to place your ear on your shoulder, pause for one second, then return to the starting position. Repeat those two actions, alternating them and performing each one four times, working entirely to the left side. Now follow the same sequence to the right side.

Neck Exercise 5: **THE CHIN TUCK**

To start: Stand or sit erect.
The action: Keeping your head level, slowly tuck your chin in (not down) as far as possible. Keep staring straight ahead. Don't look up or down. Hold that position for a slow count of four, then relax before repeating.

Once you are comfortable with this exercise you can increase its effect by gently pushing on your chin with one hand after you have achieved your maximum tuck. Apply a gentle but firm degree of extra pressure.

Chin tucks can also be performed lying down as a method of relieving acute neck pain. Don't use a pillow. Lying on your back, slowly draw your chin in while you face the same spot on the ceiling to keep your head from tilting. Hold that position for a few seconds, then relax before repeating.

Strengthening Exercises for the Neck

These next four exercises pit one set of muscles against another. While they require a degree of firm pressure, you should *never* exert yourself to the point where your neck begins to quiver, since that movement will irritate the discs and facet joints in your cervical spine and probably cause pain. Once again, the key is moderation and slow, smooth movements.

Neck Exercise 6: THE BACKWARD PRESS

To start: Place your hands behind your head and clasp the fingers together securely.
The action: Tense your neck muscles by pushing your head back against your hands. Maintain the pressure to a slow count of eight. Relax before repeating.

Neck Exercise 7: THE FORWARD PRESS

To start: With your fingers pointing upwards, place the palms of your hands against your forehead.
The action: Press your head firmly forward against your hands to place tension on your neck muscles. Maintain the pressure to a slow count of eight. Relax before repeating.

Neck Exercise 8: THE LEFT SIDE PRESS

To start: With your fingers pointing upwards, place the palm of your left hand against the left side of your head just above your ear.
The action: Press your head firmly to the left against the hand. Hold this pressure through a slow count of eight. Relax before repeating.

Neck Exercise 9: **THE RIGHT SIDE PRESS**

To start: With your fingers pointing upwards, place the palm of your right hand against the right side of your head just above your ear.

The action: Same as for Exercise 8, but to the right instead.

Leg Exercises

In presenting exercises for your legs – principally to strengthen your thighs – I am not straying as far from the topic of back care as you might imagine. To protect your back from unnecessary strain, you need to use your legs as much as possible. Therefore, strong legs make for a healthy back.

Try these simple exercises to strengthen your legs:

Leg Exercise 1: **THE HALF KNEE BEND**

To start: Stand erect, with your feet comfortably apart, and place your hands on your hips.

The action: Keeping your feet flat on the floor, slowly bend your knees. Half way down, pause momentarily. Now straighten your knees slowly until you have returned to your starting position. Relax before repeating.

To get the most benefit from the half knee bend, perform it slowly and smoothly. If you descend quickly you are relying on gravity to lower your body instead of using your thigh muscles. By performing the movement in a controlled way, you introduce a constant muscular tension that builds the strength you need.

Leg Exercise 2: **THE IMAGINARY CHAIR**

To start: Stand with your back against a smooth wall, feet slightly apart and your arms at your sides.

The action: Press your back firmly against the wall and slide your body slowly downwards until your thighs are parallel to the floor. Don't move your feet forward; keep them directly below your knees. Don't press your hands onto the front of your thighs; that takes much of the load off your leg muscles. Hold this position as long as you can, then return slowly to your starting position.

This exercise is harder to do than it sounds. If you can remain seated in your imaginary chair for more than thirty seconds, you're doing well. Try a few seconds the first time and work up from there in subsequent sessions.

Back Exercises

As you will see, the back exercises I recommend here are separated into more than just flexion (forward bending) and extension (backward bending) routines. Each of these categories is divided, in turn, into exercises that stretch and others that strengthen. In all, there are four categories to choose from, according to your basic problem and your stage of improvement. The exercises that are best for you when you are recovering from an acute attack may need augmenting or replacing later on, when your trouble has healed and you are ready for a program of regular maintenance, as indicated by that designation in my comments on the application of each exercise.

If a particular exercise seems to increase your symptoms it's not right for you. For example, if you are Type Two, in an acute stage, a flexion exercise will probably cause pain. That simply means you are not ready for it. You should avoid flexion routines at that stage and try some other exercises recommended on my list. When the disc has healed you will be able to add forward bending (flexion) to your long-term program.

On the other hand, there is no need to progress automatically. If the first group of exercises you try makes your back feel better, stay with them and ignore the others. Sooner or later most people should gain additional flexibility, and if you feel you can handle some of the other exercises without pain, go ahead. But if they aggravate the situation, don't continue. The idea is not to do all the exercises but to find the ones that are right for you.

I recommend the same approach to the variations described for making individual strengthening exercises more difficult (and hence, for those who can do them, more rewarding). If the Level 1 version of a routine provides the relief you're looking for, don't feel that you must push on to Levels 2 and 3. Just count yourself lucky that you quickly found what you were looking for – and stay with it.

While it's often true, as you might assume, that the more strenuous exercises offer speedier improvement in your condition, they also pose a greater risk of discomfort or pain. And so, if you do decide to progress, protect yourself by adopting an increased amount of caution. Start the first routines of each session gently, avoiding violent and extreme movements. Just remember: while none of these routines will harm you, they can cause needless pain – and perhaps discourage you from continuing. Knowing when to do the various exercises is vital. You must gauge your progress carefully. As you will see in the comments on each exercise, some can be performed safely and usefully at "any time," while others are designated as suitable only "after recovery, for long-term maintenance," when your acute pain has resolved.

FLEXION (FORWARD BENDING) EXERCISES

Flexion exercises are designed both to strengthen the abdominal muscles that help support the back, and to increase flexibility by opening up the small joints along the spine while stretching the structures in the backs of the legs, notably the hamstring muscles. Traditionally it was believed that abdominal strengthening helped by increasing the body's ability to maintain a rigid column of air within the abdominal cavity. This column, often compared to a thick-walled balloon, becomes an additional support for the weight of the upper torso. A newer theory suggests that powerful belly muscles pull on strong fibrous sheets that encircle the trunk, creating tension near the spine and making the low back rigid and strong. Regardless of which theory is correct, strong abdominal muscles play an important part in reducing low-back pain.

Flexion exercises increase the load on the anterior column of the spine. If your pain is Type Two, that is from a disc, repeated flexion may increase your symptoms, and this type of exercise program should be stopped. If, however, the problem is primarily in the posterior column, that is Type One pain, you'll find flexion exercise routines lead to a gain in mobility and a decrease in discomfort. This is a subtle process, though, and you'll achieve your goal best if you go about these exercises gently.

For patients with resolving discogenic problems who are once again able to bend forward without pain, and are starting on a program that includes flexion exercises, the physical therapists at the CBI recommend alternating these exercises with equally strenuous extension maneuvers.

Strengthening the abdomen takes time, but it offers great rewards. As you do your flexion-strengthening exercises, you will notice that they require less and less effort and are associated with less and less back pain.

Performing some flexion-strengthening exercises incorrectly places extra stress on your neck and is a common cause of neck pain. Remember, you should bring your neck and shoulders forward as a single unit, keeping your chin tucked.

Flexion–Stretching

Back Exercise 1: **KNEES TO CHEST**

To start: Lie on your back in a crook position; that is, with your knees bent and your feet flat on the floor. Rest your arms at your sides. Adopt a pelvic tilt.
The action: Holding the pelvic tilt, draw both knees up to your chest. Maintain that position for a slow count of eight, and then return your legs to their original position. Relax before repeating.

Suitable for:
Type One – any time.
Type Two – after recovery, for long-term maintenance.
Type Three – after recovery, for long-term maintenance.
Type Four – any time.

This is an anti-gravity exercise designed to increase the flexibility of your spine and open up the facet joints.

If you have very weak abdominal muscles, try an easier version of this exercise by drawing up one bent knee at a time. The leg remaining on the floor helps steady the low back and maintains the pelvic tilt.

Back Exercise 2: ANKLE TOUCHING

To start: Sit on a chair and slump forward, with your feet on the floor, your knees bent, and your legs slightly spread.
The action: Bend forward slowly at the waist until your chest is on your knees. As you do, run your hands down the inside of your legs until you reach your ankles. Straighten up before repeating.
A more demanding variation: Instead of starting with your feet flat on the floor, extend your legs and rest your heels on the floor with your feet wide apart. This increases the pull on the back of your legs.

Suitable for:
Type One – any time.
Type Two – after recovery, for long-term maintenance.
Type Three – after recovery, for long-term maintenance.
Type Four – after recovery, for long-term maintenance.

Back Exercise 3: "TYING MY SHOE"

To start: Stand with one foot up on a low stool directly in front of you, with the straight leg bearing most of your weight.
The action: Bend forward until your chest touches the raised knee and your hands reach the raised foot.

Repeat this action four or five times, then reverse your position so that your other foot is on the stool.

Suitable for:
Type One – any time.
Type Two – after recovery, for long-term maintenance.
Type Three – after recovery, for long-term maintenance.
Type Four – after recovery, for long-term maintenance.

(continued on page 308)

Forward bending increases the load on the front of the spine, so proceed carefully. You may not be able to reach the final position in this exercise, but go as far as you can without producing a recurrence of your typical pain. By keeping one leg straight, you place tension on the nerves and muscles along the back of that leg. Keeping the other leg bent with your foot up on the stool reduces the pull on the rest of the back. If you have more stiffness or soreness in one leg, do a few extra repetitions with that leg straight, to help limber it up.

Back Exercise 4: **TOE TOUCHING**

To start: Stand with your legs straight but relaxed (not stiff), your feet comfortably apart, and your arms at your sides.
The action: Bend forward slowly at the waist, while allowing your arms to dangle loosely in front of you, until your upper body is horizontal and your back is slightly rounded. Now bring your trunk up again to the starting position. Relax before repeating.

Suitable for:
Type One – any time.
Type Two – after recovery, for long-term maintenance.
Type Three – after recovery, for long-term maintenance.
Type Four – after recovery, for long-term maintenance.

I always hesitate to recommend this exercise – not because it isn't good when done properly but because it is too often abused. I suggest you keep the following points in mind at all times:

• Toe touching should *never* be done violently. While you are unlikely to damage yourself seriously, you may pull a muscle or cause other needless strain or pain.
• You should not try to touch your toes while standing with your legs stiff and your feet together.
• It doesn't really matter whether you actually touch your toes. The idea is simply to stretch the muscles and nerves in the low back and down the backs of your hips and legs.
• The horizontal position should not be sustained. Straighten up as soon as you have felt a comfortable amount of stretch. People

with Type Two or Type Three pain must be particularly careful.

• Although the first few flexions may produce a little pain, the exercise should get easier and less painful with each repetition. Increasing discomfort means that toe touching should be discontinued.

Flexion–Strengthening

For some flexion-strengthening exercises, I define three levels of difficulty which depend on the position of your arms. Level 1 is the easiest position, Level 3 the hardest, and the progression from easy to difficult goes this way:

Level 1: arms extended over your legs.
Level 2: arms folded across your chest.
Level 3: hands over your ears, elbows out to the sides.

Note that in Level 3, the hands are *not* behind the head, since that position could allow you to pull your head forward and place unwanted stress on your neck.

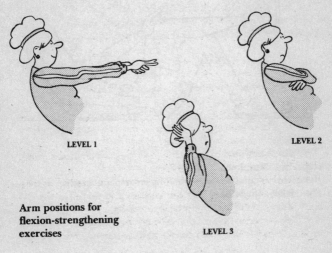

LEVEL 1

LEVEL 2

Arm positions for flexion-strengthening exercises

LEVEL 3

Back Exercise 5: **THE CROSS-OVER KNEE PUSH**

To start: Lie on your back in the crook position; that is, with your knees bent and your feet flat on the floor. Adopt a pelvic tilt: tighten your abdominal muscles and flatten the small of your back against the floor by rolling your hips forward and contracting the muscles in your buttocks. You can raise your buttocks slightly but do not push with your feet.

The action: Holding the pelvic tilt, bend your left knee and draw it toward your stomach. Keeping your arm straight, place your right hand on your left knee, raise your head and shoulders. Be sure to keep your chin tucked to avoid unwanted strain on your neck. Now use your right hand to push firmly on your left knee until you feel your abdominal muscles contracting. Hold the tension as you count slowly to eight. Relax momentarily and repeat the action four more times with the same arm and leg. Lower your left leg to the crook position, raise the right leg, and perform the pushing action with your left hand – counting, relaxing, and repeating as before.

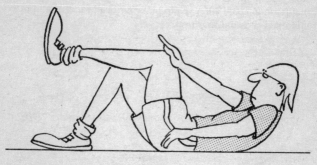

Suitable for:
Type One – any time.
Type Two – any time.
Type Three – after recovery, for long-term maintenance.
Type Four – any time.

Back Exercise 6: **THE ROLL-UP**

To start: Lie on your back in the crook position. Adopt a pelvic tilt. Tuck your chin to avoid neck strain.

The action: Holding the pelvic tilt, roll your body up, raising your head and shoulders forward and then bringing both knees up toward them. Now reverse the action, lowering your head and shoulders first, then your knees. Pause before repeating.

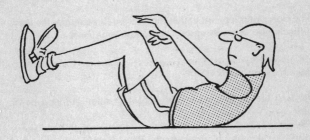

The roll-up can be done at any level:
Level 1: arms extended over your legs.
Level 2: arms folded across your chest.
Level 3: hands over your ears, elbows out to the sides.

Suitable for:
Type One – any time.
Type Two – after recovery, for long-term maintenance.

Back Exercise 7: **SUPINE LEG SPREADING**

To start: Lie on your back with both legs straight out on the floor. Adopt a pelvic tilt.

The action: Holding the pelvic tilt, bend both knees toward your chest, straighten your legs in the air, and lower them until they form a forty-five to sixty-degree angle with the floor. Now spread your legs apart and bring them back together eight times. Lower your legs. Relax before repeating. (continued on page 312)

Supine leg spreading can be attempted at three levels:
Level 1: arms extended over your legs.
Level 2: arms folded across your chest.
Level 3: hands over your ears, elbows out to the sides.

Suitable for:
Type One – after recovery, long-term maintenance.
Type Two – any time.
Type Three – after recovery, long-term maintenance.

The closer your legs are to the floor during this exercise the more
difficult it becomes. Be careful not to lose your pelvic tilt.

Back Exercise 8: **THE SIT-UP**

To start: Lie on your back in the crook position. Adopt a pelvic
tilt.
The action: Holding the pelvic tilt, raise your upper body slowly
until your shoulder blades clear the floor. Hold that partly raised
position to a slow count of eight. Lower yourself to the floor. Pause
before repeating.

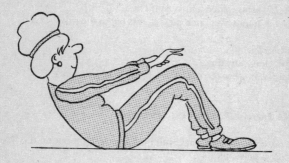

The sit-up can be attempted at three levels:
Level 1: arms extended over your legs.
Level 2: arms folded across your chest.
Level 3: hands over your ears, elbows out to the sides.

Suitable for:
Type One – any time.
Type Two – after recovery, long-term maintenance.
Type Three – after recovery, long-term maintenance.

Many people make the mistake of performing the sit-up starting with their legs straight out (or almost so) and their feet hooked under a piece of heavy furniture. That's not a bad exercise for your hips and thighs, but it doesn't help your belly muscles much. Electrical studies of muscular action have shown that with the legs held down, the action of bending at the waist takes place mainly by flexing the hips. With the feet free, the only way to perform the sit-up is to contract the stomach muscles. Keep your knees bent and try to hold your feet flat on the floor. Until you gain enough strength in your stomach you may notice that as you begin to raise your upper body your feet rise slightly in a counterbalancing action.

The sit-up is the ultimate exercise in its category. If you are going to do only one flexion-strengthening exercise, this is the one to do. Remember to keep your head and shoulders working as a unit. As you sit up, don't force your head forward or pull yourself up by putting your hands behind your neck. As I have already said, many people bring on neck pain by doing their low-back exercises incorrectly.

Another mistake people make with the sit-up is failing to sit up far enough. In a proper sit-up, your shoulder blades must completely clear the floor. Often people will raise their head and shoulders slightly, and then stop as soon as they feel tension. That's not enough. One way to guarantee that you sit up far enough is to lie on a mark made on the floor just above your waist. If someone watching you can see the mark under your body, you know you've risen far enough.

Many people complete their sit-ups to a full upright position. I don't believe there is anything wrong with this, although some physical therapists worry that it may increase the disc load unnecessarily. One thing we do agree on is that the final thirty degrees or so of elevation is easy to achieve, so, in fact, this last part of the full sit-up adds little benefit and makes the whole exercise less efficient. If that is your style of sit-up, you can improve your efficiency by sitting back very slowly and maintaining a strong abdominal contraction all the way to the floor.

Back Exercise 8A: **THE SIT-DOWN**

To start: Sit on the floor, bring your knees up and hold them with your hands.

The action: Maintaining a grip on your knees, lean back gradually. When your arms are fully extended, use them to pull yourself towards your knees again. Pause before repeating.

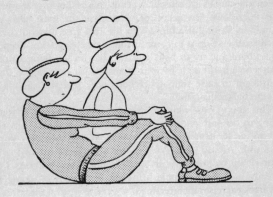

Suitable for:

Type One – any time.

Type Two – after recovery, for long-term maintenance.

Type Three – after recovery, for long-term maintenance.

This is the easiest sit-up of the three. It's a good way to get started if you find you have virtually no strength in your abdominal muscles, since your arms will provide the strength you need to sit up. Be patient; it can take months to develop your belly muscles. As they grow stronger, you'll find you can perform the sit-down by leaning back all the way to the floor and coming up again. Thus, with practice and increased muscle strength, the sit-down becomes the sit-up.

Back Exercise 8B: **THE BENCH SIT-UP**

To start: Lie on your back on the floor with your feet and the calves of your legs resting on the seat of a chair, sofa, or bench. If you're doing this correctly, your legs, thighs, and trunk will form a "Z"; your thighs should be vertical and your lower legs parallel to the floor. Adopt a pelvic tilt.

The action: Holding the pelvic tilt, perform the sit-up as described, making sure your neck and shoulders move as a unit and your shoulder blades clear the floor. Pause and relax before repeating.

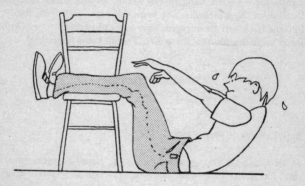

The bench sit-up can be attempted at three levels:
Level 1: arms extended over your legs.
Level 2: arms folded across your chest.
Level 3: hands over ears, elbows out to sides.

Suitable for:
Type One – any time.
Type Two – after recovery, for long-term maintenance.

The purpose of this variation is to further eliminate action of your thigh muscles, thereby placing an even greater load on the belly muscles themselves. It's the most difficult form of sit-up and is not for everyone. You should attempt it only if you're in generally good physical condition and find the standard sit-up lacking in challenge, even at Level 3.

EXTENSION EXERCISES

Extension exercises have two basic purposes. One is to strengthen the paraspinal muscles, located along your spine and felt as two ridges running down your back. The other is to increase flexibility by putting your facet joints through movements opposite to those done in forward bending. Because extension exercises increase the load on the facet joints they are usually uncomfortable for patients suffering from Type One pain.

For those suffering from a pinched nerve (Type Three) with significant leg pain, lying in extension can sometimes alter the location of the symptoms. The worst pain may shift from the leg into the back – an encouraging sign many physical therapists look for as an indication that the patient's condition is improving.

Extension–Stretching

Back Exercise 9: **PRONE LYING**

To start: Lie on your stomach. Put your hands together under your forehead. Turn your head to one side if you feel more comfortable that way.
The action: Lie there and count to ten. That's it – just lie there! Continue for as long as fifteen minutes at a stretch.

Suitable for:
Type One – after recovery, for long-term maintenance.
Type Two – any time.
Type Three – any time.
Type Four – as a possibility (see my comment below).

This one may sound like a heaven-sent instruction to some, and a real put-on to others, but it has its purpose: when you lie on your stomach, you automatically arch your back. And, as you may realize, that's exactly why this exercise is right for Type Two but unwise for Type One sufferers in the acute phase, when they typically can't arch their backs without pain.

Use any surface you find comfortable – a bed, a long couch, a well-carpeted floor; there is no advantage in choosing a hard surface (and no extra points for martyrdom). If you find this passive exercise position comforting, do it as often you like – while listening to the radio or conversing with visiting friends who are prepared to accept your eccentricities.

Most people with Type Four pain (spinal stenosis) do better on flexion-stretching routines, but a few find extension-stretching more helpful. I don't routinely recommend extension exercises for Type Four pain, but if that's your trouble, and you haven't been able to obtain benefit from flexion-stretching, you might try some extension-stretching and see what it does for you.

Back Exercise 10: **RESTING ON YOUR ELBOWS**

To start: Lie on your stomach and prop yourself up on your elbows.
The action: Hold that position at least to a slow count of ten – or for as long as you feel comfortable.

Suitable for:
Type One – after recovery, for long-term maintenance.
Type Two – any time.
Type Three – any time.
Type Four – as a possibility (see comment under Exercise 9).

This position, popular with children while watching television, is obviously just a variation of Exercise 9, but it increases the extension effect. My comments there also apply here.

Back Exercise 11: **THE "SEA LION" PUSH-UP**

To start: Lie on your stomach on a firm surface, with your forehead on the floor, your palms down, and your hands beside your shoulders.
The action: Gradually push yourself up with your hands and arms, raising your trunk from the waist up, while the rest of your body and your legs remain on the floor. Hold for a count of eight and then slowly lower your body again. Pause before repeating.

(continued on page 318)

Suitable for:
Type Two – any time.
Type Three – any time.

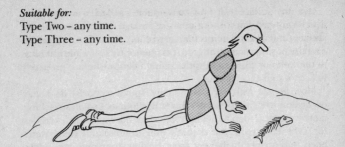

This may be the closest you ever come to looking like a sea lion sunning itself on a rock. Like the two previous exercises, this one will seem mild to anybody used to heavy workouts, but it's an active method of putting your spine through a full range of extension without straining your back muscles.

Back Exercise 12: **ARCHING BACKWARDS**

To start: Stand erect with feet comfortably apart and your hands on the small of your back.
The action: Gently arch backwards to look up at the ceiling. Try not to bend your knees. Maintain this position for a count of eight. Pause before repeating.

Suitable for:
Type One – after recovery, for long-term maintenance.
Type Two – any time.
Type Three – after recovery, for long-term maintenance.
Type Four – as a possibility (see comment under Exercise 9).

As you will probably notice, this exercise is the action you have often performed instinctively whenever you stand up to stretch after sitting for a long time. As with flexion-stretching, you should perform this movement to the point of resistance – and then just a little more.

Like the flexion-stretching exercises, this movement should become increasingly easy for you with repetition and certainly not more painful. You should become gradually aware of an increased mobility. Moving any stiff joint will be painful at first, and it's important to assess the change in pain rather than simply reacting to that first twinge. If you don't feel any benefit after several sessions, try another exercise on the list.

Extension–Strengthening

As I did with the flexion-strengthening exercises, I have provided three levels of difficulty for some extension-strengthening exercises, as determined by the position of the hands. With extensions the hand positions are roughly the reverse of what they were for the flexion exercises. Level 1 is still the easiest, and Level 3 the most difficult:

Level 1: hands clasped behind the small of your back.
Level 2: hands clasped behind your neck.
Level 3: arms extended over your head.

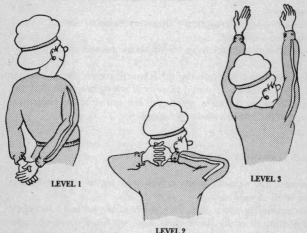

Arm positions for extension-strengthening exercises

Back Exercise 13: **HIP EXTENSION**

To start: Lie on your stomach. Put your hands together under your forehead. Turn your head to one side if you feel more comfortable that way.

The action: Bend one knee to a right angle, then, keeping that position, raise the front of the thigh off the floor. Hold the leg in the air for a slow count of eight. Repeat four times, then switch to the other leg and follow the same procedure.

A more demanding variation: Instead of bending your leg, keep it straight and lift from the hip. By extending your leg you create a longer lever, which makes the exercise more difficult.

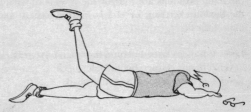

Suitable for:
Type One – after recovery, for long-term maintenance.
Type Two – any time.
Type Three – after recovery, for long-term maintenance.

Extending your hip (moving it backward) causes the paraspinal muscles to tense. Repeated movement strengthens not only the muscles of the buttocks, which are the principal hip extensors, but also the muscles along your spine.

Back Exercise 14: **TRUNK EXTENSION**

To start: Lie on your stomach with your hands clasped behind the small of your back.

The action: Tuck your chin, then slowly raise your head and chest until they clear the floor. Hold them up for a count of eight. Now lower them gently, then pause and relax before repeating.

Trunk extensions should be started at the first level of difficulty but can be done at all three levels:

Level 1: hands clasped behind the small of your back.
Level 2: hands clasped behind your neck.
Level 3: arms extended over your head.

Suitable for:
Type One – after recovery, for long-term maintenance; arm position at Level 1 only.
Type Two – any time.
Type Three – after recovery, for long-term maintenance.

Back Exercise 15: **TRUNK AND LEG RAISING**

To start: Lie on your stomach and bend your knees.
Clasp your hands behind the small of your back.
The action: Tuck your chin and then raise your head and upper torso slowly while lifting both legs until your thighs clear the floor. Hold for a slow count of eight. Pause and relax before repeating.

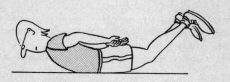

All three levels of difficulty are physiologically possible, but few people can manage Level 3 (arms over head), and even fewer should try. The three levels, again, are:
Level 1: hands clasped behind the small of your back.
Level 2: hands clasped behind your neck.
Level 3: arms extended over your head.

Suitable for:
Type Two – any time.

You can make this exercise even more difficult by keeping your legs straight as you lift them from the hips.

No one with Type One, Type Three, or Type Four pain should attempt this exercise; Type Two should use it carefully.

Back Exercise 16: **THE HORIZONTAL LIFT**

To start: Lie face down on a firm bed or table, with your lower body and legs on the surface and your upper body hanging, head down, over the edge.

The action: With a companion holding your legs down, raise your upper torso until your whole body is extended straight out. Hold the position for a slow count of eight, then slowly lower your body. Pause before repeating.

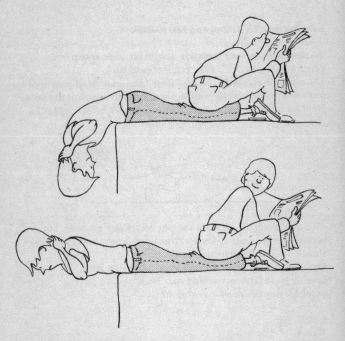

The horizontal lift can be done at any of the three levels of difficulty:

Level 1: hands clasped behind the small of your back.
Level 2: hands clasped behind your neck.
Level 3: arms extended over your head.

Suitable for:

Type One – after recovery, for long-term maintenance.
Type Two – after recovery, for long-term maintenance.
Type Three – after recovery, for long-term maintenance.

Just as the sit-up is the best flexion exercise for strengthening your abdomen, The Horizontal Lift is the best extension exercise for strengthening the paraspinal muscles. Lifting the weight of your upper body provides a real challenge.

Another advantage of this exercise is that it strengthens without requiring you to over-extend, since you are moving only from a forward-bent position up to neutral. This is especially helpful for Type One victims because they can develop their back muscles and still avoid forcing their facet joints into a painful, compressed position.

DR. HAMILTON HALL'S BACK EXERCISE CHART NO. 1
FOR THE RECOVERING PATIENT WHO IS JUST GETTING STARTED

| | FLEXION (forward bending) | | EXTENSION (backward bending) | |
TYPE OF PAIN	Stretching Exercise	Strengthening Exercise	Stretching Exercise	Strengthening Exercise
Type 1	1. Knees to Chest 2. Ankle Touching 3. "Tying My Shoe" 4. Toe Touching	5. The Cross-Over Knee Push 6. The Roll-Up 7. The Sit-Up 8. The Sit-Down 8A. The Sit-Down 8B. The Bench Sit-Up	None	None
Type 2	None	5. The Cross-Over Knee Push 7. Supine Leg Spreading	9. Prone Lying 10. Resting on Your Elbows 11. The "Sea-Lion" Push-Up 12. Arching Backwards	13. Hip Extension 14. Trunk Extension 15. Trunk and Leg Raising
Type 3	None	None	9. Prone Lying 10. Resting on Your Elbows 11. The "Sea Lion" Push-Up	None
Type 4	1. Knees to Chest 2. Ankle Touching	5. The Cross-Over Knee Push	9. Prone Lying* 10. Resting on Your Elbows* 12. Arching Backwards *as possibilities see pp. 316-317	None

DR. HAMILTON HALL'S BACK EXERCISE CHART NO. 2

LONG-TERM CHOICES FOR KEEPING IN SHAPE

TYPE OF PAIN	FLEXION (forward bending)		EXTENSION (backward bending)	
	Stretching Exercise	Strengthening Exercise	Stretching Exercise	Strengthening Exercise
Type 1	1. Knees to Chest 2. Ankle Touching 3. "Tying My Shoe" 4. Toe Touching	5. The Cross-Over Knee Push 6. The Roll-Up 7. Supine Leg Spreading 8. The Sit-Up 8A. The Sit-Down 8B. The Bench Sit-Up	9. Prone Lying 10. Resting on Your Elbows 12. Arching Backwards	13. Hip Extension 14. Trunk Extension (Level 1 only) 16. The Horizontal Lift
Type 2	1. Knees to Chest 2. Ankle Touching 3. "Tying My Shoe" 4. Toe Touching	5. The Cross-Over Knee Push 6. The Roll-Up 7. Supine Leg Spreading 8. The Sit-Up 8A. The Sit-Down 8B. The Bench Sit-Up	9. Prone Lying 10. Resting on Your Elbows 11. The "Sea Lion" Push-Up 12. Arching Backwards	13. Hip Extension 14. Trunk Extension 15. Trunk and Leg Raising 16. The Horizontal Lift
Type 3	1. Knees to Chest 2. Ankle Touching 3. "Tying My Shoe" 4. Toe Touching	5. The Cross-Over Knee Push 7. Supine Leg-Spreading 8. The Sit-Up 8A. The Sit-Down	9. Prone Lying 10. Resting on Your Elbows 11. The "Sea Lion" Push-Up 12. Arching Backwards	13. Hip Extension 14. Trunk Extension 16. The Horizontal Lift
Type 4	1. Knees to Chest 2. Ankle Touching 3. "Tying My Shoe" 4. Toe Touching	5. The Cross-Over Knee Push	9. Prone Lying* 10. Resting on Your Elbows 12. Arching Backwards *as possibilities see pp. 316-317	None

INDEX

DONE DEAL

"But your dialect . . . where are you from?"

"Vestfold."

"Huh? Is that in Texas?"

"I have no idea where this Tax-us is. Vestfold is in Norway. I am a Norseman. A Viking."

"I see." Now they were getting somewhere. Among his other mental problems, this guy thought he was a Viking . . . although, come to think of it, he did resemble a Norse god. She made a few quick notes on her pad.

"We were negotiating our love slave contract when—"

"I never agreed to negotiate any such thing," she interjected . . . perhaps too indignantly.

"I have much experience in the bedsport, of course."

"Of course," she replied and immediately regretted her sarcasm.

"Now, I cannot claim great finesse in the more refined bedsport . . . no flowery words or hand holding or such . . . and, in truth, I do not favor kissing all that much, but I have been told my endurance is remarkable. That and my size."

"Well, this love slave business would never work, I can tell you that right away," she informed him with a nervous laugh, "because most women like kissing."

"Do you?"

"Uh . . . well, yes. Of course."

He seemed to consider her faltering words, the whole time staring at her with those luminous blue eyes. Finally, he said, "Agreed."

"Agreed? What does that mean?" she practically shrieked.

He arched an eyebrow at the panic in her voice. "I agree to give kisses, and you agree to give . . . well, some things I want . . . nay, *need*."

TRULY, MADLY VIKING

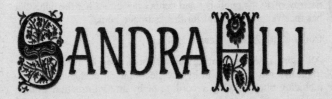

SANDRA HILL

LOVE SPELL BOOKS   NEW YORK CITY

A LOVE SPELL BOOK®

July 2000

Published by

Dorchester Publishing Co., Inc.
276 Fifth Avenue
New York, NY 10001

ISBN 0-505-52387-6

*This book is dedicated to my good friend, Katie Raiser,
who died in the course of my writing this book. Katie's
unfailing courage inspired all of us who were privileged
to know her. She was an aspiring romance novelist whose
dreams were dashed by the ravages of a deadly disease.
Here's hoping Katie is sitting on a cloud somewhere,
finally pain-free, polishing off a splendid manuscript.
Better yet, wouldn't it be nice if Katie were the angel-
muse working through the fingers of some budding
novelist out here today? God bless you, Katie.*

TRULY, MADLY VIKING

"Most men are within a hairsbreadth of being mad."
—Diogenes, 412-323 B.C.

****

"I have weathered huge waves willingly
and fought winds through many sea-
miles to make this visit to you."
—Egils Saga, circa 13th century

Prologue

998 A.D., Summertime in the Norse lands

Jorund Ericsson stared blankly at the huge grave mound. It was large enough to hold a longship and all the personal belongings necessary for the occupant to lead a good life in the afterworld.

A year and more he had been gone to the East-lands, fighting the wars of the emperor of Mikle-gard. A lifelong warrior-for-hire, he had been part of the elite Varangian Guard, made up of hand-picked Vikings from many nations. On the jour-ney home, he had idled time away by standing under the banner of the Norse king Olaf Tryggva-son, who was on the offensive again in Britain, spreading sword dew in his wake like a bloody wave. For Olaf, who happened to be Jorund's paternal uncle, this represented but a brief respite from the ongoing territorial struggles with the Danish king, Sven Forkbeard.

Some said fighting was a Viking way of life. 'Twas true.

With no apologies, Jorund acknowledged being a lord of swordplay . . . a mercenary, but not without principles; he stood only with those chieftains whose goals and standards he shared. Following this life path, he saw death as a constant companion and had long since lost count of the bodies that had fallen under his sword, or those of his comrades who now resided in Valhalla.

Still, he had never expected to find *this* upon his return to his homeland.

In his distress, his eyes darted here and there about the grave site, soon catching on the burial stone, where sticklike runic symbols spelled out:

> Here lies Inga Sigrundottir,
> Wife of Karl Jorund Ericsson of Vestfold,
> Daughter of Jarl Anlaf of Lade.
> She lived but twenty and three winters.
> Died she in the great famine,
> In the year nine ninety-seven.

Jorund choked back a gasp. There had been no great love betwixt him and Inga these six years since their forced marriage. Nonetheless, grief and great shame overwhelmed him at her death eight months past. A man protected those under his shield, lest he be a *nithing*, a man devoid of honor. He should have been here to safeguard her well-being, whether from the dangers of man or nature.

But then his gaze moved to the left, to the two small conjoined grave markers that read:

Greta and Girta Ingadottir,
Firstborn twins,
Beloved daughters.
They lived but five years.
May Freyja hold them to her eternal bosom.

Jorund dropped to his knees and put his face in his hands. He was not an emotional man. Once, amid the din of battle, he'd cleaved a man to the teeth with his battle-ax and ne'er felt a moment of remorse. He could not remember the last time he had yielded to the woman-weakness of crying—mayhap as a child when one of his brothers had hurt him in rough play—but tears welled in his eyes now.

The thought of Inga lying in the cold earth brought him regret that one so young should journey from this earth before her time. Regret . . . that was all. He was the one who had suffered most from Inga's renowned machinations, which had led him reluctantly to her marriage bed, but he bore her no ill will. She had not been a bad woman at heart.

Thoughts of his daughters, on the other hand, brought fierce pain to his chest and constriction to his throat. He had not wanted marriage. He had not even wanted children—but, oh, when he'd held them for the first time, bloody and blue with wrinkled skin, after they emerged from their mother's womb . . . well, he'd loved them on first sight. Seed of his loins they had been, but so much more than that.

The last time he'd seen his girls, they'd not yet celebrated the fourth anniversary of their birthing day. His longship had been pulling up

15

anchor in the fjord in front of his vast homestead. Inga had been standing at the bank, along with his father and mother, Jarl Eric and Lady Asgar; his brothers, Rolf the Shipbuilder and Magnus of the Big Ears; and the family retainers. Greta and Girta had come dancing down the hillside at the last moment, their blond braids swishing back and forth, their hiked-up *gunna*s wrinkled and dirty from some youthling game or another. And they had been giggling. Odd that he should recall that now. But then, he reminded himself, was there a sound more heart-touching in the whole world than that of a giggling child . . . even to a hardened warrior such as himself?

"Don't forget to bring me ribands, Father," Greta had called out to him . . . as if she hadn't reminded him enough times the night before amid sticky kisses and little-girl hugs. "All the colors of the rainbow . . . please." That last word she'd added upon seeing her mother frown down at her for the girl's lack of politeness. Inga, daughter of a high jarl of Lade in northeast Norway, had placed great importance on courtly manners.

"And silk slippers from a harem," Girta had added gaily, ducking as her mother reached out to swat her with an open palm for her impertinence.

"A harem, indeed!" Inga had snorted, but then she hadn't been able to help herself and grinned at the child's outrageousness. Girta had been known for her saucy tongue.

Jorund smiled to himself at the sweet memory, even as a strangled cry escaped his closed air passages.

"My son."

Jorund jerked upright as he felt a palm on his shoulder. Standing, he turned to see his father.

"I need your help, Jorund. Yours and that of your brother, Magnus."

"This is not the time," he choked out, waving a hand to indicate the burial mound.

"There is no better time," his father said wearily. "There is naught you can do for Inga and the girls now. Nay, do not scowl at me. 'Tis true."

Suddenly Jorund noticed how much his father had aged in the time he'd been gone. Was it the famine and all the human losses? Or something else? He furrowed his brow in question.

"Your brother, Geirolf, is missing and feared dead."

"Oh, Father! He's probably just delayed on one of his voyages." Rolf was a shipbuilder who often tested his vessels on extended journeys before selling them to high-placed nobles from many lands.

"Not this time," his father insisted. "Whilst you were gone, I sent him on a quest that I hoped would end the famine here in Norway, but then his dragonship sank after a violent sea battle with that misbegotten cur, Storr Grimmsson. His body was never found." He paused, then added, "I need to be sure, one way or another."

"You think Rolf may still be alive?" he inquired, suddenly alert, though still stunned by this latest news.

"Some seamen from Storr's crew told us, under torture, that Geirolf was last seen in the waters . . . *alive.*" His father shrugged with uncertainty. "You

17

and Magnus must travel to Iceland and mayhap even beyond that to Greenland . . . the region where Geirolf was last seen alive."

"Iceland!" he exclaimed. This was no small favor his father beseeched of him. "No!"

"But—"

"*Nei þýðir nei*," he practically shouted. Then, more softly, "No is no."

His father merely stared at him, making him feel like a child again . . . a selfish child.

Jorund was torn. Should he stay here in Vestfold and suffer penance for his failing of Inga and his daughters? Or should he leave his homeland to help his father, and perhaps expiate his guilt?

"I beg of you, my son. Put aside your sorrow for now and grant me this boon. 'Twas I who sent Geirolf into harm's way. The guilt is weighing me down so, I can scarce think or speak."

Jorund knew exactly how his father felt. Soon he nodded.

This was a mission he could not refuse.

Chapter One

Autumn, 998 A.D.
Beyond Iceland

"Look, Jorund, look! There she blows . . . *again*. Hmmm. Mayhap that is the fair Thora's way of blowing kisses at you. Dost think—"

"Magnus," Jorund Ericsson warned his brother with a disgusted shake of his head. "I have heard more than enough of your nonsense today. I suggest you go take a seat at one of the oarlocks and row off some of your excess vigor."

He was standing at the rail of his longship, *Fierce Warrior*, honing the blade of his favorite sword, Bloodletter. Magnus was standing next to him, honing his tongue. Unless Magnus had a plow in his hands, or a mead horn in his mouth, or a wench in his bed, he tended to think it was his mission in life to bedevil his brother. It was no exaggeration to say that Magnus had an opinion on every bloody topic in the world.

"Now, now, do not be overmodest, little brother," Magnus advised, puffing his chest out, which was a sure sign he was about to expound at length . . . on some triviality. His long, blond hair was pulled off his face with a leather thong tied at the nape, which drew attention to his uncommonly large ears. For years, Magnus had claimed that his large ears were a sign of other . . . well, attributes that were equally pronounced, but Jorund could hardly credit that.

And what did he call me? Little? In truth, he and Magnus were of the same immense height, though Magnus was bullish in stature, being a farmsteader by trade, while Jorund carried the leaner-muscled body of a fighting man. And they were a mere nine months apart in age. So *little* hardly applied. *For the love of Odin! What importance is there in whether my brother deems me big or little? My mind must be melting in this unseasonably hot sun. And that is another thing . . . who would think the sun could be so hot in Iceland? Perchance we have strayed farther than—*

"One and all can see that the fair Thora has developed a passion for you," Magnus blathered on. "And not just the blowing of kisses. You must admit she has been following you about for a sennight and more. Wagging her tail at you like a Hedeby whore. Besotted she is, for a certainty."

He sliced a glare at his brother. "What makes you think she is blowing kisses?" He knew that it was a mistake to react to any of Magnus's jibes. Still, he blundered on, "Mayhap she is just blowing air."

"Like breaking wind? Now there's a thought." Magnus grinned. "Mother always told us when we were growing up that females do not break wind, leastways not in public . . . just old men and bad boys. Ha! I suspect Mother was laughing behind our backs with that mistruth. Either that, or I warrant she was never in close quarters with Fat Helga, the goatherder, after a night of eating *gammelost*." He tapped his chin with exaggerated pensiveness.

Jorund groaned. *When will I ever learn? I can predict what he is going to say now.*

"Do females make a habit of trying to attract you with farts?"

I was correct. "What a ridiculous notion!" Jorund snarled, then realized that Magnus was chuckling under his breath. "Aaarrgh!" he said. Carrying on a conversation with Magnus was like talking with one of his dumb cows. His coarseness knew no limits, his earthiness coming, no doubt, from his dealing so much with . . . well, earth. Not that Jorund was unaccustomed to coarseness, being surrounded as he was by soldiers whose every other word was apt to be an expletive of the foulest nature. He'd uttered a few himself.

But, really, his brother had fallen into the most annoying habit of late—teasing him. *Holy Thor!* Who ever heard of grown men engaging in such youthful games? Life was too serious—and fleeting, as he well knew—and their mission was too important for frivolity. It was probably boredom, or frustration at being lost at sea. Well, not quite lost, just a mite off course.

Ignoring his brother's smirking face, he looked

off into the distance, where the magnificent killer whale the sailors had named Thora was indeed performing her ritual dance. It was to her that Magnus had attributed blowing kisses, of all things.

Just now, her sleek black-and-white shape leaped into the air with a spectacular flourish, a maneuver that had come to be known among seafarers as breaching.

The whale, at the height of her impressive leap, gave the false appearance of standing on her tail fins on the surface of the water for several long moments. Then she twisted her sleek body into a perfect arc with an agility remarkable for her size and dove back into the salty depths to swim swiftly beneath the waves she had created. If she followed her previous routine, she would be repeating the performance another two or three times, ofttimes varying the act with backflips, all accompanied by boisterous squeals and chirps and rapid clicking noises, before swimming off a short distance to watch and follow their sailing vessel.

There was no escaping the killer whale. They had tried to elude their unwelcome companion by rowing fast with a strong wind at their backs, and still she kept up. Surely the killer whale must be the fastest animal in all the oceans.

They knew it was a female because of her comparatively small size to the male of the species, though this friendly beast was still nigh as big as his dragonship. Well, perhaps that was an overstatement. At the least, she had to be four times his body height from mouth to tail.

There was no question in Jorund's mind—

though he would never acknowledge it to his brother—that it was himself the animal had developed an affection for. The whale had been shadowing them for more than fourteen days, coming closer and closer. But that wasn't how Jorund knew that the whale was following *him*. He knew because the whale was talking to him. Amazing as that sounded, even if only to his own ears, Jorund had taken to communicating with a killer whale. He talked to the whale in his head. And the whale talked back to him.

Languages of other countries had always come easily to him. And not just Norse and English, the language of the Saxons, which were very similar. He was also fluent in the tongues of Frankland, Byzantium, Baghdad, Rome, and Cordoba. But never had he been known to speak with animals. No one did, that he knew of, except perhaps the gods. And he was no god.

Where did this voice in his head came from?

When it was late at night and his men were asleep, he would stand at the prow of his long-ship and converse with a killer whale, of all things. Good thing Magnus was unaware of this insanity, or he would *really* have something to tease him about.

Was he going mad? Were the events of the past year too much for his brain to bear? Or was it the cumulative effect of years and years of bloodshed finally crushing down on him? Stronger men than he had gone berserk.

How can this be? he had asked Thora yestereve. It was an indication of his sorry state that he sought advice on his mental condition from an animal.

Click, click. Squeal, squeal. Click, squeal, click, squeal, the whale had answered him in ever-changing patterns. In other words, *Men question too much. Listen with your heart; speak with your heart, my friend.*

I ask for help, and you give me riddles, he'd wailed silently. *I don't understand.* He need not speak aloud for the whale to hear him—another amazing happenstance.

With her usual clicks and squeals and chirps, Thora had told him, *You will; you will.* Then, just before the whale had swum off, she'd added, *Open your heart, man. Only then will there be no barriers of country or animal . . . or time.*

Time? What has time to do with this?

"Jorund, has your mind gone awandering again? Are you all right?"

Jorund blinked and reined in his thoughts. His brother's big paw of a hand was resting on his shoulder with concern.

Am I all right?

Nay, I am not all right.

"I'm fine," he said.

But he was not fine, he soon found out.

Bam! Bam! Bam!

"*Bld hel!*" he and Magnus exclaimed at the same time, then repeated, "Bloody hell!" A number of his sailors, who followed both the Christian and Norse religions, were making the sign of the cross on their broad chests. All of them stared gape-mouthed out to sea.

Bam! Bam! Bam!

Thora was using her huge tail fins to whack the far side of the longship.

Bam! Bam! Bam!

She must be playing with them—some kind of strange killer whale game—for it was clear she was not employing full force; otherwise the vessel would have tipped over. Even so, the impact of the powerful tail hitting the wood sides was enough to set the boat rocking side to side. A little harder and the wood might splinter.

Jorund tried to listen in the way the whale had taught him. There was a loud, grinding noise in response, almost like a rusty door closing, and he thought he heard her say, *It is time, Viking*.

"Time? What time?" Jorund asked.

"Huh?" Magnus tilted his head in question.

Jorund realized that he must have spoken aloud and felt his face heat with embarrassment. Magnus would make great mock of him if he even suspected his brother was communicating with an animal.

The whale swam off a short distance and floated atop the water, just watching him with her big, beady eyes. And the groaning noise continued.

"Jorund? Are you all right?" Magnus repeated with concern.

He nodded.

"Something odd is happening here," Magnus contended. "You have not been yourself since learning of Inga's and the girls' deaths."

"I do not want to speak of that," he said icily. "Best we pull anchor and get rid of this bothersome whale. If we cannot move quickly enough to lose her, then we must kill the beast."

He thought he heard a squealy voice in the distance say, *Ha! I would like to see you try.*

Closer at hand, Magnus was not about to drop the subject. "Some people think a man must talk

25

of his heart-pain, lest it eat away at his innards . . . turn him mad with grief."

"Are you implying that I have gone berserk?"

Magnus pursed his lips and tugged at one of his big ears pensively. "Mayhap. Leastways, a little barmy."

Jorund grunted with disgust.

"Oh, I know you harbored no great affection for Inga, but your daughters . . . well, 'tis clear they held a special place in your soul."

"Have a caution, Magnus. You go too far," he warned.

But as always, his brother failed to heed sound advice and blathered on. "I know that I would surely tear out my hair in mourning if I lost my son . . . or daughter."

"And which son—or daughter—would that be?" Jorund asked with a hint of humor. It was hard to stay angry with his well-meaning brother.

"Any one of my sons . . . or daughters," Magnus answered, lifting his chin defensively. His brother followed the old custom of *more danico* and had two wives, in addition to three current mistresses . . . or was it four? All told, his seed had produced eight sons and five daughters . . . all with big ears.

Jorund made a *tsk*ing sound at his brother, whom he loved dearly, despite his nagging ways.

"I will work out my own problems in my own time and way," he told Magnus. "For now we must make haste and try to outrun this killer whale." They had anchored offshore in a small cove the night before so that they could draw fresh water from a stream on a nearby island. There were no human inhabitants that they could see. Still, they had slept aboard ship as a precaution.

Turning away, he gave orders to his crew to pull up the anchor and man their sea chests. His longship, built by his brother Rolf, was not an overlarge vessel. There were thirty-two oar holes on each side, manned by as many men who sat on their own personal sea chests rather than benches. Next to them were another thirty-two seamen, who would relieve them when their arms grew weary.

"It won't come up," a seaman soon informed him. "The anchor must have caught in some seaweed when the whale bumped us."

In the meantime, the whale was back to prodding the ship with its tail fins and snout. *Enough of this nonsense!*

Jorund said a foul word and began to remove his clothing—mantle, tunic, skin boots, *braies*—knowing he was going to have to dive below and try to loosen the tangled anchor. He could have sworn he heard a high-pitched peal of laughter, but when he glanced about the longship, he saw naught but his sailors staring back at him with worry.

"Becalm yourselves, men," he told them. "We will soon be on our way. I am an excellent swimmer and have great fame for holding my breath underwater. Leather-lunged, my father used to say of me." He was not boasting, merely stating a fact to put them at ease.

Once he was naked, except for his sheathed sword, which was attached to a wide belt at his waist and secured to his thigh with a leather thong, he dove into the water. It was surprisingly warm near the surface. Though the sea became colder the deeper he went, it should have been frigid near Iceland. He would have to ponder that puzzle later. *Even so, 'tis icy enough to shrivel even the grandest cock into a nub,* he thought with a shiver.

And what makes you think yours is so grand? he heard the whale remark with a laugh.

Oh, God! You again? Jorund commented dryly to himself as he sawed with his sword at the seaweed wrapped around the rope and anchor. He soon discovered that there was no way he could disentangle the metal anchor from the grassy tentacles. The more he tossed aside, the more seemed to appear in their place. He would have to cut the rope.

Stealthily, the whale had swum underwater and was watching his endeavors with interest.

For some reason he felt no fear . . . just disgust that this animal was causing him so much trouble.

Putting his sword back in the scabbard, he swam to the surface and took several deep gulps of air.

Magnus and all the seamen were staring over the side rail at him. Seabirds were whirling overhead in anticipation of some tasty morsel. He hoped it was not him.

"Is it free?" Magnus asked.

Jorund shook his head, still breathless. When he was able to speak, he informed his brother, "It's that special seal rope that Rolf insists on using. It will take me a little longer." Many ship owners bought the prized seal rope in the markets of Birka and Hedeby. Known for its sturdiness, it was cut in one single strip, like a spiral, from the hide of a seal or walrus. Unfortunately, it was difficult to slice through with a sword.

With one last deep inhalation of air, Jorund dove under the briny depths again. As expected, the whale was waiting for him. This time, as he sawed away with haste, the whale began a new game— butting Jorund's bare arse with its big nose. That was all he needed . . . a randy she-whale!

Finally the rope broke free. He sheathed his sword and was about to swim back to the surface when the whale shot forward and took him in her mouth, his head sticking out one side of her mouth and his flailing legs out the other side. He could feel the whale's massive teeth pressing against his stomach and buttocks, but Thora must be holding him with extra gentleness, for the teeth did not pierce his skin.

"Unteeth me, you lackbrain whale."

The only response was a chirping laugh.

He should have been mortally afraid. He was not.

At first he laughed silently at the great trick. The skalds would be telling this saga forever-more. No doubt there would even be a praise-poem honoring Jorund, the warrior who rode in the cradle of a killer whale's mouth and lived to tell the tale. Soon his mirth disappeared, how-ever, when he realized that he could not hold his breath much longer and that the whale was swim-ming at great speed . . . *away* from the longship. Once, when the whale came to the surface briefly, Jorund noted with distress that the longship was already far away . . . much too far for him to swim back. Unless the whale returned him.

But no. Thora had other plans.

With a squeal and a chirping noise of glee, the whale submerged again, and all of Jorund's silent screams and flailing limbs could not dissuade her.

Soon water rushed into his nostrils and all the orifices of his body. He could no longer hold his breath and took in great swallows of seawater. As his long hair came loose from its queue and swirled about his face, blinding him, a light-headedness overtook him, which was not altogether unpleasant. And he thought, *So I will break the raven's fast thus—by sea, rather than battlefield? So this is how it ends?*

Not quite, the whale answered. *The Fates have other plans for you, Viking.*

Chapter Two

2000 A.D. Galveston, Texas

> "Star light, star bright,
> First star I see tonight,
> I wish I may, I wish I might,
> Have my wish come true tonight."

Maggie McBride was about to enter the bedroom of her daughters, Suzy and Beth, when she heard them reciting, in unison, the childish rhyme. She'd already tucked them in and given them their customary good-night kisses, accompanied by the usual tickle. It wasn't surprising that the minute she'd departed, they'd jumped out of their beds, up to some harmless mischief . . . and it was no big deal, really. Maggie had learned to pick her battles when it came to her kids.

With a smile, she stepped back into the hall, then peered around the doorjamb to see them leaning out their bedroom window, gazing at an especially bright, flickering star. Their young, nine-year-old voices carried a breathy tone of wistful belief in the magic of the constellations as they repeated the old nursery rhyme.

Was I ever that innocent? Did I ever believe in miracles?

Shimmying their tummies back on the windowsill, they stood and adjusted their respective nightshirts—Suzy's a shocking pink image of Ricky Martin, and Beth's a rendition of Keiko, the killer whale—no less an idol to her than her sister's rock star *du jour*. Aside from their opposite personalities and interests, the girls were identical twins, both flashing brand-new shiny braces on their teeth and both sporting long mops of naturally curly hair, which was braided for sleep now into single tails down to their shoulder blades. They'd inherited their bad bites and honey blond locks from a father they'd never met—Judd Haskell. Maggie's hair was coal black and straight as a pin . . . and thanks to a recent hair adventure gone awry, *G. I. Jane* short. But they did have her cornflower blue eyes.

"My wish was that Mom would *finally* find a husband," Suzy confessed to her sister. They still hadn't noticed her standing in the hallway.

Beth nodded gravely. "Mine, too."

Maggie cringed. *Not again!*

"I am *not* spending one more Christmas at

Grandpa Haskell's farm, I'll tell you that," Suzy declared vehemently. "All he does is give us sermons on how bad it is here in the city, and how we should come live with him and Grandma. As if! And no disrespect or nothin', but I'm tired of all those stories about our dad before he died in that skydiving accident. What was a doctor doing skydiving anyhow? You'd think he was a saint the way Grandpa talks. 'If your father was alive, this . . .' Or, 'If your father was alive, that . . .' Sheesh!"

"If he was so wonderful," Beth pointed out, "how come he never married our mom?"

"Right," Suzy agreed.

Maggie barely stifled a gasp. How did they know that Judd had refused to marry her when he found out she was pregnant? Having a wife and family never would have fit into his high-risk, free-as-a-bird lifestyle. She prayed God they were unaware of an additional fact: that he'd wanted her to get an abortion. No, there was no way they could find that out. She'd never told anyone. Soon after that horrible meeting, Judd had died, the result of one of his never-ending adventures.

"And Grandma is no different," Suzy went on. "She keeps harping on single mothers, as if it's Mom's fault she had to raise us alone."

"I know," Beth said with a groan. "Last time, Grandma was quoting statistics she heard on some TV commercial about how daughters who are raised without a father often don't finish high school, and lots and lots of them get pregnant before they're sixteen."

Beth and Suzy exchanged a look at that last bit of information. "Gross!" they both exclaimed at the same time. Boys weren't even of interest to them yet, let alone sex or anything leading to babies.

"But, you know," Beth offered thoughtfully, "I betcha we could make Mom search for a dad a little harder if *she* believed all that stuff. She keeps saying school is so important."

"And I betcha we could stay home this Christmas if there were a dad in the house," Suzy added.

"Yep, a dad wouldn't let them badger Mom into giving in. He'd tell them"—here Beth's voice dropped into a low, masculine tone—" 'Sorry, folks, but the girls can't come for Christmas this year. We're a *family* now, and we need our girls to stay home for a *family* Christmas. My girls have gotta help me go out into the forest and chop down a tree. Maybe we'll even chop us a load of firewood to bring back in the pickup truck.' "

"That would be so perfect," Beth commented, "especially if there was snow. A dad, a real tree, a fire with our stockings hanging on the mantel, and snow!"

The audible sighs that followed were poignant with dreaminess.

As distressed as Maggie was over this wistful conversation, she had to smile. There were no forests in their neighborhood. An artificial tree had done them nicely for nine years now. They had no fireplace for that truckload of wood or the stockings. Nor was her driveway big enough for her Volvo *and* a truck. As for snow in Galveston for Christmas . . . *Forget it!*

Despite her half smile, she felt like weeping.

"Mom keeps saying she's happy the way things are," Suzy complained.

I am. I am. Oh, it gets lonely on occasion, but let's face it: I'm thirty-two years old, and I'm not about to give up my hard-earned independence at this late date. It's taken me too long to get where I am now. Besides, I gave up on the Prince Charming dream a long time ago. If only my two munchkins would give up on the perfect-dad dream.

"But *I'm* not happy, you know. Not one bit."

"Me neither," Beth agreed.

Maggie's heart went out to her two precious daughters. There *was* a hole in their lives without a father. She knew that. But sometimes no father was better than a bad father. And Judd would have been a terrible father, no doubt about it. Besides, she'd done a darn good job playing mommy *and* daddy to them, and raising herself up by the bootstraps as well to the point where she could now proudly proclaim herself Dr. Margaret McBride, psychologist.

"Mom is so beautiful. Just like Demi Moore," Beth added. "Everyone says so. Even with that haircut. And especially since she got that rad belly-button ring. I still can't believe she did it. She could get any man she wanted."

Maggie didn't know about getting any man she wanted, especially since she couldn't remember the last time she'd had a real date. But she was with the girls on one thing: she couldn't believe she'd gotten the belly-button ring, either. It was so out of character for her.

When Maggie was a young girl, she had developed earlier than her friends and was the brunt of many taunts from adolescent boys based on the mistaken belief that big breasts meant hot babe. Of course, the rest of her body had eventually caught up with her breasts—though she was far too curvy for her taste, despite constant dieting—but she'd never gotten over the habit of overcompensating for her endowments with full-cut clothes and an almost prissy social lifestyle. Until recently, that was.

The haircut had been her idea . . . a breaking free of the old when she'd received her doctorate degree last spring. Who knew the beautician would go so wild?

The belly-button ring, on the other hand, had *not* been her idea. It was the price she'd had to pay for losing a bet with her daughters, who had amazingly come through with straight *A*s for two semesters, and completed a daily regimen of household chores. Dr. Spock would have been horrified at her lack of parenting skills in using a bet to motivate her daughters. It was worth it, though. Not because of Beth, who loved school, but because of Suzy, who usually cruised along, content with *C* grades. And having the dishes done and the laundry folded without an argument had been nine months of heaven.

The belly-button ring could be removed.

"Yep," Suzy agreed.

Huh?

"Mom *is* so beautiful she could get any man she wanted," Suzy continued.

Oh. That.

"Even Ricky Martin."

The two girls giggled at that outlandish prospect: Maggie the psychologist and Mr. Teenage Heartthrob. Actually, that wasn't quite true . . . he appealed to lots more than adolescent girls.

"The only thing is, Suz, remember our match-making effort last year with the assistant manager of Shop 'n' Save. Whooee! It was a disaster from the get-go," Beth reminded her. "I thought Mom would like a younger man. She *is* cool . . . for a mom. And Spike was, you know, major cute! Go figure."

"But eighteen?" Suzy grimaced in remembrance. "Mom about swallowed a bird. She was soooo mad!"

Maggie clamped a palm over her mouth to keep from laughing out loud. Spike—the little snot—had taken one look at her belly-button ring and invited her to the drive-in. *Ha! Not in this lifetime!*

"That fiasco came right after we tried to fix her up with Rita's vet," Suzy remembered.

Rita was their ten-year-old, twenty-pound Persian cat. This was the same vet who'd made an astute observation about Rita one day; "Your cat doesn't stray far from her food dish, does she?"

"Who knew Dr. Cheswick was gay?" Beth whispered the last word.

I did. The minute I saw him.

"And then there was the state trooper who visited our school."

"Yeah." Beth sighed. "He had the neatest buzz cut."

It *was* an attractive haircut. And George *was* handsome as all get-out. Too bad his political views on guns and minority groups had clashed with hers on the first meeting.

Suzy giggled at some remembrance. "How about the priest you brought home for dinner?"

"How could I know he was a priest? Sheesh! He was wearing a jogging suit," Beth said defensively, "and to-die-for Nike Air Jordans."

37

Now, that one was hugely embarrassing.

"Well, Christmas is only three months away. She leaves us no choice," Suzy asserted, straightening her narrow shoulders with resolve. "If she can't find a dad for us on her own . . . well, maybe"—she motioned her head toward the heavens outside their window—"God can help."

Beth brightened with understanding. "Right. How can Mom get mad at God?"

"Exactly. She couldn't possibly blame us." Suzy blinked innocently at her sister.

Maggie thought about stepping into the room and setting the girls straight, but somehow she couldn't burst their bubble. They had plenty of time to learn that dreams came true only in the movies.

Before hopping into their beds, they each took one last look at the wishing star, then gasped. Maggie stifled a gasp, too.

It almost seemed as if the star winked at them.

Then their attention was diverted elsewhere.

"Oooh, Suz. Look. Look at that new formation of stars over there. Doesn't it resemble a . . . a whale?"

Suzy smiled widely at Beth from her matching poster bed. "That has to be a good sign."

When Maggie entered her own bedroom a short time later, she couldn't help herself. Drawn to the large, double-hung windows, she glanced up at the sky.

The new stars were gone.

The next day

"Mother! He's bald!" Suzy exclaimed the moment Dr. Harrison Seabold was out of hearing range. With a grimace of distaste, she added, "Your first date in, like, forever, and you had to pick a baldy?"

"Susan Marie McBride! Shhh!" Maggie cautioned her daughter and darted a quick glance at her boss's departing back to make sure he hadn't overheard. They'd just entered Orcaland, the marine park that was part of the huge amusement complex on Galveston Bay known as Marine Kingdom. Harry had gone off to buy snow cones for the four of them. "Besides, he's not my date," she added.

"It's not polite to say *bald* anymore," Beth corrected with an air of one-upmanship. "He's follically challenged."

Suzy and Beth were dressed identically today—something they usually avoided with a passion—in jeans shorts and white T-shirts proclaiming *Twins Rule*. And they were both in a snit . . . something to do with a star and a father-hunt and their mother not cooperating. Even if she hadn't overheard their conversation the night before, Maggie would be able to tell that the girls were up to something. They were so transparent. She narrowed her eyes at them. If they were seriously starting that husband/daddy business again, she was going to wring their cute little necks. Really.

Besides, she'd already decided as she lay sleepless last night to have the biggest, best Christmas ever for the girls this year. At home. Case closed. No need for a daddy, after all. Snow and a fireplace were out of her realm, but if they really, really wanted a live tree, who said she couldn't handle that herself? *I am woman. Hear me chop evergreen.*

Suzy made a nose-wrinkling face at Beth. Beth lifted her pert nose in the air with a superior sniff and twitched back at her.

"You think all men should look like Ricky Martin," Beth continued. "How many posters of him do you have on the wall on your side of our bedroom? Huh? Huh?"

"Not as many as you have of Keiko the killer whale," Suzy countered. "Besides, you like Ricky Martin, too."

"Not as much as you."

"I just think it's stupid for us to go to the marine park *again*. I'd rather go on a roller coaster. We've already seen all there is to see at Orcaland." The last of her comments was directed at her sister with some hinted meaning. Presumably, there were better father prospects in an amusement park than a marine park.

Beth was very sensitive about her feelings for Keiko . . . for all killer whales in captivity, actually. Her precocious daughter even operated her own Web site for youths interested in the plight of the whales. Normally, with such criticism from her sister, she would launch into her pat adolescent lecture on the tragedy of the orcas. Instead, today she took a deep breath and explained, "What Suzy was trying to say, Mom, when she made that comment about Dr. Seabold being bald, is that we were sort of surprised that you would pick a bald man for a dad . . . I mean date."

"Don't start—"

"Okay, I admit the Shop 'n' Save guy was a bit young for you," Beth went on, "but isn't this going overboard in the other direction? I know you're always saying that it's what's inside that counts, and that brains are more important than brawn, but still—"

"He's not my date," Maggie interjected—again.

"Brains? Well, duh!" Suzy countered, ignoring her mother. "How many brains could a guy have when he parts his hair at the ear? He'd better hope the wind doesn't blow. And he certainly shouldn't go on any roller coasters." She threw in that last with a huge sigh as if it would be the greatest tragedy in the world—a dad who couldn't go on roller coasters. *Horrors!*

The twins contemplated Harry's admittedly hopeless comb-over hairstyle and grinned at each other. Instead of hiding his shiny pate, he was calling attention to it. You'd think a man with all his credentials in the psychiatric field would know better. *Men! And they say women are vain!*

The girls were really very close to each other, but their tempers had been riled today by the unseasonably hot temperatures for early October, and frustration over their matchmaking failures. And truthfully, they had been to this particular marine park at least a dozen times this year alone.

"Did you see those shorts he's wearing?" Apparently Suzy was still fixated on Harry as a daddy prospect. "They're *plaid.*" She said *plaid* as if it were something revolting like homework. Beth enjoyed school; Suzy put up with it.

"Hey, who named you the fashion police? I'm no fashion plate, either," Maggie interjected, pointing to her knee-length denim skirt and

41

cropped, short-sleeved Liz Claiborne sweater of faded blue.

But the girls weren't paying attention to her. Instead Suzy was continuing with her tirade against Harry's shorts. "Even worse, they're madras plaid. Talk about being lost in the sixties. Well, I'm not having a father who wears plaid, and that's final. Not to mention white socks and sandals. Gross!"

"You think everything is yucky if it doesn't come from The Gap."

"You think everything is yucky if it doesn't smell like a stinkin' fish."

"Whales are not fish. They're mammals."

"Fish, mammal, whatever . . . they stink."

"Oooooh!" Beth growled.

"Oooooh!" Suzy growled.

"Why don't you take a chill pill?"

"Why don't you try and make me?"

Whatever spirit of comradeship the two had been sharing fell apart then. Another moment and they would be rolling on the ground like a pair of puppies. Time for a mother intervention.

"That's enough! Both of you!" Maggie chided. Dropping down to a bench, she gathered them to either side of her. "Behave yourselves. Harry is a very nice man. I invited him to come with us today because he's worried about the clinic and whether it will close down under the new owners. He needs a distraction, not two smart-mouthed girls making fun of his appearance."

"Mom, we won't have to move if the clinic closes, will we?" Beth asked anxiously. Leave it to one of her daughters to hone in on the least pertinent point in her tirade. Obviously she was worried about a possible separation between herself and Gonzo, the star orca at the marine park, not the possible loss of her mother's job. Maybe this obsession with killer whales had gone too far. But that was a question she'd have to address later.

"I wouldn't mind moving to Houston. They have an awesome roller coaster at Rodeoland. It's not as good as the Vomit, though."

The Vomit? Maggie mouthed, then recalled that was the nickname for the Comet, the roller coaster at the amusement park affiliated with Marine Kingdom. Suzy adored roller coasters; Beth could take them or leave them; Maggie avoided them as much as possible. But that was incidental now. She pulled her attention to the present. "We are *not* moving, regardless of what happens with the clinic," she assured them. "But back to what I was telling you. I've taught you girls better than to make mean remarks about people's appearances. Remember how you felt when Joey Pisano called you Metal Mouth the first day you came to school with braces? And the Tin Grin Twins?"

Both girls nodded, and their faces flushed with shame that they'd been guilty of the same transgression.

"Listen, my sweeties, never judge a man—or woman—by what you see. You'll be wrong every time, I guarantee."

"But Mom . . ." they said simultaneously.

"And one last thing. I heard you girls last night. Forget about miracles. The only miracles in this life are the ones we create ourselves."

Suzy and Beth hung their heads—with remorse or disappointment, she couldn't tell. And, despite all her logical words, Maggie felt a twinge of regret that she'd come down so hard on them.

"Hey, toots," she teased Beth, tugging on her braids. "Don't we have a date with some orcas?"

The smile Beth plastered on her lips was clearly forced.

"And how about you, my little salsa princess? Maybe we could fit in one roller coaster ride before we go home today."

Suzy, too, forced a smile.

Maggie could see that the subject wasn't closed . . . not by a long shot. Obviously having a father was far more important to them than whales or scary rides.

Sometimes Maggie wished dreams really could come true.

They were sitting on the bleachers at the inner curve of the oceanarium that comprised the marine park. The oceanarium was a huge, five-acre inlet leading out to Galveston Bay. The orcas were prevented from escaping captivity by a net wall at the mouth of the inlet that stretched from the bottom of the water to ten feet above the surface. Because this particular sea pen was located outside the killer whale's normal habitat, there were special cooling tubes running along the bottom, and salt was added to the water.

They were watching Gonzo go through his paces, along with two baby killer whales, Mork and Mindy. The babies, which were the size of pickup trucks, performed only rudimentary tricks, like backflips and leaps into the air for food, but Gonzo was a real pro . . . and a ham, to boot. He sailed through hoops. He lobtailed the

44

crowd, splashing large amounts of water on them with his flukes, better known as flippers. He plopped himself up onto a platform. He squealed and chirped and generally appeared to be having a good time. He might be one of the top predators of the seas, but here at Orcaland he was a pussy-cat—letting the trainers ride on his back or put their heads inside his mouth where three dozen deadly teeth shone whitely in the bright sunlight. Maggie could see why Beth had developed such a strong affection for Gonzo—and all killer whales, for that matter.

Just then she heard Beth gasp.

"What? What?" she asked, quickly morphing into mother mode.

Beth was still gasping for breath and pointing out to sea, beyond the oceanarium. *Holy cow!* There was an enormous killer whale swimming just beyond the nets . . . circling and circling, blowing mists of spume, diving and coming up in geyser splashes of water.

It was not usual for free whales to approach the oceanarium because they did not roam the warmer, salty waters off of Texas, but this one must have been drawn by the other whales in captivity and the prospect of food. Or was this magnificent animal in distress?

As it began spyhopping—leaping out of the water almost in a perpendicular position—Gonzo did the same thing. They were mirroring each other's actions. Their loud chirps and whistles and squeals echoed across the inlet like eerie aquatic bullhorns. It appeared as if they were communicating frantically with each other.

That wasn't the most remarkable thing, though.

There was a man riding atop the killer whale. And he appeared to be holding on to the whale's dorsal fin for dear life.

But wait. Was he steering the mammal as if its fin were the rudder of a boat? Could this be a new addition to the marine park, staged as a grand entrance? *Wow!*

Or—*Oh, my God!*—was it a wild killer whale on the rampage?

The fine hairs stood out all over Maggie's body, and her intuition kicked in big-time. She knew— she just knew—that man was in real trouble.

"Slow down!" Jorund yelled to Thora.

Hold on, was the whale's only response as she blew enough spume out of her blowhole to drown a small village, and shot through the ocean like a rock from a catapult.

With the wind created by the beast's excessive speed, most of the substance landed on her reluctant passenger. Jorund tossed his hair back off his face and spit several times with distaste. Whale spume tasted as revolting as rancid lutefisk.

Jorund was so angry he could scarcely think or breathe.

And, yes, he had to admit it: he was so bloody frightened he might just wet his *braies*. If he were wearing *braies*, that was. And if he weren't already wet.

Apparently he had not drowned, after all. But in some ways he wished he had.

"I'm going to slice you up into the world's

46

biggest pile of whale blubber once we stop," he yelled at Thora. "I'm going to make enough whale soup to feed a nation. I'm going to make hatchets out of your teeth. I'm going to make a necklace to hold your ugly pig eyes. I'm going—"

Jorund never finished his sentence, because Thora performed another one of her quick dips in the ocean, which required her passenger to hold his breath.

When he came up again, Jorund continued his harangue: "And furthermore, the next time you decide to break your fast on shark, would you mind eating with your mouth closed? Your breath is enough to curdle milk."

Be quiet, Viking. We're almost there, Thora said with her usual chirps and squeals.

Jorund still couldn't believe he could understand whale talk. But that was neither here nor there. "Almost where?" he asked. Just then he noticed the huge net rising up high above the waves ahead.

She wouldn't, Jorund thought.

Thora increased her speed till the air whistled in Jorund's ears and his hair whipped back.

She would.

Before Jorund could blink, or say a silent prayer to the gods, Thora dipped down into the ocean and came back up in a truly impressive leap into the air. At the peak of her high jump, just before bending her massive body over into an arc for its return to the water, Thora shook herself, causing Jorund to lose his grasp on her top fin. With a scream of terror, Jorund flew through the air, over the net fence, and into the water beyond.

47

It's up to you now, Viking.

"What?" Jorund gurgled, still underwater.

Your fate.

Aaarrgh! Riddles again . . . whale riddles!

When he finally swam to the surface, his sword banging against his thigh, Jorund turned. Thora was nowhere to be seen.

Then, twisting toward the shore that was visible in the distance, Jorund saw a most amazing sight. There were people—many of them—and several whales, and melodic music in the air that sounded like *Oompapa, Oompapa, Oompapa* . . . and strange objects of many vivid colors twirling about in circles and on huge metal loops in the air.

Jorund began to swim toward the shore, even as he sighed deeply. There was only one explanation: he must have died, after all. Although he felt at peace, a sadness swept over him that he had not completed his father's work. *Ah, well! What must be, must be.*

This must be Asgard . . . Viking heaven.

With a rueful chuckle, he expressed a silent wish that his personal Valkyries would be buxom. After what he'd been through these past months, and having been wedlocked to a flat-chested woman, he deserved a well-endowed goddess. Mayhap his brother Rolf would be waiting on the shore to welcome him. Yea, if his brother had indeed passed to the other side before him, Rolf would ensure that there were big-breasted wenches aplenty to warm his bed furs.

Jorund had been swimming steadily shoreward, arm over arm, with his face in the water. He looked up now, jerked his head back, then looked again.

"Oh, holy Thor!"

Chapter Three

The man and the three captive orcas were swimming underwater now, blurrily visible in the blue water, heading straight for the bleacher area. When they were about thirty feet away, man and beasts dipped deep into the water, then came spyhopping up into four spectacular perpendicular leaps.

It was one thing to see a two-ton animal skyrocket from the water like one of God's blessed creatures. It was quite another thing to see a huge male, all sinewy muscles encased in a flawlessly proportioned body, perform the same remarkable feat, whipping a swath of long blond hair back off his face at the pinnacle of his surge.

It was especially remarkable because the man was naked. *Naked!* He wore nothing but a—*Oh, good Lord!*—was that a sheathed sword attached to a belt at his narrow waist and secured with a leather thong to his thigh? No wonder sirens could be heard in the distance; soon police would be swarming in like killer bees. No wonder there were screams of "Stand back! Stand back!" from a single security officer, who was having trouble getting through the crowd of three hundred or so spectators. The amphitheater further thwarted their progress, with no place for the spectators to exit, except where police would have to come in.

Bare seconds passed before the man came down from his leap and landed on his feet, standing in shoulder-high water. Then he began to walk up the sloping bottom toward them, the water revealing his nude body inch by glorious inch. With the lazy indifference of a man comfortable with his body, he reached up with both hands and finger-combed his long hair—surely a champagne blond when it was dry—off his face. Although his jaw was covered with several days' growth of whiskers, it didn't detract from his appeal at all. Despite his relaxed attitude, his eyes were wary.

Is this part of the act? If so, I'm impressed, Maggie thought, fanning her suddenly hot face with an Orcaland program.

"He's a trespasser!" one man in the crowd accused. "Put him in the slammer." The guy's stout body sported a T-shirt proclaiming, *If Swimming Is So Good for Your Weight, How Do You Explain Whales?*

"Ha!" the blond god exclaimed. He stood in water up to his waist now, at least fifteen feet away. "The first person who tries to slam me will be missing an essential body part. Besides, there is no such thing as trespassing in Valhalla." The man's voice carried over the crowd in a strange foreign accent.

"This ain't Vail, fella," a cowboy-clad, gray-haired man commented in a heavy Southern drawl. "This heah's Texas. You're 'bout two thousand miles off course. Ha, ha, ha!"

"Tax-us? Many lands require scutage, but ne'er have I heard of a country that asks to be taxed." The hunk just shook his head in confusion.

"Threatening an endangered species . . . the jerk!" another man called out. To Maggie's amazement, it was an outraged Harry, sitting beside her.

"I have not threatened anyone . . . yet," the stranger asserted. "And, in truth, I never 'jerked' anyone that I recall."

"Indecent exposure . . . arrest the man for public nudity," a middle-aged lady demanded as she peeked through the fingers that covered her eyes. Her T-shirt said, *All Men Are Idiots, and I Married the King*. Her bored husband sitting next to her wore a T-shirt that said, perhaps appropriately, *Sometimes I Wake Up Grumpy; Other Times I Just Let Her Sleep*. Maggie couldn't tell for sure if the "grumpy" lady was pleased or disappointed that the blond god stood in place momentarily, and was still covered to the waist by the murky water.

"Now I know that I have arrived in the strangest land of all. Since when has nudity become a crime?"

"A weapon . . . the maniac is carrying a weapon. Duck, everyone, duck!"

51

"Duck? What duck?" The man twisted his neck this way and that. Then he shrugged as if to indicate there was not a duck in sight.

Maggie was becoming as confused as this man appeared to be.

There was chaos all around them. Police and security guards were attempting to run forward, guns raised, but their progress was impeded by the capacity crowd, which was standing, inadvertently forming a barricade, some cheering, some screaming with fright, still others calling out their opinions. Even mild-mannered Harry, who claimed a longtime interest in orcas, was yelling with outrage at the interloper, whom he perceived as a threat to Gonzo, Mork, and Mindy.

But Maggie and her two daughters sat stone still, mesmerized by the spectacle unfolding before them.

"And you wanted to go roller coasting," Beth told her sister.

"This is better than *Jerry Springer,*" Suzy offered with awe.

But Maggie had more important things on her mind as she continued to gape at what had to be the most gorgeous man she'd ever seen—one of God's perfect creations, superbly formed and wonderfully wild, just like the orcas.

More than that, Maggie sensed an eerie connection between them . . . a connection that was getting stronger the closer he came.

"Cool!" Beth exclaimed.

"Ditto," Suzy added. Then: "So that's what a too-too looks like."

"Eeew. It looks like a fat worm."

"I didn't know men had hair *there.*"

It was then that Maggie registered the fact that her daughters, too, had been staring at the nude man, openmouthed, like every other female in the park. Even though his privates had been visible for only a few seconds, Maggie's maternal instincts kicked in. "Cover your eyes," she ordered.

Suzy looked at Beth. Beth looked at Suzy. They both looked at their mother—and laughed. "Yeah, right," they said simultaneously, and did just the opposite. Their eyes were glued to the man emerging slowly from the water, his step confident.

When he reached the bulkheads, he raised himself on braced arms, causing veins to stand out on the ropy muscles outlined under skin deeply tanned by the sun. As he panted to regain his breath, water drops glistened on silky chest hairs. *Lordy, Lordy!* She noticed the intricately etched arm rings that encircled his upper arms. Were they a new male fashion accessory . . . gold arm bracelets more suited to ancient warriors than modern man? If not, they should be.

Thank goodness, his more intimate body parts were now hidden by the bulkhead as he surveyed the crowd before him, as if searching for someone in particular. Maggie saw confusion in his eyes, which opened wider and wider as they moved along the rows of people gawking at him like a freak at a sideshow. He was either a really good actor, or he was a man who'd fallen into a situation he did not understand.

Either way, this was a day Maggie would not soon forget.

* * *

Jorund was totally confused.

Well, he supposed that was understandable. Entering Asgard, land of the gods, would muddle even the most clearheaded warrior.

Still, it passed all bounds, this sight that he beheld. If this was the otherworld, then the land of the gods was mightily overvalued. Where were the walls made of golden spears and the roof of gold shields? Supposedly, Valhalla, hall of the gods, had 540 doors, each big enough to allow eight hundred armed men through side by side. Furthermore, he saw no gilded longships, nor groaning boards overladen with plentiful foods and tuns of ale.

Jorund blinked with bafflement.

Not a god was there in sight—not Odin, nor Thor, nor any of the lesser deities, not even the mischievous Loki . . . and for a certainty, missing were the beautiful Valkyries that were supposed to escort brave warriors into Valhalla.

Most important, he saw no one who even remotely resembled his brother Rolf. That at least was good news. Apparently his brother was still alive.

Too bad Jorund was not.

Best he gather his wits about him and study the situation. He should pull himself up onto land and walk among these curious people who were gaping at him as if he were the strange one. However, he was much aware of his nudity, and did not relish displaying his manly parts before one and all—impressive though they might be. He was little inclined toward modesty, but he would be a lackwit not to mind being the only one unclothed . . . and vulnerable.

An idea came unbidden to him. What if this

were a test? Mayhap this was just the outer portal to Valhalla—not unlike the Christian limbo, leading to heaven. Mayhap he must endure some ordeal in order to finally enter the hall of the gods. Could being naked in a clothed crowd constitute an ordeal?

Without hesitation, he levered himself up onto the narrow, wharflike ledge, pretending unconcern over his nudity. Standing, legs braced apart, hands clasped behind his back, he harbored a passing vain concern that his staff might be all shriveled up, as male genitals were wont to be when in cool water, but he resisted the impulse to glance downward. Instead, with practiced nonchalance, he looped his thumbs in his leather belt and slowly scanned the crowd.

On his initial survey of the staring faces, he noticed children. In a blink he grabbed a large toweling cloth off the ground near his feet and wrapped it about his hips, leaving an opening on his sword side. It was one thing to exhibit bold arrogance before adults, quite another to show himself to children. He was not a pederast. Who knew there would be children in Asgard? But he supposed it made sense. There had to be a place for all the young persons to go.

But, oh, that brought another thought to mind: would he be seeing his own precious dearlings here . . . Greta and Girta?

No, it was impossible. Where did these fanciful ideas come from? No doubt he had salt on the brain from all that time spent underwater. His brother Magnus would call it pickling of the brain, though most Vikings did it with mead, rather than brine, and were known as aleheads.

Enough of this nonsense! He was a warrior . . . one of the finest in all the Varangian Guard. Where were his well-honed instincts? Why was he standing about waiting for something to happen? Every good soldier knew it was best to take the offensive.

He inhaled deeply and let all the sounds of this unfamiliar place seep into his pores. Some part of him had already suspected that foreign tongues were being spoken here, yet he'd been able to understand—and speak—moments ago. At first all the words had seemed to blend together, like endless, raucous chatter. No matter. He would do what Thora, the killer whale, had instructed him: *Listen, Viking. Listen with your heart.* Well, he did not know about listening with his heart, but he opened his mind as best he could and concentrated with all his might. Soon the words began to separate, like wheat from chaff.

"Armed and dangerous," one man shouted in an accusing manner.

"Well, of course I'm armed," he snapped back, and was surprised, just as he had been moments ago, that the words coming out of his mouth were in this strange language. "And you had best hope that you do not learn firsthand just how dangerous I am."

The man who had shouted stepped back, even though he was separated from Jorund by the several hundred people sitting and standing in the bench area. The man exchanged glances with some men behind him who wore identical clothing—dark blue *braies* and long-sleeved, collared *sherts* of a lighter hue. Silver, starlike, metal emblems flashed on their chests, and on their

56

heads were ridiculous round hats with hard brims, which were the oddest helmets he'd ever seen. They would be no protection at all in a real battle. By the looks of their livery, these men must be the royal *hird* for the king of this land, or guardsmen to one god or another, if this indeed were Asgard.

More important, the men carried metal implements in their hands, which they pointed in his direction. He sensed that they were weapons of some type.

Surreptitiously, he loosened his sword from its scabbard, making ready to defend himself, if necessary. He would not attack unless he was provoked, but it was always best to be prepared when in hostile territory.

It appeared the armed guard was having trouble spearheading a way through the mob, so he had a few more moments to study the situation. Stepping back slightly, he began to examine the people standing and sitting in the arena.

What manner of dress was this that people wore here? The arms and legs of many of the women and children were bare, as were those of some of the men. He supposed it was in deference to the heat. Still, it appeared odd to him. The majority of the men, besides the guardsmen, wore short-sleeved, collarless *sherts* with indecipherable messages on them, like *Just Do It, Forget about Your Gardens; Show Me Your Busch, Houston Oilers,* and *My Wild Oats Have Turned to Shredded Wheat.* Later he would have to ponder this bizarre business of people wearing words on their bodies, like human books. In addition, these people wore *braies* made of coarse-woven blue fabric similar to sailcloth, and high-heeled leather boots.

High-heeled boots on men! Are the men of this place demented? Do they not know how ridiculous they look? Do their toes not hurt and their ankles not ache at the end of a day spent in men's work?

His keen eyes were scanning the front row now, left to right, when his attention snagged on one particular person, then doubled back for closer inspection. Initially, he'd thought it was a diminutive, dark-haired male because of the short haircut in the Frankish mode, which exposed the nape and ears. But no, no male had the curves this person did. Full, rounded globes filled a collarless, knitted *shert* that had short sleeves and stretched barely to the waist. From the arch of her hips to just above the knee she was covered by a garment of the same blue fabric as some of the booted men.

But then she stood, as if involuntarily, and raised a hand to her hair nervously, which cause the *shert* to lift and the bottom garment to recede, leaving a band of bare skin exposed. It was that area between her *shert* and her lower apparel that caused his breath to catch and his heart to skip a beat. In that region where smooth skin gleamed with a summery glow was the most enticing belly button he had ever seen—and he had seen more than a few—pierced with a small golden ring. It was not the first such ornament he'd ever viewed, but most of them had been on houris in Eastern harems.

He couldn't help smiling. In fact, another part of his body was starting to show its appreciation, as well. He had to be thankful now for the toweling cover over his nether parts.

Jorund raised his eyes and met the direct gaze of the woman with man-hair. Her eyes were wide and blue as a springtime sky in the Baltic, fringed by black lashes that curled up prettily. Her nose was straight, her cheekbones high and her mouth full and rosy red. It was the kind of mouth that led a man to wicked thoughts, especially in combination with that belly ornament.

She did not return his smile, but instead continued to stare at him as if hit by a thunderbolt.

He knew how she felt. Ripples of some odd connection were assailing him as well.

He inclined his head to her and said, "M'lady."

She nodded back at him, but instead of saying, "My lord," in response, the normal expression when returning a salutation, she exclaimed, "Good Lord!"

He wondered if she were one of the Valkyries sent to welcome him. If so, he would not protest—not even with that man-hair. Her body was the type meant to please a man—rather, him in particular—of that he was convinced. He held out his hand to her as he recalled that the Valkyries were to take the chosen warriors by the hand and lead them into Valhalla.

Instead of stepping up to him and leading him off, the woman plopped back down into her seat, dazed with bewilderment.

"Mother! That man is flirting with you," someone said, diverting Jorund's attention away from his Valkyrie.

"I am *not* flirting. I was merely . . ." Jorund's

words trailed off as he got his greatest shock of the day. The person speaking had been a young girl, no more than eight or nine, and her identical twin sat next to her. At first he thought it was Greta and Girta, but soon decided he was mistaken. The two girls with honey blond braids and a slight dotting of freckles on their small faces were older than Greta and Girta had been, and their hair was a darker shade of blond than his daughters', and they wore strange metal jewelry on their teeth.

But, oh, look at that! One twin had ribands tied at the ends of her braids—multicolored ribands, in all the colors of the rainbow. The other wore cloth shoes of a bright red color . . . not silk harem shoes as Girta had requested, but close enough, to his way of thinking.

Was it a cruel jest of the gods? Or was it a sign? He had no time to ponder further. His attention had been distracted by the woman and two girls, but not so much that he didn't notice the moment that the soldiers broke through the crowd. They were rushing at him now, weapons raised. In fact, one of the weapons made a loud popping sound. He felt the whiz of air just past his ear, not unlike that of an arrow in flight, and then noticed the splintering of a lettered board behind him.

"No shooting, you fool! Hold your weapon," one of the soldiers yelled at another, who responded, "I thought he was reaching for a weapon."

He hadn't been, but he was now. With well-honed instincts, Jorund drew his sword from its scabbard and prepared to fight off the assault—

though why they should be assaulting him was unknown to him at this point. There were at least ten of them, but he had been outnumbered before. He could handle this.

"Halt!" one guardsman yelled. "Drop your weapon."

"Use the stun gun," another guardsman suggested.

Jorund had no idea what a "stung one" was, but he was taking no chances. When he did not comply, but instead took the battle stance, crouching with his sword at the ready, another guardsman raised a weapon of a different kind. In the blink of an eye, Jorund felt a sharp pain in his shoulder, which radiated down his arm to his fingertips, causing him to momentarily loosen his grip on his sword. Shocked, Jorund saw that there was no blood, and yet he felt as if he'd been struck by lightning. In that split second of inattention, the guardsmen jumped on him, knocking him to the ground.

In a daze, Jorund realized that he had been bested. It was humiliating that he—the most noted warrior in all the Norse and Saxon and Frank lands—should be struck down by such weak specimens, but there it was.

Even as he fought against the overpowering waves of dizziness that he sensed would lead to loss of consciousness, he was somehow able to hear and understand the words Greta and Girta sobbed pitifully: "Mother, help him. Please. You have to help him." *Ah, good girls! That's it, intercede on my behalf.*

But, no, he reminded himself, they were not

Greta and Girta. These were merely twins who resembled his dead daughters. And he needed no intercession from children. If only he could stand. For some reason, though, he was not even able to lift his arms.

"Shhh! He's a stranger," the mother answered in a voice that he recognized, even in his foggy, limp condition, as husky and deliciously sensual.

"No! No, he's not a stranger!" one of the twins wailed. "He's *the one*."

"He is not *the one*," the mother said indignantly.

"Which one?" he tried to ask, but, though his lips appeared to move, no words came out.

"Don't let them hurt him," the other twin cried. "He's not dangerous, Mommy. He's just mixed-up."

Mixed-up? That's an understatement.

They were all standing about, peering down at him as he lay ignominiously on the ground—the twins, the mother, and several guardsmen.

Finally he heard the woman with the man-hair tell the guardsmen in an authoritative voice, "I'm a doctor. I work at the Rainbow Psychiatric Hospital."

She's a dock whore? And she works in a hospitium? Amazing!

"This man is clearly under mental duress. He's my . . . uh, patient."

Man-tail door-ass? Pay-shun? I do not think I care to be described thus. He wasn't sure of the meaning of those words she'd used to describe him, but they must not be good, since the two girls gasped and the guardsmen growled with displeasure. But then, maybe not, he thought, when the girls turned to their mother as if she'd granted them some great favor . . . like his life.

He tried to speak up in protest, but his lips would not move. However, he was able to raise his eyelids to half-mast and assess his surroundings.

"Release him to my custody," the dock whore demanded.

That he understood. How ferocious she sounded! She really must be his personal Valkyrie. He had to smile at that, or at least try to smile.

That was when another man emerged into his line of vision—the strangest creature in this strangest of lands. The man wore *braies* that reached only as far as his thighs and a patterned and colored *shert*, but most unusual was his hairstyle. Bald he was on the top—like Jorund's cousin, Arnaud No-Hair—but this fellow chose to grow his side hairs excessively long on one side and fling them over his pate like a drape. No doubt it was the custom of some minor tribe in this land.

The man with the hair drape spoke to the woman with man-hair. It appeared as if he was arguing with Jorund's Valkyrie. How dared he! But when Jorund tried to rise to her defense, his brain spun woozily, and he dropped back, weak as a blood-drained warrior after a fierce battle.

The dock whore and the man with the hair drape stared down at him, still debating some issues that sounded like *unethical, illogical,* and *emotional.* The woman began to drop down on her knees at his side, but a burly guardsman held her back. "He needs my help. You didn't have to hurt him," she accused in a loud voice. "He was just . . . confused."

"Confused? The psycho had a sword," the

guardsman yelled back at her. "And he's not hurt, just temporarily stunned."

He could hear a loud, high-pitched noise in the distance, like a violent tornado at its most destructive peak—but no, this was no storm approaching. Instead, white-clothed men rushed forward and lifted him onto a canvas pallet. To his satisfaction, it took four of the white-dressed men to lift him.

"Take him to the Rainbow Psychiatric Hospital," she told one of the newcomers.

The leader of the white-dressed men glanced at the head guardsman, who shrugged as if Jorund were a problem the guardsmen would just as soon not handle. "You'd better put him in a strait-jacket, though," the chieftain said. "When the effects of the stun gun wear off, he's going to be really pissed."

Jorund tried to focus on these foreign words, as the orca had instructed him, but his brain was too muddled right now.

"Maggie, do you think this is wise?" the hair-drape man whispered to Jorund's Valkyrie.

"Yes, I do. My instincts tell me that he's not dangerous, just disoriented. And you know my instincts are good, Harry. You've told me so dozens of times."

Her name is Mag-he. A woman with man-hair, whose name is Mag-he?

"But, Maggie . . ." Hair-drape pleaded. "He's clearly disturbed. Don't you think the state hospital would be a better place for him?"

"No, Harry," Mag-he asserted. "As mental-health professionals, we have a responsibility to assume care for a disturbed individual, especially since we're the caregivers on-site. After all, he hasn't hurt anyone."

Although he somehow understood the language, Jorund failed to understand everything that the woman was saying. Still, he liked when she grew assertive in that sexy voice of hers, especially when it was on his behalf. With an irrelevance totally out of place in this bizarre situation, he couldn't help wondering how that voice would sound when she was being assertive in other situations, like bedplay.

Now, where did that thought come from? I haven't been interested in a woman in that way in a long, long time.

Hair-drape took charge then, to Jorund's surprise. He addressed the guardsman in an unexpectedly imposing voice. "I'm Dr. Harry Seabold, director of the Rainbow Psychiatric Hospital." He took a small square of parchment from a leather object that must have been hidden in a flap of his short *braies* "Officers, I'm assuming responsibility for this man."

Who? Me? Well, then, this is a new turn of events. Jorund concluded that he must have been assigned two Valkyries—a male and a female one—and both of them dock whores. He had never heard of such before, but he supposed it was possible.

Even as he was succumbing to the weight of unconsciousness, he thought he heard the twins whisper as one to their mother, "Thank you, Mommy."

He amended his earlier thought then. He must

have four Valkyries: a man, a woman, and two children. Maybe he was a more favored warrior with the gods than even he had imagined.

"And you won't be sorry, Mommy," one of the twins said with childish earnestness, "because we've decided"—she paused for dramatic effect, as young girls often did— "he really is *the one*."

The woman with the man-hair and the sex-voice groaned in the most beguiling way.

And Jorund decided he was going to like being "the one."

Chapter Four

Two days later . . .

"How was school today?" Maggie asked her girls as they sat down at the kitchen table to eat a late dinner.

It was a nightly ritual that Maggie insisted upon, even though their eating habits were divergent, to say the least. Rita, their ten-year-old, twenty-pound, white Persian cat, sat queenlike on the floor between Suzy and Beth, just waiting for a scrap to fall her way.

"Great," they both answered through mouthfuls of food.

"Didn't you have a math test today?" she asked Suzy.

It was Beth who responded. "I got a ninety-five."

Maggie sent Suzy a motherly glower, and Suzy sent Beth a sisterly glower.

Suzy colored and tried to change the subject. "How is *he* today?"

Maggie didn't need a name to know who Suzy was referring to.

"You know I can't talk about my patients," Maggie replied firmly, but she wasn't about to let Suzy escape so easily. "How did you do on the math test, Susan Marie?" Her daughter knew she meant business when Maggie used her full name.

"I got a seventy-two," Suzy admitted. "Sheesh, who cares about percentages anyhow?" Then the little imp added, "Maybe we need a new bet to make me study harder."

"Yeah, the house has been looking a little dingy since Suz and I stopped helping out," Beth contributed. "Yep, another bet would do the trick."

Maggie raised her eyebrows skeptically. "What? So I can be forced to get tatoos—or something worse—this time?" Maggie asked with a little laugh.

"Nah, we had something else in mind," Suzy said, exchanging a meaningful look with her sister.

Something else?

"There are some things in life worth getting dishpan hands over," Beth pointed out woefully.

Some things? Like what?

"Or homework fatigue," Suz added with an exaggerated woe-is-me expression.

Suzy didn't have to tell her what that "something else" entailed. Maggie already knew. The "something else" was roughly six-foot-four and bone-meltingly gorgeous.

"Nurse Hatcher said he hasn't talked at all in

the two days he's been at the hospital. She calls him a stud muffin." Beth giggled as she relayed this information.

Gladys Hatcher . . . our head nurse . . . calls him a stud muffin? Maggie gasped. "Nurse Hatcher has been talking to you about a hospital patient?" As good a nurse as Gladys was, this constituted cause for dismissal.

"Oh, she didn't tell *me*," Beth was quick to correct. "Suz and I overheard her talking to another nurse this afternoon when we were waiting for you to leave work. The bench we were sitting on was right outside the nurse's lounge, and the window was open, and, well . . ." Beth shrugged as if she'd been helpless not to eavesdrop in such a situation.

Maggie was going to have a talk with Gladys about this breach, even if it was unintentional. Anyone could have been passing by, including representatives of the Medic-All Corporation, which was currently in negotiations to purchase Rainbow.

"Mom, we've been talking, and, well . . ." Beth glanced at Suzy, then took a deep breath before continuing. "We think you should let us talk to him."

Maggie went slack-jawed with incredulity. But only for a second. "Absolutely not! No way! Don't either of you even think of approaching this man."

"But Mom," Suzy pleaded. "You already told the police he's not dangerous . . . just a little mixed-up."

"That's beside the point," she declared indignantly. "In fact, you girls stay away from the hospital until further notice. If I'm late picking you up at school, you stay in the after-school day-care program till I arrive."

"Day care!" they cried simultaneously. "We're not children."

"You're not adults, either. And while we're on the subject, there will be no more fixating on this stranger as . . . as . . ."

"A dad?" Beth offered.

Maggie put her face in both hands and groaned.

"Or a husband?" Beth added with a dramatic sigh.

Maggie groaned a little louder. She knew her little girls like a book, and she had to put a stop to this nonsense—*now*. "He is not '*the one*,'" she told them emphatically.

She didn't have to look up to see they weren't buying it . . . not one bit.

Five days later . . .

"How are you feeling today? Hmmm? Are you ready to talk?" a female voice inquired sweetly. "Now don't be afraid. We just want to help you."

Afraid? Who's afraid? A soldier's fear is his doom . . . I need no—

Jorund cracked his eyes open to mere slits.

The wench with the man-hair and sex-voice was back. *Again.* The one responsible for his current dilemma. And she was speaking to him in the same slow-paced manner he'd become accustomed to this past sennight, as if he were a child . . . or a lackbrain.

He had thought for one insane moment back at the whale place that she might be his personal Valkyrie. *Ha!* He'd soon rid himself of that foolish notion. It was more likely he'd landed in Niflheim, and this was the beginning of his eternal damnation.

He'd spoken a few words on first setting foot in this foreign land, but not once since. They could question him till all the warriors went home to Valhalla, but his lips were sealed. A fighting man knew to hold his silence in the enemy camp . . . leastways till he assessed his foe's strengths and weaknesses. Thus far—for seven whole days and nights—he'd managed to remain mute under the torment of their endless questions.

He was waiting till they removed his ankle restraints and the peculiar *shert* that forced his arms to wrap around his body. They put the restraints on him when anyone entered his cell only because he was deemed dangerous. *Sharp thinking there.* And it took four good-size men to hold him down every time they put that binding *shert* on him . . . a sadistic torture device, if he'd ever seen one.

He had learned much in the prolonged period of quiet, but there were still so many questions. He supposed he would have to talk soon.

"What's your name?" she persisted in the husky voice that could turn a man's bones to butter and his thoughts to . . . well, certainly not butter.

The wench pulled a short stick from her pocket, which she used to write on a stack of parchment on her lap. Glancing sideways, he was able to discern some of the letters she formed, thanks to this mystical capacity he seemed to have developed for understanding her language. *Silence syndrome.*

It was hard to concentrate on the meaning of the words or the magic stick, however, when his eyes were drawn to her crossed knees, where sheer hose covered nicely formed legs, exposed from thigh to oddly enticing, high-heeled shoes. Vikings had long held a tradition of attaching descriptive words to a name, like Gustov Tree-Feller, or Sigurd the Beautiful, or Halfdan of the Wide Embrace. So, to his mind, she was the wench of the man-hair, sex-voice, *and* comely legs.

A shoe dangled from the toes of one foot, which swung up and down rhythmically as she wrote. Was she nervous? Or deliberately trying to disconcert him? Or—and he felt a jolt in his lower belly—was she excited by him?

When he failed to answer, she tried a new approach . . . one he'd heard dozens of times from her. "My name is Dr. Maggie McBride."

Muck-bride? Did that mean she was a soiled bride? Soiled in what way? Well, of course she was soiled. She proudly proclaimed herself a dock whore. He smiled to himself. Some men might be put off by that, but Jorund preferred women with a bit of tarnish on the gilt.

He was still confused by the bride name, though. Was she a recent bride, or hoping to become one? *Ha!* Aroused or not, soiled or not, she would not snare him into the bonds of matrimony. He'd made that mistake once already.

And there was another curious thing. While this wench called herself a dock whore, the other women who came into his cell, big as you please, without even knocking, called themselves Norse. There was Norse John-son, Norse Fill-ups. Some men also took on that Norse appellation. Oddly, none of them had any of the characteristics he

would usually associate with the Norse race—
blond hair, height, or exceptional appearance.
Even stranger, they were all dressed in white,
right down to white shoes that squished when
they walked. No true Norseman would wear foot
coverings that announced his arrival. It would be
like shouting, "Here I am. Lop off my head."

But then, there was the wench's reference on
the parchment to silence sin-drone. He had no
idea what a sin-drone was, precisely, but he was
fairly certain it was not a desirable trait. Everyone knew a drone was a male bee. And he'd
noticed a flower garden below his window one
day, teeming with honey bees. Mayhap this was a
land of bees, just as there were said to be god-
lands of bears and wolves—and, yes, even killer
whales. The gods of this land must favor the
buzzing insects. But sin-drone . . . sinful bees?
That was hard to comprehend. How did one
know when a male bee had erred? When it
pricked the wrong queen bee?

There was much to puzzle over in this new
land.

He pressed his lips together more tightly and
cast the wench his fiercest glare.

She just smiled.

She must be simple. Or exceptionally daring.
Either way, Jorund was contemplating the best way
to kill her . . . assuming that he was not already
dead. He was still uncertain whether he had landed
in some new mortal land, or the otherworld.

He had narrowed his mental list to some particularly creative extermination methods after a
full seven days of being held prisoner in her dungeon. At least, he assumed it was a dungeon with

its barred window and locked door, though its white walls and metal fixtures resembled no torture chamber he'd ever seen. No actual physical tribulations had been levied yet, except for the Norse people pricking him on occasion with a needle and taking his blood in a little glass vessel, but there had been indignities aplenty. The most outrageous of these involved a metal trencher slipped under his bare buttocks on a regular basis for the relief of certain bodily functions. The white-uniformed dragon who performed this function had the face of a battle-ax. Her name was Norse Hatch-her, not Hatch-it; still, an appropriate name.

What was not appropriate was her other name . . . Glad-ass. Norse Glad-ass Hatch-her. Now, he had met a few women in his time for which the appellation would fit—like that high-priced strumpet from Cordova with the pretty heart-shaped arse. But Norse Hatch-her had a backside the size of a warhorse. He could not fathom anyone giving her the glad-ass description.

Every time Norse Hatch-her came into his chamber, she asked with a snide grin, "Does the stud muffin have to tinkle today?" After hearing the din of his piss in the metal trencher, he could pretty well guess what a tinkle was. But the other . . . What was a stud muffin? On occasion people referred to horse droppings as horse muffins, and for a certainty, some horses were put out to stud. Was the dragon calling him a horse's arse?

At first he felt a rise of anger at the insult. But then, it wouldn't be the first time he'd been called such.

Norse Hatch-her may have been the one to

shove down the loose *braies* that covered his lower half, forcing the cold metal object under him, but a good warrior knew that, in the end, the leader was responsible for his soldiers' actions. It was this brassy female sitting before him now who would bear the brunt of his anger . . . in good time. It was she who had instructed the guardsmen at the whale place to bring him here.

"Can't you at least tell me your name?" the wench urged.

Jorund refused to answer.

"Well, can you tell me why you were nude in a public amusement park? I really don't think you came there with violence in mind, despite your sword, but there has to be a reason for your . . . well, exhibiting yourself before a crowd at Orcaland. If you'd only talk with me about your nude display, perhaps we can . . ."

On and on the dimwit female blathered, with most of her words unfathomable to him. Still, one message came through to him: *She thinks I'm a pervert.*

He heard the sound of his own grinding teeth.

"Most psychologists sit back and listen while the patient talks. It's hard to do that when you won't cooperate."

Sigh-colic-jest? Another big word for Jorund to add to his list for later unraveling. How could the wench be a dock whore and a jester at the same time? Was she a humorous strumpet?

The whole time she talked and he pondered, the magic stick continued to skim across the parchment, leaving foreign scribblings in its wake. He would like to examine the sorcerer's instrument at a later date.

While she wrote, he used the opportunity to study her lips, which were full and wantonly kiss-some, especially with that rose-colored, glossy substance that glistened on them. Oh, that is just wonderful, he chastised himself. Now he would have to think of her as the wench of the man-hair, sex-voice, comely legs, *and* kiss-some lips. Said lips were pursed now as she tapped her witch-stick on the parchment, perusing something she had written.

Aaarrgh! What difference did the temptation of her lips make? He was going mad with all this inactivity. *Concentrate, Jorund. Concentrate.*

He half-reclined on the bed, his head supported by down pillows that were softer than any he'd ever rested upon, even in the Eastern harems. His posture was relaxed, but inside he was poised to pounce at the first opening. Unfortunately, he'd tried once with Norse Hatch-her. Thus the ankle restraints, in addition to the seamless *shert*. Who knew a female could be so strong? Or could spout such foul language? Grudgingly, he admitted that the Amazon would make a good warrior in battle . . . not only wielding a battle-ax, but a pike and a battering ram as well.

The woman sitting before him now was another matter. He could break her slim wrists with a snap of his fingers. He could lift her by the waist and toss her over his shoulder. He could press her to the bed, and . . . Well, he could do things to her.

Her eyes caught his then, as if she sensed his carnal thoughts. The air nigh sizzled between them, like heat flashes in a lightning storm. He

was aware of an intense attraction to her...
something far beyond her physical attributes. He
could tell she was attracted to him, as well...
and was just as puzzled as he.

He shook his head to rid it of these alarming
thoughts. And she did the same.

*Focus on something else. Do not be diverted. A
weak link in a man's armor can be his undoing.*
Jorund noted that at least the wench was alone
today—*Thank the gods!* Sending a defenseless
maid into his chamber was akin to sending a pal-
try kitten into a wolf's lair, assuming he could
finally manage to break free of his restraints.
Missing today was her comrade-in-arms—the
man with the bald head covered oddly with his
swath of side hair. The man was a dock whore,
too—Dock-whore Sea-bold. Jorund refused to
contemplate what a man would be doing as a
dock whore, and on the bold seas, no less. He
reminded Jorund of Dagfinn the Dumb, one of
his soldiers who'd once tried to braid his nose
hairs... all for the sake of male vanity.

Jorund thought he had it figured out. After
watching for hours on end that black box in the
corner with the illuminated face, he was coming
to understand the language of this land rather
well, even down to reading some words, as he
had those on the Lady Muck-bride's parchment.
People here spoke English, though vastly different from the Saxon English with which he was
familiar. More important than teaching him the
language, the box was giving him views into
many other worlds... Genoa City, Cross Creek,
Springfield, Port Charles, Pine Valley. Then there

were Sesame Street, Nashville, Mayberry. Speaking of the latter, Jorund was more than a little amused to realize there was a man—or was he a god?—named Barn-knee Fife with ears as big as his brother Magnus's. His brother was twice the size of the Mayberry world's guardsman, but they were both bumbling idiots.

Every time a Norse came into the room, she turned a tiny wheel on the box, which gave him a peephole of sorts into a different world. He kept watching, hoping that one of these times he would see his own Vestfold.

It was surprising, really. Norse legend said that when a fighting man died, he went to Valhalla, hall of the gods in Asgard. Apparently there were many other worlds, and many gods he'd never heard of . . . like Victor New-man and Bill Clin-town.

Surprising, too, was the way in which the gods could view what was happening in other worlds. He had always pictured Odin or Thor—even the Christian One-God—gazing down from the heavens to observe what mortal beings were doing. But apparently they must all have these magic boxes to do the job for them. *Amazing!*

"Well, since you're not talking, I guess that ends our session for today." She stood and ran a palm swiftly over the front of her garment, presumably to smooth out the wrinkles, but what she accomplished instead was the jarring of another memory: a belly ring . . . that was it. Jorund suddenly recalled seeing a gold ornament piercing her navel the first day he'd encountered her at the whale place. With an inward groan, he amended her name list. So now she was the wench of the man-hair, sex-voice, comely legs, kiss-some lips, *and* naughty navel.

Releasing a long sigh, presumably at his stubborn silence, she tossed her shoulders back, as if to show that two people could be stubborn. But her posture caused her breasts to jut out against the white silk of her *shert,* and they were magnificent, round and uplifted; he even imagined he saw the hard points of her nipples. Oh, it was too much! Soon her name list would require a skald of exceptional memory to recite, as in the wench of the man-hair, sex-voice, comely legs, kiss-some lips, naughty navel, and magnificent breasts. Mag-he Man-hair. Dock-whore sex-voice. Mag-he of the kiss-some lips. The combinations were endless.

She noticed the direction of his gaze and *tsk*ed her disapproval as she folded her arms over her chest, hiding her breasts from his view. It was a useless exercise, really, because the image was already planted in his head. "I'm really disappointed in you . . . whoever you are," she informed him sadly.

He tried not to look guilty. Men throughout time had been viewing women's physical attributes with appreciation. Why should she make him feel as if he'd failed her in some way by noticing she was a voluptuous woman?

"My daughters are the ones who begged me to help you," she told him in that low, raspy sex-voice that he was growing overly fond of. "They still ask about you every day. You've touched them in some way." She sighed again. "I can't even tell them your name." Spinning on her high heels, she then proceeded toward the door.

A fierce constriction took place in the region of

his heart. The twin girls, who resembled his own daughters, had interceded on his behalf? They had been touched by him just as he had been touched by them?

Finally, he was beginning to see some reason for his deliverance to this strange land.

Was it not possible that these girls had called to him . . . that they needed him for some reason? Mayhap—*Oh, please!*—he was being given a second chance to make up for failing his own twin girls. That prospect tantalized and terrified him.

"Wait!" he called out suddenly.

She turned slowly, surprise showing on her face at his first word in a whole sennight.

"My name is"—his eyes darted between her and the black box in the corner, still distrustful of speaking and revealing too much—"Alan Spaulding."

"I see." She murmured something that sounded like "Celebrity delusions, too." She quickly made some words on her parchment before addressing him again, this time with a smile. "And you come from Genoa City, right? How do you feel about that?" Despite her recognizing his lie, she sat back down and waited expectantly for him to talk.

"Mayhap that was a slight mistruth."

"You mean a lie?"

He shrugged with resignation. "My name is Jorund."

She smiled widely, and somewhere deep inside him, he felt a melting sensation.

"Well, it's so nice to meet you, Mr. Rand. Do you object if I call you Joe?"

Joe? He glanced back over his shoulder before he realized that, of course, there was no one else in the room. "Am I your prisoner?"

"Prisoner?" Her eyes went wide, but then she must have realized that it was a natural assumption on his part, considering he was in a torture *shert* with ankle restraints and bars on his windows. *Possible bondage fantasies*, she wrote on her parchment.

He raised his chin indignantly, though secretly he wondered exactly what a bondage fantasy was. It brought up mental images that were . . . well, fascinating.

"Of course you're not a prisoner, Joe. You'll be released once we're certain of your safety."

Hah!

"How do you feel about that?"

How do you feel? How do you feel? I feel rotten. "I'll tell you how I feel. Captive I may be, for now, but I want you to know, I won't be a slave to any man . . . or woman."

"A slave?" she sputtered. "What would I do with a slave?"

"Precisely," he answered. But then the mischievous god Loki whispered in his ear, and a tantalizing idea tugged at him. With as much casualness as he could garner, he remarked, "Except in your case I might consider being your . . ." He deliberately let his words trail off.

He wasn't really serious. Leastways, he did not think he was. Jorund was a man little bent toward humor. And the teasing taunt he'd thrown out to the wench was so out of character it fairly boggled his already boggled mind. It must be the confinement, and the shock of his death or whatever the hell had happened to him, even the influence of his frivolous brother or the damned orca. Or mayhap the blame could be laid on the first temptation he'd felt in a long, long while.

"What?" she prodded finally. "I want you to be free to speak your mind, Joe. Nothing is out of bounds in the psychologist/patient relationship. So tell me. You might consider being my . . . what?"

"Love slave."

Chapter Five

"Love slave?" Maggie squeaked out.

As a professional, Maggie shouldn't have been shocked. Patients made outrageous suggestions to her all the time. But when the proposition came from a compellingly handsome man with pale blond hair, translucent gray eyes, and suntanned skin . . . well, Maggie had to admit to a teensy bit of temptation.

She would have to be extra careful not to cross that ethical line between patient and doctor . . . even if the patient was drop-dead gorgeous, despite the fact that he wore boring blue hospital-issue pajama bottoms, ankle restraints, and a white straitjacket. Even his bare feet, which were huge—a narrow size thirteen, she would guess—were surprisingly sexy.

She had to smile at that latter whimsy. Yep,

there were strange goings-on inside Maggie these days, if she was getting turned on by feet. Actually, the psychiatrist in her had a ready, logical explanation: on a big, strong man like Joe, his bare feet appeared vulnerable and open to ... well, touch—as other parts of his covered body were not.

Her face flushing with heat at the mere thought of *touch*, Maggie experienced a twinge of guilt as she glanced at the restraints that were put on him whenever she entered his room. They were necessary, though, even with a security guard posted outside the door, because he fought confinement. Fighting back was a natural reaction, of course, but it proved that he could be dangerous, until hospital experts could complete a diagnosis.

He was lounging on the bed now, his back propped up by two fluffy pillows and his long legs spread out on the narrow mattress, crossed at the ankles. His posture said he was relaxed, but the tension of the corded muscles in his neck said he was ready to pounce at the first opportunity.

He nodded in response to her question, which she'd already forgotten with all her musings. Oh, yes, she'd exclaimed at his ridiculous love-slave proposition.

"Yea, a love slave." He spoke slowly, with a strong foreign accent. Clearly English was not his first language. "Release me from these restraints, and we can negotiate an agreement."

She shook her head and pulled her chair closer to the bed, pencil and notepad at the ready. It was time she got a more complete background on this guy, now that he'd finally deigned to speak. "I can't release you till we're certain you won't harm others, or yourself."

"Why would I harm myself?" he scoffed.

She shrugged. "Lots of people do."

He looked skeptical at that statement.

She smiled as some of his words flitted through her brain. "You would actually negotiate a contract to be a . . . love slave?" Her face heated up over those last words.

To her dismay, his intelligent eyes registered her embarrassment, and he winked. *Oh, my God! He winked at me. Whoa! Since when is a wink an erotic signal? Maybe my girls are right. Maybe I really do need a man. No, no, no. That's the last thing I need.*

Maggie also saw the way his eyes scanned her body, from the top of her short hairdo, over her silk blouse, short skirt, and sheer stockings, down to her high heels. The jacket that matched the skirt hung on a wall peg back in her office. She was attending a seminar later today.

Joe liked what he saw—Maggie could tell by the brief flicker of his eyelids and the dilating of his pupils, especially as his gaze paused over her breasts—and she had to force herself not to react, either in anger or withdrawal.

It had taken Maggie years to become comfortable with her body. As a young girl who had developed much earlier than her friends, and as a young woman who had always had a curvy, voluptuous figure that made males think she was "easy," Maggie had gone out of her way to dress in a manner that would hide her figure, and to behave contrary to her sensual nature. But she was changing—her short, saucy hairdo and the belly-button ring being the most recent signs—and she no longer dressed repressively. If people wanted to form the wrong opinions of her, that was their problem, not hers. She didn't wear slut clothes, but then she didn't dress like a librarian, either.

That didn't mean she felt entirely comfortable under the carnal scrutiny of this handsome fellow. But she wasn't dying of mortification, either.

She held her chin high in defiance, and he chuckled, as if he understood . . . which was impossible, of course.

She hoped.

"You would actually negotiate a contract to be a love slave?" Even as Maggie repeated her question, she wondered why she was pursuing this line of questioning. In her own defense, psychologists were taught to go with the flow of the patient's dialogue . . . to lead unobtrusively, when necessary, but mostly to follow, without censorship.

"Yea . . . if it would bring me closer to freedom."

"Have you ever been a love slave before?"

His eyes shot wide at her question. "Nay. Have you?"

"No," she answered with a nervous laugh. "And I'm not interested now."

His only answer was the disbelieving lift of his eyebrows. He flicked his tongue briefly over his full lips, as if to signal that, even if she wasn't interested, he definitely was.

Lordy, lordy!

This had to be a joke, but he displayed no sign of humor. In fact, the chiseled features of his fine face lacked the laugh lines that should have been etched about the mouth and eyes of a man his age—about mid-thirties. If the eyes were the windows to the soul, his bespoke grimness, not a life filled with smiles.

Who was this man? The Orcaland people claimed they'd never seen him before. A police search of his fingerprints had brought up nothing. No family or friends had shown up claiming a missing person. He seemed to be a man without a past.

Maggie shifted uncomfortably, not wanting to bring up the love-slave subject again. But then she chastised herself: no topic should be taboo in the therapy relationship. With that in mind she asked, "Exactly how would you negotiate a love-slave contract?"

She expected him to laugh, or at least grin, but his expression was somber. "On your side, there would be the promise of freedom. On my side would be the promise of bed pleasuring."

A ripple, like an erotic shock, rushed through Maggie with stunning force. And that was amazing, really, because, while she'd made great gains in her insecurities about her body, she still harbored strong inhibitions about her sexuality. Case in point, her girls' father, Judd Haskell, who'd once said she was "as exciting as nailing a bowl of mashed potatoes."

"I see." Maggie blinked several times to clear her head under the intense survey of the man half reclining on the bed before her. He saw way too much. "Define freedom," she encouraged.

"I'd rather define bed pleasuring." A slight grin tugged at his lips, and Maggie thought he might

Sandra Hill

not be without a sense of humor, after all. Perhaps it was just buried beneath the surface . . . or whatever pain had caused his breakdown.

"You talk in such an odd way," she commented. "I can't quite place the dialect."

"Hah! You think I talk oddly? You should hear yourself . . . and I do not just mean that sex-voice."

Sex-voice? Oh, he must be referring to the huskiness. That was another part of her body makeup that had contributed to her early reputation as easy. Leave it to this fellow to home in on it, right off. "My voice has sounded raspy like this since I was a child. A severe throat infection," she said, more defensively than she'd intended. "But your dialect . . . where are you from?"

"Vestfold."

"Huh? Is that in Texas?"

"I have no idea where this Tax-us is. Vestfold is in Norway. I am a Norseman. A Viking."

"I see." Now they were getting somewhere. Among his other mental problems, this guy thought he was a Viking . . . although, come to think of it, he did resemble a Norse god. She made a few quick notes on her pad.

"We were negotiating our love-slave contract when—"

"I never agreed to negotiate any such thing," she interjected, perhaps too indignantly.

"I have much experience in bed sport, of course."

"Of course," she replied, and immediately regretted her sarcasm.

Either he failed to hear the sarcasm in her voice, or he chose to ignore it. *Good.*

"Now, I cannot claim great finesse in more refined bed sport—no flowery words or hand-holding or such—and, in truth, I do not favor kissing all that much, but I have been told my endurance is remarkable. That and my size." Her only response was a gurgle, which he must have taken for a compliment because he continued, "And, of course, all Norsemen know the secret of a woman's S-spot."

"Don't you mean G-spot?" Criminy, was she the one going crazy here? What would prompt her to encourage him with questions like that?

"I know naught of a G-spot, but all Vikings know that the S-spot is far superior to any other sex spot." The lack of expression on his face gave her no clue as to whether he was serious or not.

"Well, this love-slave business would never work, I can tell you that right away," she informed him with a nervous laugh, "because most women like kissing."

"Do you?"

"Uh . . . well, yes. Of course." *Oh, good heavens! My tongue has developed a mind of its own.*

He seemed to consider her faltering words, the whole time staring at her with those luminous gray eyes. Finally he said, "Agreed."

"Agreed? What does that mean?" she practically shrieked.

He arched an eyebrow at the panic in her voice. "I agree to give kisses, and you agree to give . . . well, some things I want—nay, *need*."

Like what? she desperately wanted to ask. Luckily her good sense returned, and she bridled her tongue. Enough was enough on this dangerous subject. "I am not in need of a love slave, thank you very much. We should get back to the subject at hand—the client interview."

"Is that what this is? An interview?" He frowned. "By the by, m'lady Muck-bride, are you married?"

She shook her head in confusion. What had her marital status to do with anything? *Oh.* He must be worried about potential conflicts with another man in the event she agreed to the love-slave business . . . which would be when hell froze over. "No, I'm not married."

"I thought not. No offense, m'lady, but wedlock will not be part of our love-slave agreement."

It took a moment before her fuzzy brain absorbed the fact that he was declining a marriage proposal from her. "You . . . you . . ." she sputtered.

"Am I dead?" he asked suddenly.

"Wh-what?" Now that question really surprised her. "Why would you ask a question like that?"

"Well, the anchor of my longship got tangled in the seas somewhere beyond Iceland, and—"

"Iceland!" she exclaimed. "Joe, you are apparently lost."

He frowned. "Why do you address me as Joe?"

"Because you told me your name was Joe Rand. Oh . . . do you mean that I'm being too familiar? Do you prefer I call you Mr. Rand?"

"Nay, I prefer that you address me by my real name. Johr-rund," he sounded out for her. "Jorund Ericsson."

She put a hand over her mouth to hide a smile at her mistake. "Jorund. What an unusual name! But nice . . . very nice! I think I'll just call you by your nickname, though—Joe."

"Joe the Viking?" He pursed his lips pensively. "Somehow it does not have the same luster as Jorund the Viking, or Jorund the Warrior." Then he flashed her an irresistible grin.

She grinned back at him.

"I know I was—am—lost," he confessed. "But it was that damned Thora who caused me to end up here."

"Thora?" For some reason, the thought of Joe being with a woman caused her stomach to clench. *No, no, no.* She couldn't allow herself to become involved with a patient. Besides, for all she knew, he might be married. "Is Thora your wife?" she asked with as much nonchalance as she could muster.

"Do you make mock of me?"

She took that for a no. *Whew!* "Your lover?"

He snorted with disgust. "Thora is a killer whale."

"Thora . . . a killer whale? You named a killer whale?"

"I did. Well, actually, my bother Magnus and my sailors did. And, if you must know, Thora is the most irritating animal this side of the Baltic. And she has bad breath, too."

"I see."

"Why do you keep saying, 'I see,' when you clearly do not see?"

Maggie put her notebook aside and rubbed at the furrows in her forehead with the fingers of one hand. "A killer whale brought you here . . . from Iceland? A killer whale with bad breath?"

"Aha! Now you are beginning to understand."

"I see," she said.

* * *

The next day . . .

"That's it till next Monday," Dr. Harry Seabold told the people assembled around the conference table, thus calling a halt to the weekly staff meeting. "We should have more definite word within the next two weeks on the status of Medic-All negotiations with the Rainbow owners. I hope to give you a progress report next week."

"Two weeks! Well, whoopie-doo! My nurses are panicking *now*, Dr. Seabold. They need to know if they should be submitting job applications elsewhere," Gladys Hatcher insisted as she stood and gathered up her papers. "Some of them live from paycheck to paycheck. They can't afford to go even two weeks without work." Gladys was a big, brusque woman who took no guff from anyone, not even their boss, but she also had a heart of gold when it came to her "girls," the nurses working under her supervision.

Earlier today, when Maggie had mentioned her daughters' report of the nurse's overheard remark, Gladys had clapped Maggie so hard on the back she almost fell over and exclaimed, "Well, he *is* a stud muffin, honey. Ya can't deny that." Maggie had decided not to make an issue of it, for now.

"I know, I know." Harry was nodding in reply to Gladys's concerns. "But let's not overreact here, folks. Even if Medic-All buys out Rainbow, it doesn't mean the hospital will shut down, or that jobs will be eliminated."

But what Harry wasn't saying, and they all knew, was that Rainbow was a unique operation, and many of them, Maggie included, might not want to work for the hospital if it changed its procedures. Maggie knew of only a few mental clinics in the country that were experimenting with a minimal-security setting with a combination of in- and outpatient therapy for serious mental disorders, combined with work-training experience. It was all based on individualized contracts, a relaxed atmosphere, and close supervision. Their success rate had been phenomenal, but it was too soon to try it on a wider scale.

Would Medic-All be impressed with what they'd accomplished so far? After all, the Rainbow Psychiatric Hospital was a small facility of less than one hundred patients, and it was only five years old. Or would they bring their own people in and want a rubber stamp of the medical procedures followed in its other numerous facilities? Would the bottom line be dollars, or patient success?

Maggie feared she already knew the answer.

As the business manager, nursing director, activities coordinator, and other psychologists began to stream out of the room, Harry said, "Stay behind, Maggie. I have something I need to discuss with you."

Uh-oh. She sat back down in a chair close to the head of the table.

"It's about your John Doe. . . ." Harry, still sitting in the head seat, gave her a weary glance that didn't bode well for said John Doe. Today Harry wore a white, short-sleeved dress shirt, a red-striped power tie, and khaki slacks—every bit the head honcho, even with his hair comb-over, which he patted every so often, whether to make sure it was still in place or out of nervousness, Maggie couldn't tell for sure.

"He's no longer a John Doe," Maggie reminded him. "Remember, he started talking yesterday. His name is Jorund Ericsson."

Harry gave a short "whatever" wag of his hand. "We are walking on eggshells with the potential takeover, Maggie. I'm very concerned about our having a patient here at this time with no known medical insurance and—"

"So that's what this is all about? Money?"

"Damn straight it is," Harry shot right back, his face flushed with sudden anger. He was usually such a calm person, even in the face of traumatic events, which were not unusual in a hospital setting. The takeover talks must be taking a bigger toll on him than she'd imagined. "I've never refused to care for a patient who had no means to pay, but these are very sensitive times. I'll be damned if I'll jeopardize the interests of ninety-nine paying customers for the sake of one . . . one"—he stammered, at a loss for the least offensive words to describe Joe—"one nude exhibitionist who just happens to be wearing a hundred thousand dollars in jewelry."

"Huh?" Maggie homed in on the most irrelevant part of Harry's tirade. "What jewelry? Oh, you mean those brass arm rings?"

"Brass? Ha! Those are solid gold, if my guess is right, and probably antiques . . . maybe even tenth century—at least that's what Martie said when she was here yesterday."

Martie, an antique dealer, was Harry's on-again, off-again girlfriend. She operated a well-respected auction house with international connections, similar to Sotheby's and Christie's, though on a smaller scale, and she served on several museum boards. She ought to know.

"Martie says those arm bands are potentially important antiquities, whatever the hell that means. And besides that, have you looked at that sword the police department sent over? I did, before they locked it in the hospital safe. My God, Maggie, it weighs a ton, and the hilt is in the shape of a dragon, imbedded with what appear to be real emeralds. I didn't bring it out to show Martie, of course—that would be unethical. But I'm telling you, this guy should be a paying customer . . . insurance or no insurance."

Maggie's shoulders sagged with weariness. Harry was right. He'd gone out on a limb, giving in to her whim over bringing a stranger to their hospital. And how did she repay him? By giving him grief. "What do you want me to do?"

"One week," he stipulated, wagging a forefinger at her with emphasis. "You have one week to show some real progress with this guy. That's when the advance team from Medic-All will arrive for the red-carpet treatment. I expect your assurance by then that he is no danger to anyone, including himself. That means no more ankle restraints or straitjackets. I want to see some interaction with other patients. Otherwise he is being sent to the state facility, whether it is in his best interests or not. Rainbow's best interests are my main concern, especially now. I mean that, Maggie. I really do."

Maggie put up both hands in surrender. "I get the picture, boss."

The question, though, was how to translate that picture to her patient. Most important, would Joe the Viking cooperate?

* * *

The next day . . .

"I do not understand," Jorund said, pacing the room as he shook his head with incredulity. "What kind of prison is this?"

"Why kind of prison do you think it is?"

The wench was back in his chamber again, battering him with more pointless conversation, half of which he could not comprehend, when he needed to be on his journey back to his ship to rescue his brother Rolf. And—*Thor's toenails!*—he hated it when she never answered his questions, but instead tossed them back at him like a bloody parrot.

If he asked, "Why am I being confined?" she countered with, "How do you feel about being confined?" Or a simple query like, "Where am I?" would garner, "Where do you think you are?" Never could he get a simple answer to a simple question.

She wore another of those short-sleeved *sherts*, as she had worn at the orca place—crimson red this time, made of a stretchy material that highlighted the most perfect breasts, round globes that would fit nicely into a big male hand . . . one the size of . . . oh, say, *his* hand. Not that he was considering the handling of her breasts. It was just an observation, he told himself. Just as he'd noticed she was wearing men's black *braies* that clung to her rounded hips and flat belly in a beguiling way. Then, too, there were those enticing, open-toed shoes with flame-painted toenails today. He had the most alarming compulsion to suck on those deliciously appealing appendages.

He stopped dead in his tracks. Really, he had been isolated too long if he was developing a taste for toes. Magnus would love to hear of this. No doubt at the next All-Thing, the skalds would be writing praise-poems ... but to ridicule, not praise him. Instead of his being known as Jorund the Warrior, people would refer to him forever after as Jorund the Toe-Taster.

He'd best be on his guard. The wench might be out to seduce him with all these dock-whore wiles. And he might just be tempted if it weren't for her annoying nature. *What do you think? What do you think? What do you think?* he mocked her incessant refrain in his head. What he thought was that he was tired of thinking. It was long past the time for action.

Oh, the wench had released his ankle restraints. A guardsman was still posted outside the door, though, and Jorund still wore the torture *shert*. That ankle-restraint concession had been made this morn when he'd promised not to make an effort to escape or engage in any violence. Even so, it rankled that she engaged him in useless chatter when he had important business elsewhere. Besides—he might as well admit it—he wanted to get back to the black box and see if Josh was able to rescue Reva from those dastardly villains on that far island. He had some suggestions he'd like to offer Josh for retrieving his wayward wife. And—*Odin's balls!*—that Reva was a woman after a Viking's heart ... or any other body organ.

"What don't you understand, Joe?"

I swear I am going to rip out your tongue if you don't stop calling me Joe. What kind of name is that? That was what he thought. What he said was, "You say this is a hospitium?"

"A hospital . . . yes." She craned her neck to watch him as he resumed moving restlessly about the small chamber. "Actually, we prefer to call it a clinic."

"Ne'er have I seen a hospitium—or clan-hick—like this afore," he declared with a grunt. "I should know. There is one of the finest in the world located in Jorvik, near the minster. The good monks perform the healing arts there. They've sewn up my wounds on a dozen occasions. One time I nigh lost an eye."

Scanning him quickly, the wench took note of the white scar that ran from his right eye to his ear.

A distressing idea occurred to him then. "Since this is a hospitium, are those men in white uniforms who come in here . . . are they perchance monks?"

She smiled. "No, they're orderlies, or attendants."

"And the women in white—and you—surely you are not nuns?"

She laughed out loud at that. "The women in white are nurses, and I'm a doctor."

He exhaled with a loud whoosh, in relief.

The wench looked at him strangely. "You do understand that? No, I guess you don't." She paused. "This is a mental hospital, Joe."

Men-tall? Men-tall? He rolled the word around on his tongue silently. *Oh, she must mean mental, like having to do with the head.* It took him a few moments to digest that news. "Your country has special hospitiums for mad people?"

She nodded.

"Well, I can see where that might be a good idea." *I have ne'er heard of such a ludicrous idea in all my days. Next she will tell me there are separate hospitiums for battle veterans or breeding women.* Not wanting to give offense, but needing to know if he faced additional dangers from a berserk society, he asked casually, "Dost have so very many mad people here?"

She shrugged. "No more than any other country."

"We lock them up in my country . . . in dungeons, if they are available." Actually he'd seen only a few dungeons in his time, though he supposed some folks did lock up their infamous family members. They were probably Saxons, who were known to have no heart, even for their own kin. Even then, it was more likely to be a root cellar or woodshed, rather than a dungeon.

She gaped.

"Or just kill them." His third cousin Halfdan had killed his half-witted brother, Helvid, many summers ago because he'd slobbered in Halfdan's mead. "I have heard of some clans where less-than-perfect babes are left outdoors to die soon after birth. Life is harsh in the northlands, and sometimes 'tis merciful to spare the child with death when life would mean endless torture."

She gulped.

"In truth, I have heard of madhouses on occasion, but those were mostly in leper colonies."

She gasped.

But then, the implications of her words struck him on a personal level: *he* was being held captive in a madhouse. "You think I, *Jorund the Warrior*, am demented?"

"Well, I wouldn't use the word *demented*," she answered, but the flush on her cheeks told another story.

Sandra Hill

"What word would you use?" He narrowed his eyes at her and gritted his teeth.

"Troubled."

He released the breath he had not realized he was holding. "Of course I am troubled. I already told you I am lost and must needs get back to my ship in order to rescue my brother Rolf."

"I mean troubled in a more serious, clinical way. Joe, you need help to correct your disorders before you can be released back into society."

"If by disorders you mean mental ones, then you are sorely mistaken," he informed her haughtily. "I am as sane as the next person . . . as you, for example. Or that Dock-whore Hairy with the hair swag."

He saw her lips twitch with suppressed mirth at his description of her colleague.

"Tell me exactly what I am accused of so that I may convince you of my innocence, and leave this place."

"No, no, no. You aren't being accused of any crime. This is a low-security mental facility. If police thought you were truly dangerous, or a criminal, you'd be in jail, not here."

"Then why am I not free to leave?"

"For starters, you showed up stark naked in a public place."

"Pfff!" He blew air out in a dismissive manner. "I did not choose to arrive without garments, but I needed ease of movement when I dove into the waters off Iceland to disentangle my ship's anchor."

"See, that's another thing," she said with excitement, as if she'd made some great discovery. "Surely you're aware of the frigid nature of waters in that region. Your body never could have withstood that temperature for more than a few minutes."

He was trying his best to concentrate on her words and not notice that her nipples had pearled with her excitement and pressed outward from the stretchy material of her *shert*. He made a mental note to take a length or two of that fabric back to Vestfold with him. He knew a trader who could make a fortune selling it to the Eastern potentates. For a certainty, the nether portion of his body was developing a liking for all that the fabric disclosed on the dock whore. He forced himself to think of other things before he embarrassed himself.

"Well, you may have a point there," he managed to get out finally. "Mayhap my boat did go off course a mite. Mayhap it was not really Iceland, but some other country. Mayhap I was a trifle . . . well, lost."

"Oh, Joe"—she sighed—"that would be more than lost. From Galveston, Texas, to Iceland is more than two thousand miles, as the bird flies."

It was his turn to gasp now. "As the bird flies, hmmm? And how many sea miles would that be by longship?"

"I haven't a clue. Possibly four thousand miles." She laughed. "Why do you keep mentioning such archaic words as longship?"

"Huh?" Then, "What is archaic about a longship? 'Tis the way we Vikings travel."

"There you go again, referring to yourself as a Viking. I've got to tell you that I've had patients in the past who thought they were aliens from

101

another planet. One even believed he was the emperor Nero. Vikings, Romans, aliens . . . those are delusions, my friend."

He stared at her, slack-jawed with incomprehension.

"Vikings do not exist as a separate culture today," she explained slowly. "They were assimilated into the various countries where they raped and pillaged, or just plain settled."

"Oh! There *you* go," he said, mimicking her expression. "Why do so many people accept as truth this portrayal of Vikings as bloodthirsty marauders? Do you not recognize the bias of those bloody Saxon clerics who call themselves historians? Rumormongers, they are, one and all."

She gazed softly at him, as if she were a parent, and he a simple child.

For a brief moment, he entertained the possibility of slicing off her tongue afore he left this chamber. Once he regained his sword, that was.

"Perhaps this is a starting point for us to begin therapy." She inhaled deeply, as if to fortify herself. "I believe that your name is Joe Rand, as you told me originally. And I think I know what your biggest problem is."

"You do?" *Now, why did I ask her that? It's just prolonging this ridiculous conversation.*

"Yes. You have a T-type personality . . . you're an extreme risk taker. That was evident at the orca park when you made a grand entrance riding atop a killer whale. I'm not judging you, but some people might equate that with a death wish."

"I was not riding Thora by choice," he pointed out.

She waved a hand in the air as if his observation counted for naught. "Man is the only species that deliberately takes risks, did you know that, Joe? And I'm speaking of everything from finances to our very lives. Think about it. Stock speculation. Gambling. Skydiving. Car racing. Whatever. The safer our environment becomes, the more risks people intentionally take on."

The woman is barmy as a bat.

"You are a thrill-seeker," she concluded with a wide smile, as if inviting him to agree.

Barmy as two bats. "Are you a . . . what did you call it . . . a type-tea, also?"

"Oh, good heavens, no! I've got inhibitions coming out the wazoo." She squirmed on her chair, practically jumping with glee at the expectation of solving one of his so-called disorders.

"Really?" he asked with more interest than her comment evoked. What he'd really like to know, though, was where her cause-oooh was? Could it be anywhere in the vicinity of those nicely rounded buttocks that perched on the edge of her chair? And he had to wonder, if she got this aroused at the prospect of his being a thrill-seeker, how aroused would she get when it was her he targeted for his thrills?

"But, more important, you must accept this fact, Joe: you are not a Viking."

"I'm not?" For a moment there, she had him questioning himself. If he was not already mad, she would make him so. "What am I?"

"Why don't you tell me?"

"Why do you always throw my questions back at me?"

She sighed, but then seemed to take his criticism to heart. "I suspect you are an ordinary man with an ordinary job, who took on this fantasy in order to bring excitement to his life. There's nothing wrong with that, except that it's an illusion. And overindulgence in fantasies can interfere with reality."

If Jorund's arms weren't confined in the torture jacket, he would have pulled at his own hair with frustration. "I most certainly am a Viking . . . just as you are a dock whore. And I assure you, I am not, nor ever have been, ordinary."

She smiled at him in a patronizing manner he did not find one bit complimentary. "Of course you're special. I just meant that there's no need to attach fancy labels to yourself. Who you are is enough."

"Aaarrgh!" he growled, then forced himself to control his temper when he noticed the flash of alarm on her face and the darting of her eyes toward the guardsman just outside in the corridor. "Let me make myself clear: I do not consider Viking a 'fancy label.' I am a Norseman . . . a Viking born and bred. That, m'lady, is no fantasy."

"I see," she remarked in a tone he could tell was intended to placate. She did not believe him.

He decided to change the subject. "What is this why-two-key I see mentioned on the black box all the time?"

At first the wench did not seem to understand his words. "Why-two-key, why-two-key," she repeated several times, then laughed. "Oh, you mean Y2K."

"That's what I said, didn't I?"

She ignored his grumpiness and explained. "Even though the turn of the century has passed, lots of people are still patting themselves on the backs over having escaped unscathed."

"Well, that is as clear as fjord fog on a frosty Friggsday." But something else she'd said tugged at his brain. "What do you mean about the turn of the century having passed? It was the year 998 when I left Vestfold. There is a year and more till the turn of the century." He was beginning to think that perchance it was the wench who was mad, not the other inhabitants of this madhouse, and definitely not him.

"Joe!" she exclaimed with alarm. "This isn't the year 998. It's the year two thousand."

"That's impossible!"

She shook her head slowly with a telling sadness. Instead of his convincing her of his sanity, he could tell she was increasingly convinced he was demented.

He inhaled and exhaled several times to digest all that she had proclaimed. Finally he told her, "If I am not dead, as you have assured me, and if this is in truth the year two thousand, then there can be only one conclusion."

"And that would be?"

He groaned. "I've heard about this in the sagas of the Norse gods, but never did I actually think it could come true, especially not for mortal men. But what other explanation could there be?"

"What are you talking about, Joe?"

"I must have traveled through time."

Chapter Six

"Time travel!" *Another delusion!*

"Yea, time travel," Joe said. "Oh, I know it is hard to believe, and never would I have thought it possible myself. But the Norse sagas tell tales of even more fantastical events. Even the Greeks told of impossible heroes doing extraordinary things . . . like Hercules."

"Those are myths," Maggie informed him gently. "Fantasies."

Joe shrugged. "Mayhap one's man's fancy is another man's reality. Nay, do not frown at me so. I am a man who deals with the bloody face of war, ofttimes on a daily basis. Believe me when I tell you I am not given to fanciful notions, but even I would find it hard to discredit miraculous events."

Maggie arched her eyebrows at him. "Are you saying that you have experienced a miracle?"

"Hmpfh! What would you call being shot through time on the back of a killer whale?" Obviously Maggie's usually impassive face was not so impassive today, because Joe was quick to add, "Mayhap the Norse culture is more inclined to believe in the spectacular than yours. Mayhap, because of our harsh environment, we tend to have more hope in the gods . . . and miracles."

With an air of hopelessness, Maggie put her notebook and pencil aside and walked over to the window.

Maybe I should just give up now. Call the state hospital and have them come pick up Joe. Better yet, just let him go and fare the best he can on the streets. There's no way I can give him all the help he needs in one lousy week. No way! On the other hand, if we let him go now, he'll probably be out on Galveston Bay, rowing a longboat . . . or waving that sword around in the nearest McDonald's.

Crossing her arms over her chest and leaning against the windowsill, she stared out blindly through the bars, trying to figure out how to handle this latest problem . . . especially with the time constraint her boss had laid on her only yesterday.

"Why are you so sad, m'lady?"

Maggie jumped, not having realized that Joe had stepped up beside her. Although she was not short by any means, Maggie had to crane her neck to gaze up at him.

He didn't touch her at all—not that he could, wearing a straitjacket—but Maggie felt his nearness as a palpable thing. The pine scent of the hospital-issue soap he'd used to shower with that morning was a whisper teasing at her senses. But more than that, there was the scent of man . . . of him . . . erotic and compelling.

Maggie took a slight step backward, and her shoulders hit the side wall. She wasn't afraid, but she needed some distance between herself and this provocative male specimen.

"You fear me?"

She shook her head.

He contemplated that contradiction of words and physical evidence, then smiled slightly, as if he understood that it was herself she feared. She saw the moment of hesitancy in his smoky eyes, when he contemplated moving closer to test his theory, but luckily he exercised restraint.

Maggie wasn't sure what she would have done if he'd leaned in and rubbed his lips against hers. Or pressed his sex against hers. Or breathed her name. *Lordy, lordy! Pretty soon I'm going to qualify for admittance to my own mental hospital.*

"You didn't answer my question," he murmured gruffly, jarring Maggie back to reality. "Why did my mention of time traveling make you sad?"

"There is no such thing," she answered bluntly, "and if you really believe that's what happened to you, then that makes my task impossible . . . a task that now has a deadline on it."

"What task would that be?" He was leaning back against the window now, his butt propped on the ledge, his bare feet crossed at the ankles. How a man wearing a straitjacket could look so relaxed was beyond Maggie.

"Making you healthy?"

"Who says I am unhealthy?" His chin jutted out.

"Mentally healthy," she elaborated.

"Oh, that! The demented nonsense again," he scoffed.

"I never said you were demented, Joe. Just . . ."

"I know . . . just troubled. But why does my being a time traveler—"

"Your *belief* that you are a time traveler, not your *being* a time traveler," she interjected.

"Aaarrgh! If you keep interrupting, I will forget what I was going to say. Then you will accuse me of being demented—I mean, troubled—for that reason, also."

"Sorry. Continue then."

"Why does my *conclusion* that I have traveled through time affect your ability to cure me any more than my claim to being a Viking, or my arrival in your land, bare-arsed and wielding a sword?"

"There isn't enough time to work on all those problems. Oh, I'm really encouraged by your finally talking, and I'm sure we'll be making great progress, but not before . . ." She let her words trail off.

"You mentioned a deadline," he prodded.

She paused a moment, then disclosed, "I shouldn't be telling you this, but Rainbow Hospital may soon be sold. The prospective buyers will be here next week—six days from now—to look everything over, and Harry—I mean, Dr. Seabold—has given me my orders: everything has got to be shipshape for their inspection tour."

Jorund listened carefully, trying to comprehend

all that the wench said. Although he was learning the language of this world day by day, he still had trouble with many of the words. *What has she to do with ships?* Finally he asked, "And I would not fit into this shipshape?"

"You would not fit into this shipshape," she agreed.

"So what will happen if I am not . . . uh, ship-shape by then?"

"Well, the team—Dr. Seabold, me, and your head nurse, Gladys Hatcher—would sit down and decide whether to send you to a state-run hospital, or just release you."

Jorund inhaled deeply with surprise. "Glad-ass has a say in my fate?" he inquired. He would have to be nicer to the witch in the future.

"Glad-ass?" the wench choked out.

"Yea, Norse Hatch-her . . . the sadist with the bed trencher."

Mag-he tried to suppress a smile, but he saw it nonetheless.

"Nurse Hatcher is a very nice woman . . . a dedicated professional."

He lifted both eyebrows in disbelief. "Are you speaking of the same person? The Amazon with the arms of a seasoned warrior?"

Mag-he smiled. "I wouldn't describe her in quite those words, but yes."

"Well, I am informing you here and now, that hatchet-faced, bed trencher–brandishing, smart-mouthed woman is having naught to do with my fate," he told her in no uncertain terms. "Back to that other . . . all I have to do is stay here for six days and then I could be freed?"

She nodded. "Possibly."

"Well, why didn't you tell me this afore?" *Six days? That is not an overlong delay.* Really, Jorund had no desire to rush back to the place where the killer whale had deposited him. For some reason his instincts told him to sit back and study his surroundings, to try to understand why the gods, or the bloody whale, had chosen to interrupt his father's quest with this particular stop. He was convinced he would have to locate Thora in order to return to his own time. He sensed that Thora would be the key to his return home.

"Oh, Joe," she said in a voice wobbly with emotion. "Being free isn't the answer if you're not well."

He cocked his head to the side and studied her more closely. "Why do you care?"

"I don't know," she answered, clearly dismayed. Her lips were trembling and her eyes misting up.

"Oh, for the love of Freyja! Tears!" The wench was about to weep. Over him! He could not abide female tears under the best of circumstances, and definitely not in pity of him. Straightening, he emitted a low growl of outrage and jerked his restricted arms sharply to the sides—once, twice, three times. To his amazement, as well as hers, the torture *shert* split down the center.

She gaped at him.

He gaped at her, then clicked his jaw shut. It was not fitting that he should appear dumbfounded at his own incredible strength.

"How did you do that?"

He shrugged, as if it were nothing. In truth, he had no idea how he had done it. One minute he had seen her near tears, and the next minute he was consumed with frustration at his being unable to . . . what? *Hold her? Holy Thor! Best I rein in those thoughts.*

"Are you Houdini, or some kind of magician?"

"Well, I have been known to wield magic on occasion," he lied. *Ha!* The only sorcery skill he could boast was that an overendowed Saxon tart had once told him he had magic in his rod, and she had been *drunkinn* at the time.

She narrowed her eyes at him. "Have you been playing a game with me?"

"Nay." *But I'd like to. One that involves kiss-some lips, sweet, succulent toes, long legs, round breasts, and a sex-voice.*

"Just tell me this . . . have you been able to break free from that straitjacket all along?"

"I have not," he answered honestly.

She seemed to accept his answer.

In a matter of seconds, he had tossed the garment aside and was flexing his limbs to get the blood flowing again. He turned back to the wench, glanced away, then immediately turned back. "What?" She was staring at his bare chest as if she'd never seen a naked man before, though he was not really naked, since he still wore those loose blue hospital *braies* with the waist ties.

He would have to be blind not to see the interest in her eyes. He stepped closer, obeying a strange compulsion that drew him against his will. It was like the sensation one got sometimes when standing on a cliff. A person didn't want to jump or fall forward, but there was some physical pulling sensation nonetheless. Had she cast a spell on him?

"Don't touch me. . . ." she protested weakly.

"I have wanted to touch you for days," he admitted in a gravelly voice, but he restrained himself from doing so. For now, he was content to inhale her flowery scent, to appreciate the rise and fall of those magnificent breasts, to wonder at the trembling of her full, cherry lips.

"You shouldn't . . . you can't."

"Who says I cannot?"

"I do. It's unethical."

"What?"

"I'm a doctor; you're my patient. There can be nothing personal between us."

He made a snorting sound of disagreement. "I know about this dock whore/pay-shun business from *The Guiding Light*. There was this man, Dock-Whore Rick, who . . . well, never mind that. Heed me well, wench; I never hired you to be my dock whore. Therefore, I cannot be your pay-shun. Mayhap I will be Dock-whore Hairy's pay-shun. Then I can touch you all I want."

He could see that he was confusing Mag-he. *Good.* It was always best to keep a wench in a muddled condition, lest she start thinking she had a brain equal to a man's. Also, women, no matter their station, were more likely to succumb to men's baser suggestions in that state. Once he had befuddled an Irish wench so badly that she had agreed to the most outrageous things. But that had been a long time ago, and it was neither here nor there.

Jorund needed a plan. Too many baffling thoughts and feelings were hitting him from every angle. If he were in the midst of battle, he would be dead by now. Where was his legendary gift for war tactics? How had he lost his focus?

113

"Come." He directed the wench to a small metal table with folding chairs on either side. "Sit down, and let us come up with a plan for healing me."

She eyed him skeptically, the way that women were wont to do on occasion when they thought their men were up to some mischief.

He sat down, but she still stood on the other side of the room, suspicious of him. He wished she would hurry so they could get this business over with. By his count of the big, circular ticking device on the wall, *Judge Judy* would be coming on the black world box soon, and he did enjoy her saucy tongue when wielding her edicts. He was learning much about the law of this land.

The wench went to a door first, which he had learned previously was called a close-it. From it she took a *shert*, which matched his *braies*. "Put this on first," she demanded.

He was about to ask why, but he knew . . . somehow he knew. His near-nudity disconcerted her. Now that was a fact to be stored for future reference. He did as she asked, leaving the strange fastening devices undone; they were known as butt-ons. For a certainty, he intended to take a sampling of these back to his country. He knew a few merchants who would pay a fortune for knowledge of their marvelous usage.

Now that they were sitting across from each other, Jorund took a deep breath and began, "Your problem is that you must heal me within a week, whilst—"

"No, not exactly. That's the purpose of a mental facility . . . to be helping patients with problems. What we can't have is your being locked in a barred room with ankle restraints and a straitjacket. I'm not saying they aren't legitimate tools for controlling out-of-control patients, but if the need for them continues for a week or more, then that person probably belongs in a maximum-security mental facility. Not here."

He put both hands in the air in a manner that said, *What is the problem?*

She tilted her head in silent question.

"Can't you see, the problem is halfway solved? My feet are free. . . ." he teased, extending one leg and wiggling his toes at her.

Her face went prettily pink at his action, and he thought, not without some satisfaction, that mayhap she had a fascination for his feet, just as he'd experienced over her flame-colored toenails. *How odd!* That was another fact to store for future reference.

"And I no longer wear the torture *shert*. Do you see me attacking anyone? Or harming myself?"

Just then the guard must have peered through the window and noticed that he was free. He opened the door and rushed in, about to attack him—or try to. "Dr. McBride! Why didn't you call for help?"

Dock-whore Muck-bride stood quickly, placing herself between Jorund, still seated, and the burly guardsman. "Everything's all right, Hank. I, um . . . I released Joe. A little experiment. And it's working out just fine."

God, he loved it when his very own Valkyrie— even if she wasn't such, he liked to think of her so—went hostile on his behalf. He would have jumped up and defended himself if he hadn't been enjoying the sight of her in battle mode so much.

"Well, if you say so," the guardsman agreed reluctantly and left, though Jorund noticed that he left the door ajar.

"Well done, m'lady." He gave her a smart salute.

"Huh?"

"You put Hunk in his proper place."

"Huh?"

"Now that we have resolved the first two obstacles—the ankle restraints and the torture *shert*—what can be done about the bars and locked doors?"

"I think an experiment is in order. We move you to another room. No bars. And the door will be unlocked for certain periods of the day . . . not all the time, at first. At those times you will be able to go to the activities room or the workout room, where you can mix with some of the other patients. How does that sound?"

Just wonderful! I will get to exchange pleasantries with demented people. "Fine," he said, because that was obviously the answer she wanted.

"Good." She smiled broadly. "I think we'll start by having you eat dinner with the others in the dining hall."

"I hope there will be no more of that green jail-low. That provender is a torment even the vilest prisoner should not be subjected to."

Mag-he thought a moment, then laughed. "Oh, you mean Jell-O. Yes, you're right. They do tend to overdo the green Jell-O a bit. Anyhow, if the dining experience works out all right, tomorrow you can join group therapy for the first time."

He didn't even want to know what he would be doing in a group with other half-witted people. But his brain cautioned him not to protest too much, to take one step at a time, to watch, assess, then act. "So this is how you heal people?"

"Well, not exactly. Usually we draw up a contract."

"See. Did I not offer already to have a contract with you?"

She shook her head at him as if he were a mischievous child. "Not that kind of contract."

His shoulders slumped with disappointment. "You do not want me for a love slave?"

"Get serious, Joe."

"I was serious. Well, mayhap I wasn't, really. But it did pose interesting possibilities. On the other hand, you could be *my* love slave. That definitely would be of interest. What do you think?"

"I think you just took five steps forward and ten steps backward in your healing with that comment."

"So what kind of contract do you usually do?" he asked, not bothering to hide his chagrin.

"We do a mental-health diagnosis, which we discuss with the patient. Then we set up goals for how to overcome those mental problems and enter back into society as a productive member . . . though some of our patients still work with us after they've left the clinic."

"I could do that," he concluded enthusiastically.

"Wonderful." He could tell she was about to conclude their meeting, which he wasn't prepared to do just yet.

"Wait," he said, stretching out a hand to encircle the nape of her neck. The short hairs were prickly and silky at the same time against his fingertips. "Do you not conclude contracts in a particular way, as they do in my country . . .

117

especially when the contract is a man-woman one?"

"Wh-what do you mean?"

Jorund saw the small pulse leap in her throat, as if she enjoyed his touch, despite herself, and yearned for more. Well, she was about to get more, if he had his way.

"In my culture, a true Norseman likes to seal his bargains with"—he leaned forward—"a kiss."

"Liar," she whispered.

The blood in Jorund's veins was pumping so wildly, he was in no condition to protest her insult.

His lips brushed hers then, back and forth, light as a feather, but the pleasure it evoked was so intense, he moaned against her lips. Or was it she who moaned into his mouth? He could not help himself then. He deepened the kiss and slipped his tongue between her parted lips. Sweet, sweet, sweet, she was. And hot!

He drew back sharply, and withdrew his hand.

He stared at her, mesmerized.

She stared at him, mesmerized.

It was she who spoke first. He could tell that she was about to say that this shouldn't have happened, or that it wouldn't happen again, as women throughout the ages were wont to do after they had succumbed to temptation, but instead she surprised even herself by blurting out an irrelevancy.

"I thought you didn't like kisses," she whispered in that sex-voice that seeped under his skin and grabbed at his loins with a jolt.

At first he was unable to utter a word. When he did, it was in a choked growl. "I changed my mind."

* * *

The next day . . .

Joe was about to begin his first group-therapy session, and Maggie was more than a little nervous.

It had taken some convincing to have Harry agree to Joe's moving into therapy so quickly, but even he was impressed with the way the man, who still claimed to be a tenth-century Viking, was mixing in with the others. Not only had he signed the personal contract required by Rainbow, the rules of which must be obeyed or the patient would be expelled, but he had behaved himself at dinner the night before, and he'd taken to the workout room with great enthusiasm.

One of the aides reported to her this morning that Jorund had lifted weights like an Olympian, and had manned the rowing machine as if it were an actual boat. In fact, he'd given it a name . . . *Fierce Wizard,* or some such thing. In true leadership fashion, he had set two other patients, who had been lethargic about exercise thus far, to rowing in tandem. You'd think they were the potential crew members of a . . . well, a longship.

Still, it was good to see Joe being proactive about something, anything. So much progress in such a short time was hard for Maggie to comprehend, but she wasn't about to protest a good thing.

"Are you ready?" she asked on arrival at his new room, where he was waiting for her. This room was the same as the other, sans barred windows and two-way mirrors on the corridor wall. She was about to escort him to the terrace room where group-therapy sessions were held. It was a light, sunny place that everyone liked.

"I must be. ~~We have~~ only five more days to get my ship in shape." He jiggled his eyebrows at her with his little joke, which was really odd because he appeared to be a man little inclined to teasing.

It was adorable the way he deliberately misinterpreted words and phrases. At least, she assumed it was deliberate. The other possibility meant more hurdles for them to jump in his therapy. And actually, he was adorable, period. Today he was wearing a white Dallas Cowboys T-shirt tucked into a pair of tight-fitting jeans and high-top athletic shoes. His long blond hair was held back off his face with a rubber band.

"We're wearing matching *braies*," he commented as they strolled down the corridor.

She looked down, then over at him. Yes, they *were* both wearing denim *braies*, which appeared to be the word Joe used for pants. But Maggie wasn't wearing a sweater or T-shirt today, as she usually did for these sessions. Instead she wore a white cotton blouse and a blue blazer. Group-therapy day was usually one on which she deliberately chose casual clothes to fit in with her patients. But today, she suspected, she hadn't wanted to be disconcerted by any hot looks toward any part of her anatomy . . . in particular, her breasts.

"I like you better in those sheer hose you wore yesterday," he mentioned, "but tight *braies* have a certain allure, too."

As if she cared!

Okay, she hardly cared.

She was trying not to care.

Oh, lordy!

Heads pivoted as they passed, and not just

those of the women staff and patients. Men
gawked, too. Joe Rand was a sight to see. It was-
n't just his immense height or good looks. It was
the way he carried himself, as if he were someone
important. No, that wasn't quite it. It was pride,
or grace, or an innate air of leadership . . . she
couldn't say for sure which.

"Do I pass your inspection?" he asked, apparently aware of her scrutiny.

"Just checking out your new duds. Thank God
for Goodwill."

She wasn't fooling him one bit. He was enjoying her discomfort immensely. That was especially obvious when his gaze snagged on her lips,
and paused.

Was he remembering their kiss?

She had certainly been able to think of little
else. And her dreams last night had been X-rated.
For a man who disliked kisses, he'd sure known a
whole lot of ways to kiss. In her dreams, at least.

"Oh, lady, if you're thinking what I think you
are, I am not going to be able to concentrate on
anything during this group-therapy business.
Leastways, anything except how soon I can bed
you."

Maggie gasped. "I was not thinking anything at
all like that." *Exactly*. "I will tell you this, Joe:
there can be no repeat of what happened yesterday. I'm willing to overlook one kiss. You caught
me off guard. But if you try it again while you're
my patient, I'm going to have to excuse myself
from your case."

The knowing look he gave her didn't bode well
for Maggie. This Viking was going to do whatever
he wanted. And he wasn't fooled one bit by her

insinuation that the kiss had been a one-sided deal. She had participated, too. And enjoyed it immensely.

Luckily, they were interrupted then by Harry, who was on his way to a budget meeting.

"How do you do, Joe?" Harry reached out and shook Joe's hand . . . an action that Joe looked on with puzzlement. "I'm Dr. Harrison Seabold. I know we've met before, but I just thought I'd introduce myself again. Glad to see you moving around, buddy. And talking."

Joe looked at their joined hands, then at Maggie. "Is this a gesture of welcome in your land?"

"Yes. Exactly," she said, which prompted him to reach out and shake her hand, as well . . . heartily.

"How do you do?" he repeated woodenly.

"Not quite so tight," she advised, and he loosened his iron grip.

"See," he pointed out as they continued to the end of the hall. "I can adapt to your culture."

In little ways, he could. But Maggie wondered how he would handle the bigger things—like his first group-therapy session.

The others were already there when they arrived, sitting about in a circle of folding chairs.

Steve Askey was an attractive, fiftyish former professional baseball player and Navy SEAL vet, who suffered from PTSD, posttraumatic stress disorder. His alcoholism and subsequent self-destructive behavior had already resulted in a broken marriage, which had further escalated his problems. Despite being on the wagon for a year, he thought he had no future. She could see it in his posture as he slumped in his chair, staring at nothing.

Chuck Belammy, thirty, was purported to have multiple-personality disorder, except that his was the darnedest case Maggie had ever heard of. His personalities were animals: a cow who ate grass and mooed all the time, a galloping horse, a chicken pecking for kernels of corn, a rooster crowing—which could be annoying in a hospital setting—and a slithering snake. His animal personas all had names. Right now he must be Bessie, because he was making mooing sounds and chewing his cud. Actually, Chuck's "animal MPD" was a sham ... something the very intelligent young man had dreamed up to throw his doctors off track. Underneath, he hid some other mental problems that he deemed too horrible— or embarrassing—to share ... yet.

Natalie Blue, twenty-four, was agoraphobic— afraid to leave her house, even to go shopping. Ironically, she dreamed of being a country-western singer, which would be impossible if she was unable to perform before crowds. But she'd progressed tremendously in the past six months. At least now she came to them as an outpatient. There was a time when she'd been unable to leave the security of her bedroom.

Rosalyn Harris, twenty-eight, was a mousy librarian, when she was able to work. Most often she just rocked back and forth. Sometimes Rosalyn mutilated herself. Thus far Maggie had been unable to diagnose the cause of her condition, except that she had feelings of low self-worth. Rosalyn lived at home and was brought to the clinic weekly by her parents, who insisted on her getting therapy because they believed she was anorexic. Maggie thought there might be some other reason for her withdrawal . . . something Rosalyn had yet to disclose.

Harvey Lutz, a nerdy looking young man in his early twenties, was a bipolar obsessive-compulsive who had a habit of continually counting things and lining them up. Right now he was counting lint pills on his wool trousers. Every time he got to twelve, he stumbled and started over.

Fred Bernstein, a balding, middle-aged man, was delusional, hiding his problems in fantasy identities. From one week to the next, she never knew if he was some famous movie star, athlete, or biblical figure. She couldn't wait to hear why he was carrying two large, ironstone dinner platters today. The kitchen staff wouldn't be pleased to know they were missing.

Sometimes there were extra people in the group: a biker from Houston with head injuries, a chronically depressed accountant who yearned for a lost love, and various others. The wonderful thing about Rainbow, in Maggie's opinion, was that people could come and go, as their ailments required.

Maggie sat down next to Rosalyn and motioned for Joe to sit across the circle, with Chuck on one side and Steve on the other. That was when she realized that Joe wasn't beside her. Looking up, she saw him still standing in the doorway, gawking at the group as if he'd landed in . . . well, Bedlam.

But what he said was, "Is this Niflheim?"

Chapter Seven

Jorund could not believe his eyes. He'd never seen so many lackwitted people in one room in all his life. Even Viking warriors in the midst of battle who had gone berserk did not look this bizarre.

The most difficult thing to accept in this scenario was that Mag-he thought he was as demented as this lot of mush-brains. Raising his chin, Jorund fixed a glower on the female who had brought him there, and immediately eased his temper. There was a pleading expression on her face—one that begged him not to make a scene, or embarrass her in front of her other pay-shuns.

Biting his bottom lip to keep him from saying what he really thought, Jorund followed Mag-he's direction and sat in a seat across from her.

Almost immediately, he jumped when he got a good view of the man sitting next to him . . . and what he was doing.

"Bock, bock, bock, bock, bock!" the red-haired young man, who couldn't have seen more than thirty winters, was clucking as he bobbed his head like a rooster.

Jorund glanced at Mag-he, then back at the man, who greeted him with, "Cock-a-doodle-do!"

Yea, I was correct. A rooster.

"Everyone is looking good today," Mag-he said brightly.

Is she demented, too? Everyone did not look good, in Jorund's opinion. In fact, they were a sorry lot, if he'd ever seen one.

"We have a new group member today." She went around the circle and told Jorund each of their names . . . Steve, Chuck, Not-a-lie, Rosalyn, Furr-red, and Hair-vee. "I'd like to introduce you all to Joe Rand," Mag-he was saying.

They all stared at him curiously, and a woman who was as plain as a brown field mouse whistled under her breath, which seemed to surprise everyone. At least it took everyone's attention away from him.

"Did you say something, Rosalyn?" Mag-he asked excitedly.

The mouse woman kept her gaze downward, as if there were something important on the legs of her gray *braies*, which she pleated and unpleated in a jittery fashion. She refused to answer. And Jorund noticed something else: there were scars all over her forearms, like cuts from a sharp blade, and small burn marks, too.

Mag-he shrugged at the uncooperative pay-shun and was about to speak herself, but Jorund felt the need to correct something before she started.

"Ah, Dock-whore Muck-bride." He waved a hand at her to get her attention.

The nervous tapping of her wooden stick on the parchment pad told him she was tense over what he might say.

"My name is not Joe Rand. It is Jorund . . . Jorund Ericsson." While he spoke, he stood and went to each person in the circle and pumped their right hands with his right hand in salutation, repeating over and over, "How do you do?" It was a strange ritual, but then there were strange customs in many of the lands he'd visited.

She hesitated at his insistence on using his real name, then agreed with a nod of her head. "Fine, Jorund it is then . . . unless of course you go by the nickname of Joe, as well."

"I never have, in the past."

"Well, it's up to you," she said cheerily, as if it were of great import what name he answered to.

"I care not what you call me," he grumbled. "I am Jorund the Warrior. If you want to call me Joe, it is neither here nor there to me, though I think Joe the Warrior sounds mighty peculiar. By the by, am I cured yet?"

"No, you're not cured yet," she declared with a laugh, then addressed the group. "Joe has a great sense of humor. Ha, ha, ha."

I do?

"Jorund the Warrior, huh?" a man on his other side commented. "You one of them WWF crazies or something?" The man was about fifty years old with a receding hairline but a well-honed body that would do a Norseman proud. He wore the same blue *braies* as Jorund did . . . in fact, all the men, and Mag-he, too. His short-sleeved *shert* carried the words *U.S. Navy SEAL.*

It was odd this practice they had in this country of carrying messages on their *sherts*. Jorund had noticed this first at the orca place. Now not only did the man on one side of him wear words on his apparel about seals, but the clodpole on the other side proclaimed on his long-sleeved *shert, I Don't Suffer from Insanity; I Enjoy Every Minute of It.*

Back to the seal man. " 'Double-ewe, double-ewe, if?' " Jorund inquired, as if he cared a whit . . . which he did not. The whole time he was thinking, *Good Lord! One of these half-brains thinks he's a rooster, and the other thinks he's a seal. What next?*

"Cra-aaazy! I'm cra-aaazy for feelin' so lonely." Another woman, huddled in a chair in the corner, began to sing.

Jorund almost fell out of his seat at the sudden singing.

The female was young, in her twenties, and pretty in a frightened-bird sort of way. Her voice was rather melodious, but singing spontaneously struck Jorund as rather . . . well, crazy. *Crazy* was a word he had learned from the black world box in his room, which he had come to find out was called a tea-vee.

"I go out walkin' after midnight . . ." the woman sang next.

He saw no one walking, and it was definitely far from midnight. Jorund glanced around and noticed that no one paid any mind to the singer. It was as if they didn't even hear her, or mayhap they were ignoring her, to spare her humiliation.

"WWF is the World Wrestling Federation," Mag-he explained.

At first, Jorund had to think what she was referring to; then he recalled that the seal man had asked if he was in the double-ewe, double-ewe, if.

"It includes professional wrestlers who put on rather flamboyant acts in the ring."

Jorund had no idea what she'd just said.

"Like Hulk Hogan. 'Stone Cold' Steve Austin. Jake the Snake. Or Jesse 'the Body' Ventura," the seal offered.

"I knew a Norseman once who called himself Snorri the Snake; he had a special talent for fluttering his tongue that women especially liked. But he lost a leg in some Saxon battle a few years back. 'Tis hard to keep track of all the Norse-Saxon battles. There are so many of them. The English weasels are always trying to provoke us Vikings." Jorund couldn't believe he was jabbering away like a magpie.

The rooster next to him suddenly became a snake and was darting his tongue in and out of his mouth and making slithering motions with his shoulders. Everyone else was gaping at Jorund as if he'd sprouted three heads, but they didn't even blink at the snake.

Jorund knew he spoke in what they considered a foreign accent, in words they were unfamiliar with, but really, he was not the odd bead in this circle. He continued expounding: "I can wrestle, of course, but mostly I am just a Viking . . . a Viking soldier."

"A soldier!" Steve, the seal fellow on his other side, exclaimed. "Son of a bitch! Don't tell me you have PTSD, too."

Jorund gave his attention to the man, who was sitting up straighter now. "Pea-tea-ass-deed?"

"That's posttraumatic stress disorder," Mag-he interjected. "It's a syndrome that many soldiers get after active duty."

Another person with a sin-drone! Just like me.

"You were a warrior?" he asked Steve. "And you suffer from this Pea-tea-ass-deed?"

"Hell, yes. Along with alcoholism, chronic depression, a broken marriage, impotence, 'Nam shakes, flashbacks, nightmares that could turn your hair white. You name it, I got it."

"What is impotence?" he whispered in an aside to Steve.

"Involuntary downtime for your . . ." He waved a hand toward his genital area. "Former Red Sox baseball player. Navy SEAL vet. Can't get the lead back in his pencil. What a laugh, huh?"

Jorund nodded knowingly, and he did not think it was a laughing matter at all. "I know much of this ailment."

"You do?" Maggie asked with astonishment.

"Not from personal experience," he was quick to add, "but many of my soldiers suffer from this malady after a particularly gruesome battle, or after serving in too many wars."

He glanced around and saw that he had everyone's attention, even the women. Was he talking too much? He looked at Mag-he and she appeared enthralled, so he assumed he was on the right course to curing himself.

"Are you for real?" But Steve meant no insult.

He was genuinely interested in knowing more, as became evident with his next query. "And how did those soldiers get . . . better?"

"Well, the healers never did have the answers. But then, they rarely do. Just slap on the leeches and grind up a few powders. As I recall, time was the most important thing."

"It's been ten freakin' years, man!" Steve snarled.

Jorund decided to ignore his less-than-respectful tone. "The most important thing is for the man not to believe that he is less than a man. It is a natural condition that will pass, in time, if the man does not let himself think it is permanent. Unless, of course, there was actual bodily injury, like an arrow to the balls, or a battle-ax severing the cock."

Every man in the room cringed and crossed his legs.

"Then, of course, there are some potions that can help, in some cases," Jorund concluded.

"Like Viagra? That's for old men," Steve scoffed.

"Not necessarily," a new voice in the circle offered. It was Hair-vee, a young man who had been counting the lint pieces on his trousers ever since Jorund had arrived. "I tried it once."

"You did?" at least five voices asked.

"Yep. My girlfriend got it for me. Man, oh, man, I had a five-hour hard-on. Shirley was happier than a hog in a mud slide."

"You are such a bullshitter," Steve observed.

"You don't even have a girlfriend," Chuck added.

"What's vie-ag-rah?" Jorund wanted to know.

131

"You know what they say about the watched kettle never boiling," Hair-vee threw in. "Maybe you've been watching your kettle too much."

"Maybe I'll break a kettle over your head, Lutz," Steve remarked.

Unconcerned, Hair-vee went back to counting, his own teeth this time. It was not a pretty sight.

"I heard some positions are better than others for maintaining . . ." Rosalyn's voice trailed off when she saw that everyone was gawking at her.

Furr-red, the man holding the two dinner trenchers, bobbed up and down in his seat. He couldn't wait to offer, "A psychiatrist once told me that too much masturbation can make a guy get the technique down so good that no woman can please him."

"What's master-bait-shun?" Jorund asked.

"Jesus H. Christ!" Steve put his face in both hands and groaned. "Please, God, cut out my tongue if I ever decide to say anything to this motley crew again."

"My brother bought an electronic device on the Internet that you attach to your willy." Not-a-lie had stopped humming long enough to offer that sage advice. "It could tell a guy exactly how long his erection lasted, and how hard it was. Honest. Unless he got a shock, of course."

"I wish I were dead," Steve said. Then: "You people really are nuts if you think I'm gonna risk lightning boltin' my dingo."

"I think we've heard enough on this subject for today," Mag-he announced in a decisive voice, her face blushing profusely. From the blush on her face, he figured a dingo must be something sexual . . . and interesting.

"Fred, what are those lovely plates you're carrying today?" Mag-he asked.

"My name isn't Fred," Fur-red said. "It's Moses."

Oh, for the love of Freyja!

"These are the Ten Commandments," he added, contemplating the food trenchers with the same fondness a mother would show toward a newborn babe cradled in the crook of her arm.

And Mag-he thinks I am in the same class as these muddleheaded fools?

"Natalie, we haven't heard from you today, except for some singing, which was lovely, by the way."

Not-a-lie had her hands folded in her lap, where she kept wringing them nervously. But she did peer up finally and disclose, "I went to the mall with my mother this week."

"Why, Natalie, that's wonderful!" Mag-he said, and started to clap her hands together. As if on cue, everyone else started clapping their hands together, too. So Jorund joined in, as well. He assumed that this hand-clapping was a sign of approval. He had no idea what they were all approving of, but for now he was willing to go along with the crowd, especially if it would convince Mag-he that he was improving.

"I'm a sex addict," the mousy woman known as Rosalyn blurted out.

Everyone appeared stunned by her announcement. Then, one by one, the men leaned forward with decided interest to gaze at the plain wench.

"What's a sex add-hick?" Jorund asked Steve.

Steve jiggled his eyebrows. "A person who can't get enough."

133

"Enough what?"

The only response Steve gave him was a grin and a jab in the ribs with his elbow.

"Oh," Jorund murmured when realization hit. And he, too, leaned forward for a better view. The wench still looked plain as barley flour, even with her now flaming face.

"Rosalyn," Mag-he said. "You never told us *that* before. Thank you for sharing." Mag-he started to clap, and everyone joined in. The men clapped really hard.

"I wanted to tell you, but I was too . . . too embarrassed."

"Now, Rosalyn, you know that we decided at the beginning of group that there would be no judging of each other . . . that no one should be embarrassed to disclose anything. Therapy won't work if we're not, all of us, honest with each other."

"Hell, if I can admit I've got a limp wick, what the hell were you afraid of?" Steve asked huffily.

Rosalyn gave Steve a scathing glare.

"Why are you here?" Hair-vee had stopped counting his teeth and was now counting the butt-ons lining the front of his *shert*, even as he addressed his blunt question to Jorund.

All eyes swung his way.

He wasn't sure what he should say. "I'm here to be, ah, healed."

"From what?" the singer asked, then resumed humming.

Jorund mumbled under his breath.

"What?" They all strained to hear.

"I am Jorund the Warrior, and I come from the tenth century," he practically shouted.

All jaws, except Mag-he's, were open. She just seemed sad.

Then a small voice next to him that sounded very much like a horse neighing commented, "Well, whoop-dee-dee!"

Maggie was leaning over Beth's shoulder that evening while she explained her Internet Web site.

"Orcalove.com is only for kids around my age, from eight to twelve. I want other young people, all over the world, to learn about killer whales. We share information, but mostly we want to increase the number of people who care about them. If we start young enough, maybe our generation will be the one to stop the killing and capture of these creatures."

"You sound like a teacher," Suzy commented from the sofa, where she was supposed to be doing homework. Instead Maggie noticed that the TV had somehow been turned on, to MTV, no less, and that singing sensation, Ricky Martin, was swinging his hips and belting out the sexy lyrics to his stellar hit song from the previous year, "Livin' La Vida Loca." Even Maggie had to stop and look and listen when he came on. Beth, too. In no way did he resemble Joe, as Beth had stated one time, but the singer was very cute.

"So what if I sound like a teacher," Beth protested. "It's important to save the orcas."

"Yeah, yeah, yeah," Suzy commented to her sister. "Wanna dance?"

"Oh, OK," Beth said. First she saved the information on her computer screen and walked over

135

to Suzy, who was standing in the middle of the small den now, mimicking the movements of Ricky and the scantily clad dancers. The two of them were soon into the salsa beat. "Inside out, upside down, Livin' La Vida Loca," Ricky belted out, while the girls danced on, swinging their hips, lifting a leg, shaking their buns.

"Come on, Mom. You, too," Suzy encouraged.

Maggie hesitated a second, then joined them. It took her a moment to get the moves right, but soon she, too, was swinging and swaying to the irresistible beat. When the song ended with a flourish, they all fell back onto the sofa, laughing uproariously.

This was one of those moments out of time that would be impressed on Maggie's memory. It exemplified, albeit in a small way, how she and her girls were happy and contented in their lives. That was so important. More important than money, or . . . or husbands and daddies.

"Is Joe getting better?" Beth asked, as if reading her mind.

Maggie nodded. "Yes. Yes, he is. Today he had his first group-therapy session, and he did surprisingly well." That wasn't disclosing too much doctor/patient information, Maggie figured. And actually, Maggie was so proud of Joe . . . not just for his own progress, but for the sensitive way in which he'd treated his fellow patients.

"When he's better, can we meet him?" Suzy pleaded.

"I don't know. Maybe. No promises."

"You know something odd," Beth said. "I forgot to tell you this before, but my friends on the Internet have been reporting sightings of that whale that brought Joe to Orcaland. It's as if it's been hanging around, looking for him."

"Oh, I don't know about that. It could be any whale. How would they know it was this particular one?"

"All killer whales are not alike, Mom. Each has distinguishing marks and coloring. Besides, Joe's whale is odd because orcas rarely travel in the wild in this part of the country. The water is too warm."

"There's probably some scientific explanation," Maggie insisted.

"Or maybe there isn't," Beth countered.

"Why can't you just believe in the magic of it all?" Suzy wanted to know. "Why can't you accept that maybe—just maybe—the orca brought Joe here. For us."

"That would be more than magic, hon." Maggie hauled both Suzy and Beth into a hug on either side of her. "It would be more like . . . like . . ." Maggie couldn't come up with the exact words she was searching for–not fast enough, anyway. But her girls had no trouble. They finished for her.

"Like a dream come true."

Two days later, Maggie was walking outside on the clinic grounds with Joe.

He was alternately staring at the sky and over toward the highway. Though he no longer talked about it, the man couldn't seem to accept the concept of airplanes and automobiles. His face was grim with some private thoughts. Perhaps homesickness. But the home Joe insisted was his, was thousands of miles away, and a thousand years in the past.

Despite that, his progress thus far—ever since he'd started talking—was remarkable, to say the least. If he would stop insisting that he was a tenth-century Viking and tell them who he really was, Maggie would almost believe he had no mental problems at all.

The most gratifying thing about his progress was that he was helping the other patients. Dozens of the resident patients were heavily involved in exercise, and that was always good.

Many of them had already been addicted to soap operas, but now it had become a communal undertaking, directed by Joe. They watched the soaps together, then discussed them, as if these were real-life happenings. *Isn't that Victor Newman a self-important dictator? How about that hotty, Brooke Logan, with her penchant for stealing other women's men? Will Reva recover from her latest bout of amnesia?*

Joe also had a fascination with the reruns of *The Andy Griffith Show*. One of the nurses told her that Joe liked the program so much because Barney Fife reminded him of his big-eared brother . . . a Viking named Magnus.

"I'm going to have to leave here soon," he announced suddenly, sinking down on a bench near a small flower garden.

"I see." Alarm shot through Maggie like wildfire. She sat down beside him and closed her eyes momentarily in dismay.

"I left my homeland on a quest for my father. Much unfinished business awaits me. I cannot dawdle here much longer without making an effort to locate Thora and my way home. If naught else, I cannot risk being on the high seas come winter."

At first, an overwhelming sadness swept over her—that he still clung to these foolish notions. But then inspiration hit her. "I have the most wonderful idea."

"Somehow I misdoubt that your idea of a wonderful idea would coincide with mine . . . unless it involves sex."

She slanted him a disapproving frown, then continued. "I think we should go on a field trip to Orcaland. It might be just the trick to jar your memories and convince you that you aren't really a time traveler."

He just stared at her.

Disappointment that he wasn't immediately receptive dampened her enthusiasm, but only for a second when she realized he might not know what a field trip was. "A field trip is an excursion away from a facility. Not a permanent release. Just a day trip."

"So you are suggesting that you and I go to Orcaland . . . to visit the site of my time travel, and perhaps get a glimpse of Thora . . . and some answers."

She nodded hesitantly. "It wouldn't be just you and me, though. I would have to take the others in the group. I know, I know," she said excitedly. "We could stop by that traveling Vietnam memorial exhibit, as well. The Moving Wall, I think it's called. That might benefit Steve. And later, dinner at that new club, Boot Scootin' Cowboy, would give Natalie a glimpse of how her life could be if she ever realized her dream of being a country-western singer. I hear they have live entertainment there."

"Mayhap we could also stop by a farm and let Hair-vee check out the livestock for a new personality. Or perchance Rosalyn the mouse could snag a customer or two for a swiving marathon."

Maggie gave Joe a dirty look. "Your sarcasm doesn't help."

He shrugged.

"This is a good idea. A *really* good idea," she insisted. "Of course, I'll have to get permission from Harry—I mean, Dr. Seabold—first, but I don't think he'll object."

"Is he your lover?"

"Huh? Who? Harry? No, of course not." She put a hand to her mouth to hide her smile.

He exhaled with a loud whoosh, as if relieved. "Good."

Good? Why is that good? No, don't ask. It will just start him on the topic of things he and I shouldn't be discussing. But, good?

Changing the subject, she remarked, "Of course, my daughters will be upset that they can't come along. Especially Beth. She just loves killer whales and Orcaland."

Joe drew himself up stiffly. "I give you notice here and now: I am going nowhere with those girls of yours. Not now or ever. Keep them away from me."

Maggie would have been outraged at his maligning her daughters if she hadn't noticed the haunted expression in his gray eyes. In fact, she could swear they were misty with tears.

"Joe . . . ?" she probed.

He turned his face away from her.

She put a hand on his arm. "Don't you like children?"

Swinging his head, he scowled at her. "Heed me well, wench. Push me too far, and I will not be responsible for my actions."

An alarming question occurred to Maggie . . . one she should have asked before. "Are you married? Do you have a wife somewhere?"

His throat worked as if he was attempting to speak, but the words wouldn't come out. Finally he answered in a whisper of a voice, "I have no wife."

For some reason that news heartened Maggie. She shouldn't care, but she did. "Okay, one last question."

"One too many," he grumbled, looking down at his fists, which were clenched between his widespread knees.

"Do you have any children? Perhaps a little girl who resembles one of mine?"

"Your tongue outruns your good sense, you foolish wench." He stood suddenly and faced her angrily. A low growl came up from deep within before he informed her in an ice-cold voice, "Seed of my loins exists nowhere in this living world, neither male nor female." With those words hurled at her, Joe stomped off on the sidewalk leading back to the clinic.

Maggie watched him leave. Without realizing it, Joe had given her a clue that might lead to his cure. Children. There was no doubt in Maggie's mind. Children were the clue to Joe's dysfunction.

* * *

Jorund's emotions were in a roil the rest of that day.

He exercised on the rowing machine till he thought his arms would fall off. He joined some pay-shuns in a lackbrain game of Bingo. He threw a Freeze-bee in the halls with Steve, till Norse Hatch-her took the circular toy away from him. He Ping-Ponged till his head felt as if it Ping-Ponged. He ate a dinner of burr-eat-toes and salt-sa that about took the lining off his tongue. He viewed "Em-tea-vee" till his eyes burned.

Still, thoughts of his daughters would not go away. Was he cursed for the rest of his life, or may-hap all of eternity, to carry this guilt with him?

It was all Mag-he's fault. Why did she have to probe so deeply?

"What I need is about a tun of mead," he muttered.

"Isn't mead some kind of beer?" Steve asked from the open doorway. "Me, too, then. A cold beer and a baseball game would come in handy about now. Mine would have to be the nonalcoholic kind, though." Without being invited, he stepped into Jorund's room and sank down into one of the two leather armchairs in front of the tea-vee.

"Baseball? Isn't that a game where you hit a ball with a stick and run around a diamond-shaped field? One of the Norses explained it to me."

Steve gaped at him for a second, then laughed. "Hell, don't tell me you've never seen a baseball game. Man, that's purely un-American." Taking the remote control from Jorund's hand, he flicked the channels until he came to one of those baseball games, the Dodge-hers against the Red Sox, and for the next hour he proceeded to explain the game to a fascinated Jorund.

"And you excelled at this game?"

"That was thirty years ago, but yeah, everyone said I was the next Ted Williams."

"And this is what you did in life? You played games?"

Steve laughed at his apparent confusion and named some seemingly high amount of money he was paid for this occupation.

"You obviously loved this game. 'Twas in your eyes when you watched it on the tea-vee box. Why did you stop?"

"I was drafted . . . well, actually I jumped the gun because I knew I was going to be drafted."

"Drafted?"

"Uh-huh. I got the word that Uncle Sam wanted me for military service, and there was no saying no in those days. The Vietnam War was at its height. I enlisted in the Navy SEALs." He shrugged. "The rest is history."

Jorund didn't understand all that he had said. Uncle Sam, for instance. Nay-vee, for another. But the gist of it filtered through: Steve had fought in some gruesome war as a soldier of some sort, and although it had been many years ago, he still suffered the consequences.

"Did your wife leave you whilst you were away at battle?"

At first Steve's eyes flashed angrily at the intrusive question, but then his body relaxed, almost as if he was tired of holding it all in. "Nah! Shelley stuck around for twenty years. I haven't seen her for ten years. Hell, that was the last time we made love, too. The last time I was able to get it up. And a poor performance it was."

Jorund decided to ignore Steve's remarks on his sexual prowess. "Well, you are fortunate then. Many a feckless wench have I encountered in my day. Faithless women who spread their legs for another the minute their men pick up spear and shield to go off a-Viking or a-fighting."

"Huh?" Steve said. Then his thoughts reverted back to his Shell-he. "Man, I made Shell's life a living hell. Good thing we never had kids. I probably would have made them suffer, too."

Although Steve claimed happiness in not having bred children, Jorund could see the lie in his lifeless eyes. Jorund could understand this. Hadn't he disdained children all his life, too? Then hadn't he seen the mistruth of his lifelong protestations the moment his daughters were born?

"I have heard much on *The Young and the Restless* this week about divorce . . . which we have in my land, too. Did you divorce your wife . . . or did she divorce you?"

"Shelley's back in Iowa, teaching school. I figured she'd file for divorce once she met another man and wanted to get married again. I never received any notification, though, so I really don't know." He stared blankly at the screen for a long time before he spoke again. "I thought she'd find someone else right off the bat. In fact, I hope she did. Shell is so beautiful. She deserves more than a broken-down ex–baseball player." His voice cracked on that last, making it as clear as a sunny day on a northern fjord that Steve's biggest problem wasn't his impotence, or aleheadedness, or black night-frights, but the empty hole left in his life by a woman.

That was the way of it throughout time, Jorund decided. Women were the root of all men's problems.

Chapter Eight

Maggie rarely went back to the hospital at night, but the girls were attending a birthday party at a friend's house, and she just couldn't stop worrying about Joe. The anguished look on his face when she'd last seen him stabbed at her heart.

"Joe?" She stepped tentatively into his room, which was dark except for the light from the TV screen. "Are you awake?"

He didn't answer, though she could make out his semirecumbent form on the bed, arms folded behind his head.

"I came back to apologize," she said, closing the door behind her, then stepping closer to the bed, where she could see that his eyes were open and staring right at her. "I shouldn't have pushed you with all those family inquiries. It was too much, too soon. And you have a right to some privacy. When you're ready—"

Before she had a chance to finish her sentence, Joe reached out and grabbed her by the waist. "Oh, I am ready, wench. I am more than ready." In a blink, she was flat on her back on the bed, and he lay on top of her, his upper body braced on his extended arms.

"M'lady, you are driving me mad," he said in a husky growl.

"Mad?" she chocked out. With his maleness pressed against her femaleness, sanity seemed to be lacking in her as well.

"Yea, all your probing interrogations are driving me mad. Then, too, there are your kiss-some lips, and sex-voice, and eyes so blue they draw a man in and catch him unawares, and legs just the right size to wrap around a man's waist, and breasts. . . . holy Thor, your breasts would fit just perfectly in my hands. All these things are driving me mind-draining mad." He took a deep breath, one she felt against her diaphragm, then continued. "I was sane when I arrived in this godforsaken land. Why are you doing this to me?"

"Why do you think I'm doing this to you?" she squeaked out.

"Aaarrgh! Always you turn my questions back on me. Can you not give a straight answer just once?"

"Well, yes," she whispered.

"And you will answer straight and true?"

She nodded.

Maggie knew it was a mistake even before Joe uttered the delicious words, "Do you want me as much as I want you?"

Oh, this was dangerous territory for a psychologist to enter with her patient. Maggie could lose her license. But even if no one found out, she would know there was an ethical line that had been crossed, if she answered honestly with herself.

He put his fingertips to her lips. "Shhh. Don't speak. There are some things that need not be said aloud."

He lowered his upper body so that he rested on his elbows. Furrowing his fingers through her hair on either side, he cupped her head. "Why did you cut your hair so short?" he asked, even as he inhaled deeply, taking in the scent of her shampoo.

"I lost a bet with my girls."

His face jerked to the side at the mention of her daughters, as if he'd been slapped. It was she, then, who cupped his jaw and turned his face back. "Joe? What is it? Tell me why the mere mention of my daughters upsets you so,"

"You overreach yourself my lady."

"I want to help."

"What you want does not signify in this situation. You can't help . . . not with this. Leave be, I tell you. Leave be."

She realized that he wasn't ready to share his grief yet . . . whatever that grief was. "You've got to let me up, Joe. If anyone saw us, I could be in big trouble. You, too, for that matter. Remember the contract you signed with your X mark?"

"Words! Nothing but words! You gainsay me at every turn, my lady. How long do you think I will allow you to hold me off?"

"Let me up," was her only response.

At first it appeared as if he would balk, but then he said, "I will release you if you but grant me one token."

"And that would be?" she asked with a small laugh.

"A kiss."

"A kiss?"

"Yea . . . a *good* kiss."

"You said you don't like kisses."

"I thought we already cleared up that misunderstanding. I have changed my mind . . . leastways, with you. Besides, I doubt you would agree if I'd suggested a good swiving."

"Not if it's what I think it is." *This conversation is totally out-of-bounds. I am totally out-of-bounds.*

He smiled . . . another of those smiles that parted his lips and exposed his white teeth, but did not reach his eyes. "It is. But you should know that I give good swives."

"You also give good kisses."

"I do?" he said, inordinately pleased. "And with so little practice. Imagine how good I will be when we have kissed a hundred times or so."

"A hun-hundred?" she stammered. "You said one kiss."

"For now," he murmured against her lips. "One *good* kiss for now to hold me over till next time."

"Joe, there can't be a next—"

Her words were cut off with the soft caress of his firm lips against hers. Back and forth, back and forth, he rubbed till she was pliant and willing. Only then did his kiss turn into a hungry, punishing, sweet torture, an exercise in eroticism. He shaped her lips with his, then pressed

149

hard. When his tongue thrust into her mouth, she moaned, then moaned again when it began an in-and-out rhythm that caused her nipples to peak and hot liquid to pool between her legs.

Maggie went delirious with need, something she had never done in all her thirty-two years. She would die if this kiss went on any longer. She would die if it stopped.

His hands were everywhere—fondling her breasts, skimming her hips, cupping her buttocks and rocking her against his erection.

Erection! Maggie's eyes flew open, and it was as if she stood above the writhing bodies on the bed. When had her legs spread wide and wrapped themselves about his hips? When had he begun pounding against the apex of her thighs, mimicking the sex act? *Good Lord!* Maggie shoved hard against his chest, and because he was caught unawares, she was able to slip out from under him and stagger to the door, where she pressed her forehead against the cool glass and panted for breath.

Behind her, she heard a string of unbroken words in a foreign tongue, which she assumed were swear words. They dwindled down eventually to silence.

Finally, when she had calmed down, Maggie flicked on the light switch, and turned.

Jorund sat on the edge of the bed, his arms braced on his widespread knees, breathing heavily. He stared at her with barely suppressed anger. "You will bend to my will one day," he said, and he was serious. "Your days are numbered."

"This will never happen between us again," she

disagreed in a shaky voice, rubbing her fingers across her kiss-swollen lips.

He started to laugh then, and couldn't seem to stop.

"What's so damn funny?" Maggie asked huffily.

Joe wiped at his eyes with the backs of his hands. "I'll tell you what's so funny, my lady. You speak of endings, but methinks there is another direction for our relationship."

"Relationship? Relationship? We have no relationship," she shrieked.

He hit the side of his head with the heel of one hand. "Must you be so shrill? Your screeching hurts my ears. Reminds me of a seagull when it spots a tasty meal."

She gritted her teeth and clenched her fists to calm down. "Get this though your thick skull: we have no relationship."

"Ha! Think again, my lady," he declared with a droll expression on his face. "I have just realized an important fact about us."

She was about to scream that there was no "us," but restrained herself. Instead she lifted one eyebrow in question.

"I think you are my fate. I think you are the reason I was sent here."

Maggie did scream then, silently.

"Oh, my God!"

The tour of the Rainbow facilities by the Medic-All contingent had just been successfully completed, and Maggie was about to breathe a deep sigh of relief when she heard Harry's exclamation. Turning, she followed the direction of his gaze, down the corridor to the open doorway of the exercise room. It was her turn to exclaim then, "Oh, my God!"

Joe was leaning against the doorjamb, wearing black sweatpants, white high tops, and a gray T-shirt that spelled out, *No Pain, No Gain*. He was talking animatedly to a short, gray-haired gentleman in wing tips and a pin-striped business suit . . . a stranger, as far as Maggie could tell.

With trepidation, she inquired of the Medic-All PR man, George Smith, "Who is that?"

"Oh! So he decided to come, after all," George answered enthusiastically. He was already walking away.

"Who?" she and Harry said at the same time, rushing to catch up. The other six members of the Medic-All group, along with two members of the Lawrence family, which owned the privately held Rainbow facility, followed quickly behind them.

"Jerome Johnson. President and CEO of Medic-All," George informed them over his shoulder. "He was supposed to be tied up all day in meetings with the Dallas lawyers. Guess he decided to cut them short."

So this was the elusive, high-powered Donald Trump of the HMO world. He resembled a mild-mannered Mr. Milquetoast, but looks were deceiving. *Money* magazine described him as mysterious and obsessively protective of his private life. As far as Maggie knew, he'd never been photographed for the media.

Hattie Lawrence, a spoiled Houston socialite, whispered in Maggie's ear, "Who is that character?" She was staring fixedly at Joe. "He'd better not be spoiling this deal for us. We've worked too hard to—Mercy! The man is a giant . . . and drop-dead gorgeous. Please don't tell me he's a patient."

Hattie was three times divorced, with as many face-lifts, tummy tucks, and boob jobs as a thirty-five-year-old woman could sustain. Luckily, the greedy woman had only a small say in Rainbow's future. Her daddy, Jack Lawrence, also in attendance, held the purse strings. Today was not the first time she and Harry had met Jack Lawrence or Hattie, but most of the negotiations had been taking place between the Lawrence family and the Medic-All people, off premises.

"That's Joe Rand, and yes, he's a patient."

Hattie's face dropped with disappointment.

They had almost reached the exercise wing, and Maggie could hear Joe expounding to the Medic-All honcho: " 'Tis my opinion that all of your patients can benefit from a daily exercise program. You know what the Norse proverbs say: sound bodies go hand in hand with sound minds." Jorund took a deep breath and continued. "Spear throwing and hand-to-hand combat on the practice field work best, of course, but in their absence, your exercise machines provide a fair substitute. I tried to instruct the pay-shuns yesterday on swordplay, but Norse Hatch-her nigh had a fit over that. You'd think broom and mop handles were priceless objects. Dost think a practice field would be a possibility for the future?"

Oh, good heavens! A patient lecturing on mental health and fitness! A patient who thinks he's a tenth-century Viking!

And Jerome Johnson was all ears.

"Even those who live in those wheeled chairs should be working muscles that are still alive," Joe was blathering on. "Otherwise they will all atrophy . . . that's a word I learned on *Wheel of Fortune*. Oh, you watch that show on the world box, too? Anyhow, just since I've been here—about two sennights—you can see a change in some of the pay-shuns. Hair-vee Lutz, for example, has the strangest compulsion to count things. Well, now he is counting the strokes of his oars on the rowing machine."

Sure enough, through the open doorway to the exercise room, they could see Harvey counting away as sweat poured down his face and he continued to row. Appropriately, the logo on his T-shirt today read, *I Get Enough Exercise Just Pushing My Luck.*

"See Chuck over there? Today he thinks he is a puff fish, but look how energetically he is rowing. This is the first time in two years that Chuck has worked his muscles."

Yep, Chuck was puffing away like a steam engine—or a puff fish, whatever that was—as he worked the rowing machine. The bright young man wore a T-shirt that pretty much said it all: *Okay, Who Put a Stop Payment on My Reality Check?* Someday soon Maggie hoped to find out what Chuck's real problem was, because it sure as heck wasn't being a split animal personality.

"And my comrade, Steve Askey, is pressing five hundred benches," Joe was still blathering on, "or is it pressing the bench at five hundred . . . ? Oh, I didn't see you there, Dock-whore Muck-bride . . . and Dock-whore Sea-bold. Have you met my new friend, Jaw-rome Johnson? He's a Norseman, too . . . from New-arc. That's in the world of New Jar-see."

Her jaw dropped another notch.

"You will hardly credit the coincidence, but Jaw-rome is a former fighting man, too, like me and Steve, except he was a green bar-ray."

For a prolonged moment, silence hovered in the air. But leave it to Joe to break the ice even further.

"Tsk-tsk!" Joe chided Maggie and Harry. "Aren't you going to shake hands with Jaw-rome?"

Maggie's mouth clicked shut, along with Harry's, Hattie's, and Jack's.

"How do you do?" she and Harry said, shaking the hand extended by Jerome Johnson. Joe beamed as if he'd invented the ritual of hand-shaking. Then Hattie and her father stepped up as well, although they had apparently met John-son on some other occasions.

Joe appeared very pleased with himself. You'd never know he was a patient, and not a hospital administrator.

"Did you know that Jaw-rome has his own longship, Mag-he . . . I mean, Dock-whore Muck-bride?" She had warned Joe on numerous occasions that he should address her in a more professional manner. "He is going to take me on a voyage someday."

Maggie groaned mentally. How long had Joe been talking with Jerome Johnson? Much too long, apparently.

Jerome smiled softly and patted Joe on the shoulder. "Actually, I have a yacht, and it was a short cruise on the Gulf I mentioned. As a possibility, mind you, just a possibility."

"Yacht, longship, *knarr* . . . they are all boats," Joe expounded. Then he returned the favor and patted Jerome on the shoulder in a good-buddy fashion.

Maggie caught a warning glance from Harry and immediately stepped forward. "Joe, would you mind coming down to my office with me?"

Joe immediately brightened and complied. *Thank God!* He probably thought there was more hanky-panky on the menu. Not that any of it had ever been initiated by her. "I hope to see you again soon, Jaw-rome. And remember what I told you about putting whale fat on aching muscles . . . arthur-itis, you named the malady, I believe. 'Tis what my father does all the time for his creaking bones, especially after a long time at sea a-Viking."

Oh, no! Had he just accused Mr. Johnson of having a creaking body?

But Mr. Johnson just laughed. "You betcha, young man. Make a note of that, George. I want a tubful of whale lard, ASAP. I'm willing to try anything for this damned arthritis."

George was turning a strange color of pale green.

"And here is a surprise for you." Joe was talking to Harry now. "Jaw-rome loves the idea of our field trip. So you must put aside all your res . . . reservations, I think you called it."

Harry started to turn green, too.

As Maggie and Joe walked down the hallway toward her office, she was steaming, and he was beaming.

"Am I cured yet?" he had the nerve to ask.

* * *

A week later . . .

At last the momentous day had arrived. Maggie was taking Jorund and all his new comrades in madness on their promised field journey.

Jorund had to admit to being a mite fearful. In order to get from the Rainbow Hospitium to Orcaland, the first leg of their journey, he would have to ride in one of the horseless carts he had seen nigh flying down the road from his chamber window. Actually it was a huge, yellow, boxlike structure with windows and wheels, known as a bus.

"What's wrong with a good pair of oxen to pull a cart? Or a sturdy horse?" he muttered to Mag-he, who was checking names off a piece of parchment on her clipping board as the other members of the group filed up the steps of the vehicle. It was a sign of his condition that he paid no mind to Mag-he's tight den-ham *braies* and short-sleeved sweat-her that exposed a tiny bit of her midriff each time she lifted an arm in the air to wave someone new onto the death cart.

Mag-he darted a quick look of concern toward him, sensing his reluctance to join the others. "There are plenty of horses in Texas, but a bus is more practical for our purposes . . . and safer."

"So you say!" he muttered under his breath. It would not do to outwardly show his trepidation, especially when everyone, even Not-a-lie, the wench who was afraid of crowds, had already bounced up the steps. Not-a-lie was wearing the most unseemly garb: white boots, a cowgirl hat— *Who ever heard of a cowgirl? Or bragged of being such?*—and a *shert* and short *gunna*, known as a

157

skirt, both with fringes all along the edges. With that amount of skin showing, she could pass for a harem houri.

Dock-whore Hairy was behind a large wheel inside the bus. He was going to drive, not trusting Mag-he and her demented troop to go off on their own. Two of the guards, who were known as attendants in this world, would accompany them as well. Norse Hatch-her came, too—surprisingly feminine in a long, gauzy purple skirt and matching *shert* with the words, *C'mon. Make My Day.* On second thought, she resembled a giant plum.

Bracing himself, Jorund forced himself to go up the steps, feeling much as if he were walking the plank. Breathing a sigh of relief at passing that hurdle, he glanced down the rows of seats, many of which were empty, since their group numbered only twelve—their original therapy group and a few others.

"Stop touching my fringe," Not-a-lie snapped to her seat partner.

Hair-vee ducked his head sheepishly. "I was just counting them for you."

"Well, I don't need you to count them," she grumbled. "And why do you have to sit next to me? There are plenty of other seats. You're crowding me." Not-a-lie's waspish demeanor was belied by her shivering body. This outing must be an ordeal for a person with her unique anxieties.

Hair-vee got up and stared longingly toward the empty seat next to Rosalyn, the mousy woman who worked all day long with books—a lie-bear-ian, which was amazing, really. In Jorund's world, books were a rare commodity; in this world, they were as plentiful as grass. Rosalyn gave Hair-vee a glare that was as forbidding as a berserker with a battle-ax guarding a castle wall. All of the men had been trying to get on Rosalyn's good side ever since she'd announced her extraordinary longing for sexual activity.

Rosalyn's word-*shert* spelled out, *Read My Lips.* He tried to read her lips, to no avail. Apparently he was capable only of reading whale's minds.

Jorund began to walk down the aisle when his gaze snagged on Furr-red Burns-tine. He stopped dead in his tracks. The man had gone too far this time. Much too far!

Last week, at group therapy, Furr-red had arrived in the garb of a caveman. Cavemen were apparently the ancestors of all human beings, though Jorund could hardly credit that. Jorund's Viking forbears had never looked like that rendition of early man—of that he was certain. Furr-red had worn naught but a beaver skin, which turned out to be one of Norse Hender-son's winter outergarbs—a coat—wrapped around one shoulder like a Roman toga. When he bent over, everyone got a good view of his bare, flabby buttocks . . . not a pretty sight. And he'd carried a huge club, which Mag-he had immediately confiscated, claiming that it was the trunk of a newly planted crab apple tree from their back courtyard.

Today Furr-red was impersonating his idea of what a Viking warrior would look like. It was insulting, to say the least. On his head was a long, blond wig that Jorund could swear he'd seen on a scullery maid's head just yestereve. On his upper arms were two makeshift bracelets formed from strips of tinfoil, a product used in modern kitchens to save food. He wore tight sweating *braies* on bottom and a loose black *T-shert* with the sleeves and neckline ripped off, the whole cinched in at the waist by a wide, brown leather belt.

"Who the hell are you supposed to be?" Jorund demanded.

Furr-red cowered back into his seat near the window. He was nigh whimpering when he replied, "Fred the Viking."

Jorund shook his head from side to side. The man meant no harm, he decided. Still, under his breath, he commented, "More like Furr-red the Idiot."

Just then he noticed Steve, who was motioning him toward the back of the bus. He headed in that direction, passing other Rainbow comrades along the way, including Chuck the Duck. That was who he assumed Chuck was today, since he was quack-quack-quacking to no one in particular. Just as long as he didn't drop any bodily "gifts" in the bus, Jorund could care less what animal he chose to be this day or any other. Chuck's message-*shert* said, *Out of My Mind. Be Back in Five Minutes.*

Mag-he sat down in the front seat, directly behind Dock-whore Hairy. The doors swished shut. And they were off. Well, he assumed they were off. At first the bus lurched and stopped, lurched and stopped, lurched and stopped till Dock-whore Hairy got the feel of driving a bus. *Holy Thor! Not only am I riding in a most dangerous horseless cart, but I am putting my life in the hands of an incompetent driver. 'Tis comparable to going aviking with my sister Katla at the rudder.*

But they were riding smoothly now. Jorund let out a pent-up breath, although he held on to the seat in front of him as they traveled at an excessive speed out onto the road.

"What's the problem?" Steve asked, staring at Jorund's white knuckles and his face, which was, no doubt, white as well.

"Must we travel so fast? What is the hurry?" he complained.

"Huh?" Steve responded. "We're only going twenty miles an hour on this entrance ramp. Wait till we get on the highway. The speed limit there is sixty-five."

"I cannot wait," Jorund said dryly.

Steve was frowning as he studied his rigid demeanor. "You've never ridden on a bus before?"

"I've never ridden on anything that moved without animal power . . . unless it was a ship on the open seas, driven by the winds and the hard rowing of well-muscled men."

Steve shrugged his shoulders sadly. "Man, you are as screwed up as the rest of us."

"Nay, I am not," Jorund declared. "What you all cannot accept is that I really am a Viking, come here from the tenth century."

Instead of arguing, as he usually did, Steve asked skeptically, "Why?"

Jorund relaxed back into the seat. As long as he didn't look out the windows and see the landscape passing in a blur, he could almost forget where he was. He pondered Steve's question. "I do not know. I am hoping some answers will come to me today."

"At Boot Scootin' Cowboy? In a music hall?

Hell, I know a lot of guys who think they can find answers in a bottle of booze—I did for more years than I can count—but I guarantee that even a glass of beer will be off-limits to us today."

"I did not mean that music place. I was referring to the killer-whale place."

"Do you still think that a killer whale is the key to your being here in Galveston?" Steve and all the others in his group therapy had laughed this week when he'd told them the tale of his arrival atop Thora's back, bare-arsed and raging mad. Steve wasn't laughing now.

"I know it." Jorund snorted with disgust. "If I can find her, I'm certain that this puzzle will become clear." Leastways, he hoped that was the case. He thought of something else. "Mayhap you will get some answers yourself when we visit that war praise-wall."

It was Steve who turned stiff then. "I am not getting off this bus when we get to that freakin' wall. I swear, I'm not. I know Dr. McBride has all these piss-poor ideas about making a big breakthrough with me, but it isn't gonna happen there . . . or anywhere else, for that matter." He turned away and stared morosely out the window. In an undertone, he murmured, for his own benefit only, "I don't see enough of 'Nam in my dreams. I gotta see it on a damn wall, too?"

The hairs rose on the back of Jorund's neck then. In the distance, he could see a large sign that said, WELCOME TO ORCALAND. And beyond that was the water inlet that led out to Galveston Bay and the seas beyond.

Would this be the day he returned to the past?

* * *

Maggie found Joe, finally. He was sitting on a small promontory near the outer rim of the inlet, arms resting on bended knees, gazing out beyond the bay. Of course, he had defied all rules by wandering away from their group, which was still watching the Gonzo show back in the arena.

"Joe?" she inquired softly.

At first he didn't seem to hear her. Even though his lips were moving, no words came out. It was as if he were speaking some silent language. Then he turned. Maggie's heart almost broke at the bleakness in his gray eyes.

"She's not there," he told her.

"Who's not there?" Maggie dropped down to the ground beside Joe and put a hand on his shoulder in concern.

"Thora."

"The killer whale?"

He nodded. "Much as I've tried to communicate with her, there is no response."

"You . . . you talk to orcas?"

"Not all orcas . . . leastways, I don't think I can talk to them all—just my own personal pain-in-the-arse killer whale, Thora."

This was not good news. After all the progress Joe had made, believing that he could talk to an ocean mammal could be chalked up to additional delusions, along with his time-travel and Viking claims.

"Does the whale talk back to you?"

"Yea, it does. In my head."

Oh, God.

He slanted a glance her way. "You think I'm demented, don't you?"

"Of course not."

163

"You are a poor liar, Dock-whore Muck-bride."

"Well, anyhow, it's not the end of the world that you didn't have a chat with Thora today," she said brightly. "Let's view it in a positive light."

"For the love of all the gods, spare me," he replied with a groan. "You are going to start the sigh-colic-jest blathering again, aren't you?"

She raised her chin, affronted. "I don't know what you mean."

He exhaled with a loud whoosh. "All those words and phrases that say nothing: 'I see. How do you feel about that? What do you think?' Never do you answer a question directly, but always turn it back on your pay-shuns. 'Tis enough to drive a sane man mad, I tell you."

She began to ask him how he felt about that, then stopped herself short. He was right. She did have a tendency to spout psychobabble, when the philosophy behind Rainbow was to avoid the therapist-as-robot approach. Psychologists no longer needed to hide personal emotions and reactions or remain silent and unmoved in the client relationship. At Rainbow, a therapist was supposed to be free to be oneself, while remaining objective at the same time. "What I started to say about putting a positive light on this event is that maybe this is a sign—I know you are big on signs—that it's time to put aside the past and move forward."

"To heal myself?"

"Yes!" she said enthusiastically.

He shook his head. "There is no bright side in this catastrophe today . . . and, yea, it is a catastrophe. Look at this from my perspective, m'lady.

There is no winter chill in the air here, but winter has already begun in other parts of your country. On the seas I need to travel, the air will be frigid—too cold for sailing on an open longship till springtime. Have you ever tried to row a boat with ice on the oars? Have you ever stood for hours at a time in weather so wet and cold that every hair on your body turns to icicles, even the chest hairs? Of course you haven't. Can you not see that I must communicate with Thora soon, or be forced to wait many months to leave this land?"

"Is that such a bad thing?"

"Yea, it is the worst of all things. My brother Rolf is in danger. Every day might count in my completing his rescue."

Maggie thought about all his impossible words. "Assuming I believe everything that you've said, Joe, it seems to me that there must be a good reason why you were sent to this land . . . and this time." She nearly choked on that last part. "If you're going to accept that the Fates—or the gods . . . or even a killer whale—are determining your destiny, then you also have to accept that coming to Galveston was preordained."

He followed her words with interest. "I have considered all these things, and I agree that it was no mistake that landed me on these shores. But sometimes man can influence his destiny. In fact, does not your Christian religion have a saying that God helps those who help themselves?"

Maggie had to laugh at Joe's quick mind. She wished she knew who or what he really was. Aside from being a gorgeous specimen of manhood, he was intelligent and strong and a born leader. What did he do for a living? Was he a career military man? A construction worker? An adventurer, or an extreme exercise fanatic . . . like the father of her two children, who had a perfectly good career as a resident physician but had to jump out of airplanes, as well? There should be a clue in all she knew of Joe, but the answer eluded her.

"Well, enough of this for today," she said, standing and brushing the dirt off the rump of her jeans—a maneuver that Joe watched with decided masculine interest, despite his desolation over his predicament. "We have to get back to the orca show. It should be over soon."

As they were strolling in front of the bleachers toward the Rainbow group, which was watching the show avidly, Joe remarked, "I just wish that damned killer whale would get back here and rescue me, so I can rescue my brother."

Just then Gonzo swam up and flicked his huge tail fins, causing a wave of water to cover Joe from head to toe. So much for communicating with killer whales! Or maybe Gonzo was communicating, after all, in response to Joe's deprecating comment about whales. Sort of an orca version of "Screw you, Viking!"

Chapter Nine

Jorund and Steve sat alone in the bus.

In the distance, across a wide lawn, could be seen the rest of the Rainbow group staring at a stone wall, which apparently contained the names of all the dead soldiers who had fought in the Battle of Vee-yet-numb. It was a good idea, in Jorund's opinion . . . one that he intended to mention to King Olaf when he returned to Norway. Of course, they would need a wall much bigger than this one if they were going to record all the dead Vikings in battle after battle through the centuries, rather than any one war or another. In truth, there had been so many Norse wars, the skalds had lost count long ago. Some people, especially those bloody Saxon clerics who recorded English history, claimed a Viking would fight with anyone, even his own brother. It was true.

A few of the people who had come to view the Moving Wall besides the Rainbow group gave curious looks at Chuck the Viking . . . and at Not-a-lie, too, who was wont to break into song at the least provocation. Right now she was singing about a honk-key-tonk angel, her fringes swaying from side to side as she danced to her own music.

"Come, Steve," Jorund urged his friend. "You are a man of courage. Are you going to turn coward now?"

Jorund was not in a good mood, especially after his disappointing failure to locate the elusive Thora. Although he had not voiced this particular concern to Mag-he, the worry nagging at him most was the possibility that he might not ever find Thora or his way back to his own time. What would he do then?

In his present ill temper, he did not feel inclined to prod a stubborn ox like Steve to see the error of his ways. But the grief-stricken man was as close to a friend as Jorund had made in this godforsaken land of the twentieth century, and he could no more abandon him to his pain than he could his own brother, Magnus . . . or his brother Rolf, he reminded himself guiltily.

"Get lost, birdbrain," Steve responded in a most thankless manner. "The last thing in the world I have is courage."

"Did you not win that famous medal for valor? Have you not endured thirty years of inner torment? Do you not stay away from your soul mate, Shell-he, for love of her? Do you not battle with demons every night in your dreams, and come out the victor? That spells courage to me." Jorund had never been a talkative fellow, but he certainly seemed to have developed a taste for tongue flapping now. And he was good, too. Puffing his chest out, he concluded, "Betimes, survival itself is a form of triumph."

Steve gave him a level stare. "You are so full of it."

"Let me tell you a story—"

"Oh, God! Not another freakin' saga. I swear, if I hear one more tale about Sigurd and the Dragon Lady, I'm gonna puke."

Jorund lifted his chin, affronted. Well, mayhap he had been overdoing the life-lesson legends a mite, but he felt a little closer to home and his old life when he retold the poems and stories of his people. In truth, he probably sounded like his brother Magnus when he'd tipped the mead horn once too often and began to sing ribald songs . . . except in Jorund's case, he told stories. "I thought you liked my sagas."

"I was being polite, man. Hell, they might be perfectly good yarns when the poets—uh, skalds—put them together, but let me give you a bit of advice, pal: you are no storyteller. Stick to fighting, or whatever the hell it is you do."

Jorund bristled. Should he punch Steve in his sullen face? Or better yet, should he hoist him by the scrawny neck, toss him over his shoulder, and carry him bodily to the bloody wall?

It was an easy decision. He turned slowly and let a slow smile crease his lips.

"Wh-what? Why are you looking at me like that?" Steve asked warily. Then, "You wouldn't! Oh, no, you wouldn't!"

Jorund would.

* * *

"Maggie, they're safe in the bus," Harry told her. "But if you're worried about them, go back and wait there. I'm capable of handling the rest of the group, along with the aid of Gladys and the two attendants."

"No, no," she said. "I wouldn't want Joe and Steve to think I didn't trust them." Still, she glanced back toward the parking lot at the unmarked bus. Then she glanced again. "Oh, boy!"

Jorund was striding across the lawn, carrying a cursing, squirming Steve on his shoulder. He did so with ease, even though Steve was at least six feet tall and a hundred and seventy pounds.

She started to step up and chastise Jorund for creating a scene. Tourists right and left were gaping at them. In fact, Maggie saw a local newspaper photographer, who hung around the traveling wall in hopes of catching a human-interest story, sit up alertly on the park bench where he'd been waiting. His van with the Galveston *Daily News* logo was parked at a nearby curb.

But Harry put a hand on her arm. "Wait, Maggie. Let's see how this plays out."

"But—"

"Think about it. Maybe, just maybe, Joe will be the one to jolt Steve out of his self-pity. Maybe this is the breakthrough you've been waiting for."

Jorund, on the other hand, felt like breaking something. Ever since he'd landed in this world, he'd had nothing but problems. Now he, who prided himself on his aloofness, was involving himself in other people's problems as well. With a snort of disgust, he planted Steve on his feet in front of the wall, and glared at several people, who stepped away, not wanting to be in the proximity of flying fists.

"You have no right," Steve stormed, his green eyes flashing angrily. He shoved Jorund in the chest.

"Yea, I have every right. You are my friend," Jorund retorted, and pushed him back in the chest. Like two scrappy youthlings we are behaving, Jorund thought. To the side, he heard Mag-he make a *tsk*ing sound. Jorund gave Steve an extra shove in the chest and demanded, "Stop creating such a spectacle and tell me, which of these names mark your *hird?*"

"Herd? What the hell did you think I was in 'Nam—a cow?" Steve jeered.

"Nay, you have already told me you were a seal, and a *hird* is a troop, my friend . . . a troop of soldiers. Tell me, which of these fallen men were your comrades?"

For the first time, Steve faced the wall, and his face went ashen as he walked slowly along till he found the names he wanted. Tears filled his eyes, and Jorund noticed that Mag-he's eyes misted over as well. She and Dock-whore Hairy exchanged a look. Was it worry, self-congratulation, or compassion?

A visible shudder rippled through Steve's body as he moved closer and traced some letters with a forefinger. This had to be a deeply moving experience for him. One name after another he recited aloud in a choked voice. Then, in a deadened monotone, he said to Jorund, and to Mag-he and

Dock-whore Hairy, who had stepped up to form a half-circle in front of the wall, "During Vietnam, SEAL teams One and Two amassed a combined kill ratio of two hundred to one, with only forty-six deaths, and those were mostly due to accidents, not enemy direct fire. It seems obscene, doesn't it, to quote that statistic now, with all the antiwar sentiment, but damn, we were good at what we did."

"So you have reason to be proud of your work . . . despite the grief of war," Jorund told him softly, putting an arm around his shoulder. Truly, he understood the man's conflicted emotions: Steve had been trained to be a soldier—in one of the best units of the fighting men—but was horrified by all the bloodletting, some of it needless. Life was not so different between his world and Steve's. There were wars that had to be fought for noble reasons, but some wars, in retrospect, were obviously the political games of greedy kings and chieftains.

Maggie was regarding him as if he were some kind of hero, when all he'd done was comfort a man in need. How little she must think of him if she considered this to be extraordinary behavior on his part.

Dock-whore Hairy was nodding repeatedly. No doubt he thought the two of them were well on their way to being cured. Well, mayhap Steve was, but Jorund had never been demented to begin with.

"You have no idea how hard this is," Steve told him in a cracking voice. "Those men depended on me. If I'd done a better job, they might still be alive. The guilt, even after all these years, just tears me apart."

Appropriately, Not-a-lie started to croon, "I fall to pieces. . . ."

Rosalyn offered gently, "Maybe you'd like to go on a date sometime, Steve." Obviously she had another type of therapy in mind for him. They had a vulgar name for it in this new world. It was comparable to a pity-coupling in his world.

Steve appeared horrified at Rosalyn's offer.

Jorund ignored them all and continued speaking to Steve of a soldier's guilt. "Betimes you feel as if it should have been you, do you not? In truth, you question whether this life you lead isn't really your hell on earth . . . a punishment for some past wrong—though in our land we do not call it hell. It is Niflheim, land of eternal ice, ruled by the queen of the dead, Hel." Jorund shivered violently, as if actually feeling the icy atmosphere of the underworld.

Steve was staring at Jorund. "How do you know so well how I feel? How come you can put my exact feelings into words?"

"Because they reflect my own," Jorund answered with a huge sigh. "I lost my wife and two twin daughters to famine a short year ago. And 'twas my fault for not being there to protect them." All the muscles in his body sagged, and he seemed bleak with misery as he saw the empathy on Steve's face.

"Sweet Lord! I'm sorry for opening healed wounds."

"Healed? Nay, never healed," Jorund corrected. "Know this, you dunderhead: I make it a practice never to speak of my past. It is a sign of my comradeship with you that I share it now. Let us not broach the subject again."

Steve inclined his head in agreement.

But Mag-he and Dock-whore Hairy were staring at him with decided interest. And Jorund realized just how much he'd revealed . . . secrets he would have much rather kept to himself. Now Mag-he would be asking him all kinds of questions: *What do you think of your dead wife? What did you think of your daughters? What did you think of the famine? What do you think, think, think.* And he had given her that ammunition.

For the rest of their visit to the wall, Steve was somber, but no longer anguished. In fact, he shared information with those around him about how he'd become a Navy SEAL. And he had some of the men listening, bug-eyed, while he related stories about his baseball career.

"Hey, aren't you Steve Askey?" someone asked suddenly.

"Uh-oh!" Maggie exclaimed. She had been deeply touched by both Steve's and Joe's stories, but now she saw trouble approaching in the form of the middle-aged reporter, who had been sitting on the bench. He was now staring fixedly at Steve, eyes narrowed as if to boot up some distant memory.

"I'm Jack Farrington from the Galveston *Daily News*," he said, showing a press card for identification. "If you'd just give me a minute for a few questions . . . ?"

Steve backed away a step or two, as if he'd been

attacked. "No, no, you've got the wrong man." Even though he used his real name, everyone at Rainbow knew that Steve had been hiding out from his family and the public for the last ten years, and they'd respected his privacy. Apparently that was about to change now.

Meanwhile, the reporter's camera was flashing away. "Hey, Steve, I don't mean any harm. Just let me get a picture or two. I saw you play in Dodger Stadium back in sixty-nine . . . your second and last season. Man, oh, man, what a day! You hit three home runs. Some people say you were better than Mickey Mantle and Ted Williams combined . . . that you could've been the greatest baseball player of all time. Hell, that was just before you went off to 'Nam and . . ." The reporter's face went red as understanding hit. He glanced at the wall, at Steve, then back to the wall.

"I am not that man."

"Why is Steve saying he's not Steve?" Fred asked at that inopportune moment. He had been counting the names on the wall since their arrival, but apparently this was more interesting even than his obsessive-compulsive needs.

"Shut up, Furr-red," Joe said with a glare, which caused Fred to scurry back to the wall. Then he addressed the reporter. " 'Tis time for you to depart."

"Who are you to tell me what to do?" the reporter asserted belligerently.

Oh, no! Please. Don't say it.

"I am Jorund the Viking," Joe declared.

Maggie and Harry both groaned at the same

175

time, and the two attendants stood at the ready, in case there was a need to rush the group back to the bus quickly.

"Jorund the Viking?" the reporter mocked. "Yeah, and I'm Joe DiMaggio."

"Fortunate you are that I do not have my sword with me. You would be missing a tongue for your insolence."

"Ha! You don't scare me," the newshound cried out as he took one last photo, then literally ran away. He must have recognized the threat in Joe's stance, not to mention his ill-chosen words. Over his shoulder, Farrington shouted, "Hey, Steve, did you know the Baseball Hall of Fame has been trying to locate you?"

"I think Steve's had enough of walls and halls for one day, don't you?" Maggie observed to Harry.

"Should I chase him and lop off a body part?" Joe asked her then.

"No!" she shouted.

He frowned at the vehemence of her response. "Holy Thor! I was just jesting." Then he seemed to think of something else. "I have set back my healing a pace or two today, have I not?"

"Or twenty," she commented drolly.

"I need a beer," Steve said.

"I need an ale," Joe said.

"I need to get out of here," Maggie said.

Boot Scootin' Cowboy was a huge success.

Maggie had never before been to a nightclub in the daytime. But she was in one now. And she was having the time of her life. So was everyone else.

And it wasn't just because this particular club was a local country-western hangout, as well as a Galveston tourist attraction. There appeared to be a spirit of freedom and comradeship and normalcy in the patients that Maggie had never seen back at the hospital.

They had eaten a late lunch first . . . Tex-Mex all around: mesquite-grilled shrimp fajitas with guacamole salads, and strawberry sopapillas for dessert. Everyone had been permitted one beer each; they'd all declined in deference to Steve, who must avoid even a drop of liquor or fall off the wagon.

Now most of the group was up on the dance floor, alongside other patrons, learning the beginning steps of a line dance. With Brooks and Dunn belting out "Boot Scootin' Boogie," everyone was laughing and smiling, even as they tripped over their own feet. The dance instructors, a cute young blonde in a cowgirl outfit similar to Natalie's and a lean young man in jeans, a cowboy shirt, and boots, repeated the instructions over and over . . . such things as heel bounce, stomp, shuffle, camel walk, knee roll, vine right and left, pivot, and lots of scoots and touches. The "touch" call meant a smart slap on the buttocks.

Joe was sitting across the table from her, shaking his head from side to side at the group's antics, as he sipped at a soda. He was the only one who'd refused to participate in the dancing. Maggie had chosen to sit it out with him.

He repeated now what he'd said then: "Why would a grown man willingly make such a fool of himself?"

"It's fun," she declared. "Sometimes people do things just for the fun of it."

"Idiots, mayhap."

"Come on now, haven't you ever enjoyed an activity that involved laughing at yourself?"

"Nay," he answered. "Have you?"

"Of course. Rollerblading, which resulted in many black-and-blue marks on my rump. . . ."

He craned his neck to the side, as if half expecting her to drop her jeans and show him. When she gave him a sharp "As if!" look, he just grinned and took another sip of soda.

"And roller coasters, which terrify me, but I ride them anyway."

"Roller coasters?"

She explained briefly, then noted, "One of my daughters, Suzy, is a real T-type personality. She must have inherited it from her father, because I sure don't have a daredevil bone in my body. Remember, I told you that T-types like to take risks. They revel in being scared to death. My other daughter, Beth, isn't afraid of roller coasters, but she doesn't get the thrill of the thrill, like Suzy does."

She noticed a slight flicker of emotion on Joe's face at the mention of her girls, but he soon masked it. "And you think I enjoy being frightened?"

"Well, weren't you frightened riding on top of that killer whale?"

"Extremely," he agreed, "but I did not engage in that activity by choice. In fact, most times I take no unwarranted risks. A good leader never gambles with his troop's lives."

She nodded.

Then he homed in on something else she'd

said. "You mentioned your daughter's father being a risk taker."

It was Maggie's turn to bristle now. She shouldn't be discussing her personal life with a patient. But the atmosphere was so relaxed here, and she didn't want to spoil the mood by making Joe feel he'd crossed some line.

"Judd Haskell was a surgical resident at Houston General Hospital. He had only one year to go before he would have been a full-fledged doctor."

"Another dock-whore!"

"Joe, you do know that a doctor is a physician, don't you?"

"A healer?" he asked. His face bloomed a lovely shade of red. "I knew that."

She narrowed her eyes in disbelief.

"Well, I didn't know at first, but later I learned about dock-whores being healers on *The Guiding Light*. Betimes I forget, though. 'Tis such an odd name to give a healer."

Sometimes it saddened Maggie to hear Joe use such archaic language and misunderstand so much about the language and culture of America. He seemed so normal that she could almost believe he was as sane as she was. "Back to your question about Judd. He died taking a foolish risk . . . foolish in my opinion, anyway. He was skydiving, and his parachute malfunctioned."

"Skydiving?"

"Jumping out of an airplane."

Joe gasped. She had already explained to him before what an airplane was when he'd commented on the large objects seen occasionally in the sky over Rainbow. "Why would anyone willingly jump out of an air machine?"

"My point, precisely."

"And you think I am insane!" he exclaimed with a shake of his head.

Just then the rest of the group came back to the table, all laughing and talking at once. Harry had paused before a mirrored beer sign to adjust his hair drape, which must have gotten mussed during his energetic activity.

Even Steve had joined the dance lessons, much to Maggie's delight. There were so many good things that had happened today, and she considered Steve's progress the best. His willingness to step up to the Vietnam wall was well worth the field trip. He plopped down into the chair next to Joe, signaled the waiter for a cold Coke, then drawled at Joe, "Coward."

"If 'tis cowardly to avoid making a fool of myself, then I admit to being such. I never suspected you could wiggle your arse in quite such an attractive manner."

"Like my butt, do ya?"

Before Joe could answer with the smart retort she knew was coming, one of the band members announced over the loudspeakers, "We're about to begin the weekly amateur talent contest. Remember, folks, all the winners of these weekly competitions get to come back to Boot Scootin' Cowboy on New Year's Eve for the grand finale. It'll be televised on the local cable network. The top winner gets to make a demo with a major record company."

Everyone clapped.

Maggie glanced down at her watch. It was five o'clock. They should be heading back to the hospital about now. Maggie looked at Harry; they both looked at the rapt faces of everyone in their group, including the two attendants, but most especially at Natalie, who was adjusting wonderfully to the nightclub. She and Harry both shrugged, agreeing silently to wait a little while longer.

Joe stood.

She and Harry were immediately alert.

"I'm just going to the privy," he informed them with a clucking sound of disgust. "If I'd wanted to escape, I would have done it at Orcaland, or at the wall."

They both relaxed and turned their attention back to the entertainment. Even so, Maggie was uneasy till he returned a short time later.

First a sister act did a clogging routine to the tune of a fast-paced Charlie Daniels song about the devil coming down to Georgia. They were really good.

Then five boys under the age of twelve—the next Osmond Brothers, she presumed—did a rip-roaring medley of country-western hits, like "God Bless Texas," "Your Cheatin' Heart," "Stand By Your Man," and "Friends in Low Places."

A college sorority had ten of its sisters do an extremely provocative line-dance routine to the old Rod Stewart song, "Do You Think I'm Sexy?" By the sound of the thunderous applause, the crowd thought they were.

There were some duds in the bunch, too. A too-loud guitarist from Abilene. A shy piano vocalist whose voice could barely be heard over the sound of her music. A young male comedian who must fancy himself the Andrew Dice Clay of Opryland.

Just before the end of the program, the lead singer of the band took the microphone and announced, "We have one last-minute entry . . . a little songbird from right here in Galveston whose dream is to become the next Patsy Cline. Hey, a whole lot of women down in Nashville have been tryin' to take her place over the years, but who knows, maybe this will be the one. Let's give a big Texas welcome to our hometown gal . . . Miss Natalie Blue."

The nightclub burst into applause, but there was an ominous silence at their large table. Natalie was stunned, her face going as white as her cowgirl outfit, and her fingers, which had been encircling a glass, beginning to shake visibly.

"How did this happen? Who signed her up?" Maggie demanded.

As one, everyone's heads turned toward Joe, who was beaming as if he'd just pulled off a big coup. Apparently his trip to the "privy" had involved a detour. "Wh-what?" he asked, when he realized no one was tossing congratulations his way.

The applause was tapering off, and the bandleader was saying, "Hey, Natalie, where are you? Time's awastin'."

"Isn't this what you always wanted, Not-a-lie?" Joe asked.

"It's not the right time," Natalie whimpered.

"Pfff! If you're waiting till the right time, you might never get your chance. In my land, there is a saying: 'Gold given by a beggar is no less lustrous than gold given by a king.' "

"Joe, that has no relevance to this case," Maggie chided. The big lunk had gone too far this time. "You had no right—"

"I told you, your storytelling skills stink," Steve added.

"Natalie, you don't have to go there if you don't want to," Harry advised her soothingly. "I'll go up and make your apologies. We can just slip out quietly."

"No!" Natalie cried, standing abruptly.

Everyone just stared at her.

"I'll do it. I will. I'm going to do it." She looked at Joe then. "Will you walk me up there? I'm not sure my wobbly legs will carry me that far."

"For a certainty, m'lady."

Joe took Natalie to the side steps leading to the stage, where one of the band members helped her up. With a few whispered instructions, Natalie walked up to the standing microphone. By the pallor of her face and her stiff posture, she seemed to think it was a guillotine.

But then everything changed.

With the first drawn-out, clear note of Patsy Cline's "Crazy," Natalie Blue had everyone's attention. Her voice was powerful and poignant and wonderfully unique as she crooned, "Cra-aazy. I'm cra-aazy for feelin' so lonely." By the end of the song, Maggie had tears in her eyes, and she knew—she just knew—that someday people would mark this place and this day as the time that Natalie Blue began her professional career. The crowd gave her a standing ovation, shouting for an encore. And Natalie, surprisingly poised for a person consumed with a fear of crowds, smiled and eased into the piercing "Sweet Dreams."

To no one's surprise, Natalie won the competition for the day, and promised to come back for the final event. Whether she would crumble once they left the club, or revert back to her old phobias, Maggie couldn't say for sure, but at least for tonight Natalie was a big hit. And New Year's Eve would be a goal they could aim for in therapy.

Joe glanced her way and winked smugly. "You may thank me now or later."

"Oh, really." She laughed.

"Methinks I will dance now."

"Huh?"

"Yea, you may thank me by dancing with me, Dock-whore Muck-bride."

"I already told you that a doctor is—"

He chucked her under the chin. "Must you always be so serious?"

"Hey, that should be my line to you. You're the one who's always serious."

Meanwhile, Joe had been leading her toward the sawdust-covered dance floor, where Steve and Rosalyn and Harry and Natalie were already beginning to dance to, appropriately, "The Dance" by Garth Brooks.

A slow dance! Maggie realized at once, and shot a suspicious glare at Joe. Expressionless, he was holding his arms open to her, but his gray eyes, usually somber and grim, were twinkling with mischief.

"I prefer this type of dancing to the line dancing. Not that I know how, but it does not look too hard. In truth, it resembles making love, only standing up."

Maggie gasped, but she wasn't sure if it was because of his words, or the fact that he pulled her into a full-frontal embrace that involved his arms being locked around her waist and her shoes dangling off the floor. Most important, they were chest to chest, belly to belly, and, well . . . you-know-what to you-know-what. Oh, my God! she thought.

"Oh . . . my . . . God!" Joe choked out, aloud.

There was no satisfaction in knowing he shared her flash-fire arousal at their innocent embrace. No, she corrected herself immediately. There was nothing innocent about the chemistry that exploded between them at the merest touch, whether it was dancing or a scorching kiss.

"I told you this couldn't happen again," she said in a strained voice as he swayed from foot to foot . . . his Viking version of dancing, she supposed.

"Nay, m'lady. You told me we could not kiss again. You did not tell me that we couldn't dance."

"This is *not* dancing."

"It's not?" he asked, eyebrows raised in question.

"Both feet of both partners need to be on the floor to qualify as dancing."

"They do?" He stared at her, dubiously. "More's the pity."

He let her body slide down his body till her flat shoes rested on the floor. The sensations he created along the way were so intense Maggie feared her eyeballs might be rolling back in her head. She blinked once, then twice, just to make sure.

"Just holding you like this makes me breathless," Joe told her in a raspy voice. His eyes were heavy-lidded and smoldering.

Breathless? I make him breathless? Oh, why

*does it feel so good to know I can affect him so?
And, hey, is that my heart beating like a jackhammer?* "You make me blush when you look at me like that. Stop it!"

A slow grin spread across his lips. And he continued looking.

She dropped her eyes before his steady, slumberous gaze. She didn't want him to see—or sense—the hot ache that was building in the pit of her stomach. All from a mere dance.

"Your arousal arouses me," he admitted, almost as if he resented the fact, then proved it by adding, "I do not want to be aroused by you. I need to get back to my time. I need to help my brother. I need no complications."

"And I would be a complication?"

"Lady, you could be the biggest complication of my entire life."

"Even more than your wife?"

He exhaled with a dismissive sound. "My wife was never a complication. She was an arrangement. Never, ever, did she affect me as you do. Not she or any other woman."

"Bet you say that to all the wenches."

"Not even when I am seducing them into the bed sport. Well, there was that one wench in Cordoba—"

Maggie punched him lightly on the shoulder.

He laughed softly, a low, masculine sound, barely more than a growl. She loved his laugh. He did it so rarely.

"What are you thinking?" he asked.

She laughed then. "Hey, that's supposed to be my line."

"I can scarce believe I am about to ask you this

186

question. I swore, after Inga's death, that I had had enough of women . . . except for the occasional coupling, that is." He inhaled deeply, as if for courage. "I do not suppose that you would consider coming with me when I go?" he inquired tentatively.

"To the tenth century?"

"Yea, to my time and country."

How could she take such a proposal seriously? "On the back of a killer whale?"

"God, I hope not." Then he thought of something else. "On the other hand, if we were both bare-arsed naked . . ."

"You are impossible." She shook her head and smiled up at him. "No, I would not consider going with you. Keep in mind, I have two daughters who need me here."

The somber expression that immediately blanketed his face told her loud and clear that he wouldn't be bringing up time travel with her again . . . because he didn't want a reminder of her twin girls.

They continued their dance in silence then, her arms wrapped around his shoulders, her face resting against his chest. It was a beautiful moment . . . a perfect ending to a perfect day.

Why, then, did Maggie feel like crying?

The next day Joe disappeared, without warning, from the Rainbow hospital. His sword was missing, too.

Police were called and an APB put out with his description, to no avail. Other patients were questioned. He'd told no one of his plans, not even Steve, who was desolate without his new friend, especially with all the media publicity he'd reluctantly attracted as a result of the report at the Moving Wall. Area hospitals reported no injured Norsemen of his size in their emergency rooms. Maggie even searched the Orcaland site on several occasions. Nothing.

Was he lost?

Had he died? Perhaps he had swum out into the bay, hoping to connect with his special killer whale, and drowned instead.

A heavy grief settled over Maggie, and over the hospital wing where Joe had touched so many people. Suzy and Beth were devastated that they'd lost the man they had chosen as a father before they'd actually met him. She had talked to Harry about it, and neither of them could figure out what there was about this man that had affected them all so strongly.

So it was that one week passed, then a second, finally three weeks, with no sign of the mysterious man who had shown up in their lives suddenly, and just as suddenly disappeared. Tomorrow was Thanksgiving. Maggie hated negativity, but she couldn't find much to be thankful for, not with Joe missing.

Where was Joe spending his nights? Was he cold? Was he hungry? Was he alone?

That night Maggie began a brand-new practice . . . one she would never admit to anyone, not even her daughters. She was wishing on a star, and her refrain was always the same.

"Come home, Joe."

Chapter Ten

At seven o'clock that night, there was a loud pounding at the front door.

Rita jumped from her favorite perch on the window seat of the front bay window, where she had been snoozing. With a long mewling "Meeooow," she stretched and ambled toward the entryway.

More persistent knocking followed.

Maggie assumed it was Suzy and Beth coming home from church choir practice. Even though November wasn't over, rehearsals for the annual Christmas concert were already in full swing.

But why hadn't they used their keys to open the door? *Ha! Silly question.* As usual, their arms were probably too full of the backpacks and whatnot that young girls felt the need to cart everywhere they went.

She swung the door wide. "Just in time. Dinner's about ready. We're having your fav—"

It wasn't her daughters. It was Joe. And, even through the light drizzle of rain, she could see that he looked awful.

She should have been angry that he'd left the hospital without notice, and had been missing for three long weeks.

She should have slammed the door in his face for breaking his therapy contract, thus barring him from returning to the clinic as a patient.

She should have been dismayed that he'd come to her home—a no-no for mental patients and their psychologists.

Instead she opened her arms wide and hugged him tightly. She was just so glad to see him again . . . to know he was safe.

He hugged her back just as fiercely. For several long moments they stood silently on her front doorstep, locked in the tight embrace, regardless of Rita hissing behind them, and a curious neighbor, Mrs. Watkins, walking her Pekingese along the front sidewalk.

Finally she drew back and studied his haggard, whiskered face with concern. He must not have shaved since he'd left the hospital. His usually lustrous hair, which he normally tied back into a queue at his neck, was wild and matted, barely recognizable as being a pale blond color. He wore the same clothing he'd left with, blue jeans and a long-sleeved denim shirt, both of which were dirty and torn in places. Most ominous was the lethal sword that he wore in a scabbard attached to the wide leather belt at his waist. Had he used that sword on anyone or anything?

"Come in," she ordered, as she realized he was shivering.

He hesitated. "Are you alone?"

She cocked her head in question. Apparently, despite his need for care, he was reluctant to enter her house unless she was alone. Then she understood. Her daughters—her *twin* daughters—that was whom he wanted to avoid. "I'm alone."

His body relaxed visibly, and he stepped inside.

There was a loud hissing noise, and a white ball of fur hurled itself toward Joe. Maggie's forehead creased with puzzlement and her hands went out instinctively to protect Joe. Rita wasn't usually hostile. He put an arm over his face to defend himself, but Rita had already attached her front claws to his shirt and her back claws to the lower part of his anatomy. Her tail thickened, her body stiffened, and her fur stood on end. She even began to shed fur like mad.

"Don't move," Maggie cautioned Joe as she began to gently extricate Rita's claws.

"Move?" Joe choked out. "I can scarce breathe for the proximity of the beast's talons to my male parts. Be careful, lest you change my sex in a trice."

She laughed as she lifted Rita away; whispered a firm rebuke in her cat's face, which Maggie could swear wore a smirk, then scooted her away.

"What kind of wild creature was that?" he grumbled as she closed the door and led him toward her den. Rita followed after them, despite his frown. "Perchance it needs a taste of my sword, Bloodletter." He patted the weapon at his side.

"A cat," she answered. "Our pet cat, Rita. And don't you dare pull out that sword, or hurt Rita. She was only being protective of me."

"That is a cat?" The glower he gave the feline said it all. "Cats are pampered pets in the Eastern harems, but never have I seen a cat so fat. Are you sure it's not a tiger . . . a white tiger? I have heard of such, though they are rare."

Rita hissed her opinion of his derogatory remark.

"No, she's just a cat . . . our own little kitty cat."

He made a harrumphing sound at the word *little*. "You must have monster mice in this land to feed one that size."

The idea of Rita being a mouser was so preposterous that it didn't even warrant correcting. Maggie had obtained Rita as a kitten from a shelter more than ten years ago, and the animal had been spoiled from the get-go. Rita in the wild would be as much an anomaly as . . . well, Joe in a civilized setting.

"I do not like cats," he declared, his upper lip curled with distaste.

Oh, so that's the reason for Rita's aggression.

Rita meowed something that probably translated to, *I do not like you, either.* Then she scurried away, no doubt fearing that her gourmet cat food and favorite table scraps would be cut off in favor of rodent fare.

But Joe had more important things to deal with than a cat. Already his mind had moved beyond the pesky feline. He sank down onto the big, upholstered sofa, then put his face in his hands. Concerned, she sat down beside him and put a hand on his arm.

"Joe, what's wrong?"

"Everything."

"Where have you been?"

"Everywhere."

"Could you be a little more specific?"

He glanced up and smiled at her. It was such a sad smile, barely curving his lips, and never reaching his stormy gray eyes. "For three sen-nights, I have wandered the woods and inlets of Gal-vast-town Bay, trying to locate Thora, or my ship. 'Twas all for naught."

"Where have you been staying?"

"Outdoors," he answered, as if it were nothing to live and sleep outdoors. The weather was fair for November in Texas, but the nights were decidedly cool.

"Where did you eat? *What* did you eat?"

Her question seemed to surprise him. "Whatever was available."

She was still confused. He had no money that she knew of. So restaurants were out of the question. *Oh, no!* He didn't steal food, did he?

He must have sensed her thoughts. "Tsk-tsk, Mag-he. I am no thief. Nay, I snared rabbits and caught fish and cooked them over an open fire. Once, I even ate a snake. 'Twas tougher than shoe leather, but filling."

A snake? She could barely keep herself from gagging. "Why didn't you just come back to the hospital?"

"I could not. Time was of the essence, with winter approaching on the north seas. Besides, I knew that I would no longer be welcome at the Rainbow hospitium once I broke the contract."

"And now what?"

He shrugged. "I am not sure. Well, one thing I

am certain of is that I am trapped in this world till springtime. Even if I were able to locate Thora now, I misdoubt that longship travel on the Iceland route to Norway would be a wise choice."

"But . . ." Maggie started to ask where he would stay, but decided she had more immediate concerns. "Listen, you've got to get out of those damp clothes and take a shower."

"Are you implying that I am malodorous?"

"Let's just say, Old Spice won't be asking you to do any commercials. I assume they had no deodorants where you were."

"Deodorants? Hah! I was lucky to be able to wash up in the bay with sand and water."

"You'll be lucky if you haven't caught pneumonia."

"New-mown-ya? The only thing I caught in that cold water was seaweed, puny pan fish, and one flounder."

She laughed. She was just so glad to have him back. "While you're shaving and cleaning up, I'll throw your stuff in the washing machine. You look famished. By the time you're through in the bathroom, and have eaten some dinner, the clothes should be dry."

He lifted his eyebrows with interest. "You want me to disrobe? Right now? In front of you?"

"No, Mr. One-track Mind. You can throw your dirty clothes outside the bathroom. It's nice to see you have a sense of humor about this, though."

"I was not jesting." His face was already serious, but now it turned even more serious as he regarded her with an uncertain expression on his face. He was usually so confident. "Was I wrong to come here?"

She hardly hesitated at all. "No, I'm glad you came. But how did you find my house?"

"Hattie gave me directions."

"Hattie?"

"Hattie Lawrence."

Warning bells started clanging inside Maggie's already aching head. "The daughter of Rainbow Hospital's owner?"

"Yea, the selfsame one."

"But . . . how . . . when . . . I don't understand."

"She slipped me a card with her name and telephone number that day they visited the hospital. She said, 'Call me sometime, sugar.' So I did."

Oh, my God! Hattie hit on a patient at the clinic. Hah! Is that any worse than me?

"I called her tonight and said that I was released from the hospital. A small mistruth," he admitted unabashedly. "I told her I was in a phone booth with no book of numbers and could she please look up your address for me. She was very nice."

I'll bet she was. "How did you make a phone call without any money?"

"Oh, I used a phone card."

Maggie was getting a splitting headache the size of Joe's outrageous story. "You have a phone card?"

"Nay. John Lennon lent me his."

"I hate to ask this, but where did you meet John Lennon? Don't tell me he came riding in on a killer whale, too." Or in a yellow submarine, she thought.

"Of course not." He gave her an impatient frown that said she was being silly. "John Lennon is a homeless person who lives near the mission

195

flophouse . . . leastways, that is what he called it. All he asked in return for my use of the phone card was for me to give peace a chance. Is that not an odd thing to say?"

"A homeless person with a phone card? And his name is John Lennon?"

" 'Tis what I said, is it not?" he snapped churlishly. "And, by the by, once I get some coins, I would like to go back and thank him for his services. Mayhap you could even invite John to live at Rainbow Hospital. He thinks he is a beetle, you know. And since you already have Steve the seal and Chuck, who thinks he is every animal in the land, depending on the day of the week, why not a bug as well?" He smiled brightly at her, as if he'd made a brilliant suggestion.

Maggie had to smile, despite herself. Joe certainly put the fun in *dysfunctional*. *But enough of this nonsense!* She put her hands on Joe's shoulders and pushed him toward the hallway. "Go!" she ordered. "Go, take a shower."

"God, I love it when you go Valkyrieish on me. Mayhap it is my destiny to be saddled with a pushy wench."

"I am not pushy. I am not a wench. I am not your Valkyrie. And, most definitely, I am not your destiny."

But Maggie wasn't so sure about that last.

A short time later, while Joe showered noisily in the bathroom down the hall, Maggie heated up the Texas chili she'd made the girls for dinner, along with a loaf of warm sourdough bread. She glanced out the kitchen window and noticed something important . . . the first star of the night. Could it possibly be shining brighter than ever before? And that constellation over there . . . surely it wasn't configured in the shape of a whale, just as the girls had noticed many weeks ago.

No! It's just my imagination.

Still . . .

"Thank you, God," she whispered.

"Look at him. Look how handsome he is, even asleep."

"Shhhh. Mom told us to stay away . . . not to disturb him."

"He's so big. No wonder he ate the entire pot of chili Mom made for our dinner, and a whole loaf of homemade bread."

"I've always wanted a big father."

"Me, too."

"He looks a little bit like Kevin Sorbo . . . that guy who used to play Hercules on TV."

"I think he looks more like Ricky Martin."

"I think he looks better than both of them."

"I think he looks like . . . a dad."

There was a long sigh then. Actually, two long sighs at the same time.

As Jorund emerged slowly from a deep sleep, he heard voices discussing him. Whoever they were, they must be pay-shuns of the hospital if they actually thought he resembled that Greek man of strength, Hercules. Right now Jorund felt weaker than dragon piss. And had someone really said that he resembled that infuriating singer with the magic hips, Ricky Martin? Jorund would never swing his hips like that in public . . . or in private, either. It was not manly, in his opinion.

197

He cracked both eyes open to mere slits, then shot bolt upright, which caused him to almost fall off the piece of cushiony furniture called a sofa, where he had fallen asleep after a most satisfying shower and dinner. He'd been talking with Mag-he about what he would do next when his eyes had drooped shut.

He had not wanted to be here when her daughters returned. But it was too late now. Two young girls with blond braids and silver jewelry on their teeth were staring at him. Twins.

"Go away," he said in a growl.

They looked fearful, but stood their ground.

"We've been praying for you every night," one of them said.

"Me? Why would you pray for me?"

"Mom said you were lost, and we prayed that she would find you. Mom drove around the bay lots of times, trying to find you."

"She did?" But Jorund had forgotten himself. He wanted naught to do with these urchins who reminded him so much of his own daughters. "Did I not tell you to go away?"

"Where should we go? This is our house."

"Can you not go to another chamber?"

"We want to watch TV. This is the TV room."

"Where's your mother?"

"Taking a bubble bath."

Now *that* conjured up some interesting pictures.

"She's using the lilac bath salts I bought her last Christmas," one of the twins informed him with total irrelevance. At least, he thought it was totally irrelevant till the other twin inquired, "Do you like lilacs?"

"I like lilacs fine," he snapped. Just for the

meanness of it, he added a loud growl, like a grizzly bear.

The girls just giggled. They actually giggled at his fierceness.

Just as his own daughters would have done.

In misery, he informed them, "You are breaking my heart. Can you not see how painful it is for me to be around you two?"

"You don't like us?" they both asked in unison, their voices squeaky with hurt.

" 'Tis not you that I mislike, particularly. I have trouble being around young girls." To his surprise, he noticed that his right hand had been lying over his heart protectively the whole time he spoke. *Why did I divulge that? 'Tis none of my concern if their feelings get hurt at the least little jab. Oh, holy Thor, why do they not go away?*

The twins exchanged worried glances with each other, then some whispered words he could not hear. They appeared ready to depart. Finally he seemed to have gotten through to them. But why were they approaching the sofa where he still sat?

"Mom always says a hug is the best medicine for a breaking heart," one twin told him, already reaching out her skinny arms toward him.

"No!" he cried out.

But the other twin had an even more horrifying idea. "Can I sit on your lap?"

"No!" he repeated in an anguished cry.

Short seconds later, Jorund Ericsson, the most barbarous Viking in all Vestfold, wept silently into the hair of two little girls who sat on each of his knees, arms wrapped around his shoulders, faces pressed into his neck. Oh, the little-girl smell of their skin was so familiar to him he could scarce breathe.

And then . . . oh, he should have been surprised—but he was not—when a strange voice in his head made a click-click-clicking noise and a whalelike grinding. To Jorund, it seemed to say, *Now you know why you are here, Viking. Now you know.*

"Mommy, please don't send him away," Beth begged from her bed, where Maggie had just tucked her in. "It's the magic of killer whales and God and wishing stars—all these things—that sent him to us. I just know it."

"There's no such thing as magic," Maggie chided her gently. "You're old enough to know that."

"Even from God?" Beth argued. "You mean there's no such thing as miracles?" Beth blinked innocently at her.

Oh, that was a low blow. "Of course there are miracles. Joe hardly qualifies as a miracle, though." *Or does he?*

"Can't you just believe in dreams come true, Mommy? Just a teeny-tiny bit?" Suzy added from her twin bed.

"But, honey—"

"You always told us anything is possible if you pray hard enough." It was Beth who addressed her now, and it was hard for Maggie to counter that argument, especially when she was quoting Maggie's own words.

"But sometimes the answer God gives us is no," she reminded them.

"And sometimes it's yes," they both exclaimed in unison, bright smiles on their faces.

Maggie would have liked to contradict her

daughters—to tell them that reality had to be faced, that Joe was very likely a mere blip on the screen of their lives, not a permanent fixture–not to be depended on. But she couldn't get the image of Joe out of her mind . . . Joe holding Suzy and Beth on his lap . . . Joe weeping silently over them . . . Joe putting aside his own grief to comfort her precious darlings.

Needless to say, in the end it took Maggie an exceptionally long time to get the girls to sleep that night. They were just so excited.

Maggie was excited, too, but for different, more personal, and very alarming reasons. That prompted her ten P.M. call to Harry at his home.

"Joe is here," she informed Harry without preamble.

"Is he all right?" was Harry's first question. His second was, "Are *you* all right?"

God bless Harry's good heart. No recriminations. No ranting or raving about unwise psychologists or ungrateful patients. Just a genuine concern for the well-being of all concerned.

"We're fine," she assured him.

"You know he can't return to the clinic."

"I know. And he does, too. Harry, this is going to sound crazy, but—"

He laughed softly. "Odd word to come from a psychologist."

She laughed, too, but there was a hysterical tone to her laughter.

Harry must have noticed, because his voice was serious when he prompted, "You were saying?"

"I was about to say that, despite all the appearances to the contrary, I don't think Joe is mentally ill."

"Are you sure that isn't just wishful thinking?"

Maggie sighed. So her feelings toward Joe were apparent to others. "That may play some part, but my gut instinct is that there is some other reason for all these things he claims. To tell you the truth, I've felt that way from the beginning, and I just can't get rid of this sense I have that there's something more to Joe's story . . . something beyond the explanations of science and logic."

"Maggie, Maggie, Maggie. The man says he's a tenth-century Viking who was delivered to this land by a killer whale."

"I know."

"And you believe that?"

"I'm not sure what I believe. I just know that he's not insane, or deranged, or mentally ill."

There was a long pause while Harry digested all that she'd said. They both knew there were cases that defied all the textbooks, that sometimes instinct was the best measure . . . but would he accept what she said now?

"Okay," he agreed finally. "What happens next?"

"I just want to go on record as stating that Joe Rand is no longer my patient."

"Uh-oh."

Uh-oh is right. Major uh-oh! "You've already said he's not a patient at the clinic anymore. I want to establish a paper record that he's not *my* patient, either."

"For the lawyers?"

"If need be."

"Maggie, be careful. You've got children to consider."

"I'm doing this for my children . . . as well as myself. He wouldn't hurt them any more than he would hurt his own children." No matter what Joe said, she couldn't lay the blame for his daughters' deaths on his shoulders.

"Are you sure about this, Maggie?"

"As sure as I've ever been about anything in my life." And she was, she recognized with a freeing sort of ebullience.

"I wish you luck then . . . or a miracle."

Maggie suspected she'd already been handed a bit of both.

"You can stay. . . ."

Jorund glanced up an hour later to see Mag-he standing in the doorway of the den chamber. He lifted one eyebrow in question. He hadn't realized that his staying or not staying had ever been an issue. He'd just assumed . . . well, he supposed that had been presumptuous of him.

"For a while. Till . . . till we figure things out."

"What things?"

"I just talked to Harry—Dr. Seabold—and everything is settled."

"What has Dock-whore Sea-bold to do with my settling?" Understanding struck him like a lightning bolt. "I am no longer your pay-shun."

She nodded.

Despite all that weighed him down, Jorund couldn't help grinning. If he was no longer considered her pay-shun, then that opened the doors to all kinds of . . . well, possibilities.

"Don't get any ideas," she chided him. Meanwhile, her gaze kept coming back to his exposed chest, visible through his unbuttoned *shert*, which he hadn't bothered to tuck into his *braies* after his recent shower.

"Oh, I have ideas aplenty. I wonder if my ideas coincide with your ideas."

"Probably."

"Probably? *Probably?* Sweetling, you'd best not toss out such seductive words unless you plan to follow up on them."

She just shrugged, but that shrug shouted a thousand things to him . . . all of them sexual.

"Sweetling, huh?" she asked with a soft smile. "I like the sound of that." Her voice was even huskier than usual. Jorund had been fond of that huskiness from the start. Now he would like to experiment with different ways of tuning that huskiness to his own satisfaction.

"Come here, Mag-he," he said, and was surprised that his voice, too, was husky.

She backed up a step instead. "Slowly . . . we've got to take things slowly here."

At first he wanted to balk . . . to argue that going fast was the better course. But perhaps she was right. He had been assailed by so many new emotions these past hours.

"For now, let me help you make up a bed for the night." Motioning him to stand, she stepped into the chamber. The soft folds of her scarlet silk robe outlined her body as she moved, especially where it was belted at the waist. He felt an immediate jolt of awareness at the joining of his thighs. Was she wearing undergarments under the robe? Or had she come to him naked, already prepared for his lovemaking? Oh, what a heady thought that was! His entire body went hot and throbbing with the mental picture. He had been without a woman for a long time. He had been without Mag-he for a long time.

Was now the time?

As she showed him how to pull out the bed mattress that was magically enclosed inside the sofa, the scent of lilacs wafted his way, and he recalled that the girls had said their mother was taking a bubble bath. Then, taking soft pillows, bed linens, and blankets from a close-it, she began to make up the bed. Each time she bent or turned, the filmy robe clung to a different, more enticing curve of her body.

He smiled.

Turning suddenly, she caught him in the smile, and seemed surprised—then embarrassed. Did the blush that now flooded her face and neck also color other parts of her body?

"Tomorrow is Thanksgiving, Joe," she informed him as she turned her back to him and worked to smooth out the wrinkles in the blanket. That gave him a good view of her backside as she bent to the task. Holy Valhalla, the wench had more curves than a Norse fjord.

But then Mag-he's words registered, and jolted him out of his erotic musings. With disgust, he realized that he had been ogling her body like an untried youth before his first swiving. "Thanksgiving?" he inquired in as level a voice as he could manage. *Well, I certainly hope I will be having something to be thankful for, after tonight.*

"In our country it's a special day when everyone gives thanks for their bounty. In our home we

205

have our Thanksgiving feast early so we can go to the Orcaland amusement park for the last day of the season . . . weather permitting, of course."

"And?" he prompted. Why was she telling him this now?

"And I want to make sure you will be all right with that. Will you be able to stand being around my daughters? You've had a rather strong reaction when I've mentioned them previously."

He thought long and hard. It was a good question. Could he be in the company of twin girls, when his own cherished twin daughters were dead? "I think I will be all right. If I have a change of sentiment, I will take myself from their presence."

"I don't want my girls to get hurt. I mean that." The fierce expression on her face bespoke a mother's protectiveness. Just as Jorund had been aroused by Mag-he's sex-voice and her alluring robe, he was also stimulated by this aspect of her personality. "I won't hurt them."

"Not just physically. I want your assurance that you won't hurt them emotionally, either."

"How can I promise that?" he cried out. At the first opportunity, he was going to leave this time and place. The way things looked now, it might not ever happen. But then again, the window in time might open for him suddenly, without warning. How could he make pledges that might be beyond his power to keep?

"My daughters love you, Joe."

To his dismay, he groaned aloud. A warrior should not display his weaknesses, but, in this instance, he could not help himself.

"Don't ask me why or how that happened; it just did. At least promise me that you will do your best not to hurt their feelings . . . or break their hearts."

"If I have that much power, I should depart your home now. I do not want to be responsible for their joy, or their sorrow."

"It seems to me you have no choice."

He nodded, suddenly choked up. But then he thought of something else . . . something that caused his throat to clear and his heart to lift. If he was going to be stuck in this land, then he was going to commence enjoying the benefits, such as they were. He had been docile too long . . . allowing events to lead him, instead of being the aggressor like the military chieftain he was.

Mag-he stood on the other side of the sofa bed, wearing her siren robe, staring at him. There was no fear in her luminous blue eyes, just curiosity. And boldness.

Her gaze kept returning to his chest, which was bared by his unbuttoned *shert*. He smiled with satisfaction. So the wench liked his body. That was encouraging news.

She saw his smile. "I was just checking to see if Rita had scratched you badly."

He made a scoffing sound of disbelief. It was his finely honed body she was examining, not some piddling scratch.

Her stubborn chin jutted out defiantly. *Foolish wench*. Even a hardened warrior knew when to yield to greater forces.

He began to move around the mattress, a predatory rush of blood beginning to surge through his body. It was the selfsame feeling he had before every battle.

"Wh-what?" Mag-he stammered. Her shaky voice belied her brave stance. Still, not one step did she back off. He had to admire her for that.

" 'Tis time," he said, and took another step toward her.

"Time for what, Joe?" she whispered in that sex-voice of hers. He felt it all the way to his man parts, which began to thicken in appreciation. Truly, that voice of hers was going to be his undoing yet, if he were not more careful.

"My name is Jorund." Only a few more steps. Her intoxicating lilac scent was making him dizzy.

"Jorund," she rasped out. Her head was still tilted in confusion, but she had the good sense to back up one step, then another.

He followed after her, in stalking mode now. " 'Tis time," he repeated.

"For what?" she repeated, too. But now her back hit the wall.

"For unfinished business."

Chapter Eleven

Maggie's senses reeled under Joe's heated gaze.

She should look away. She tried to look away. But she could not. She was too entranced by the sensuous flame that had ignited in his smoky eyes, scorching her inch by inch, as they roamed her figure in the Victoria's Secret silk wrapper—a birthday gift from her girls two weeks ago. They'd obviously considered her frumpy old chenille robe unsuitable attire for daddy hunting.

His voice was low and raw as he whispered, "You are so beautiful."

And Maggie felt beautiful at that moment. And raw.

The man was stalking her . . . no doubt about it. She would have darted for safety if her back weren't pressed to the wall. On the other hand, maybe she wouldn't have fled. For once in her life, Maggie yearned to free the sensuality she'd suppressed for so long. She didn't want to be self-conscious about her body or worry what other people would think. She wanted to be wanton.

As Maggie stood, transfixed, he moved toward her slowly, but purposefully. Then, in a blink, he wrapped his arms about her waist, lifting her high, and walked her to the bed. Without breaking his stride, he tossed her onto the mattress and followed after her, landing between her inadvertently outspread legs.

They both gasped at the delicious contact of his sex against her sex, even through the barrier of his denim jeans and her robe. The position had been an accident, but Joe wasn't about to set aside the advantage. Instead he moved himself from side to side, adjusting himself more firmly in the cradle of her thighs. The whole time he watched her steadily, clearly wanting to witness her every reaction.

Oh, this was too embarrassing for a sexually inhibited person like herself. Could he sense the passionate fluttering that had started between her legs and moved like wildfire to all the erogenous zones of her body? Well, at least she used to be sexually inhibited. Now she didn't even recognize the wild woman who was yanking at his open shirt and tossing it aside. She could smell the clean, musky scent of his skin, but more than anything she wanted to see it, and feel it, and taste it.

"Your eagerness excites me mightily," he said as he brushed the palms of both hands over her breasts, causing them to peak through the silk fabric.

"I'm not eager," she lied. What she thought was, *Touch me, touch me, touch me, again, again, again.*

As if he heard her thoughts, he put his open mouth over the tip of one breast and began to suckle wetly through the flimsy cloth barrier with a hard rhythm.

Maggie almost shot up off the bed, except that his lower body still held her in place . . . his lower body that had a thickening ridge pressed against her in just the right place.

He took her hands and encouraged them to explore his shoulders and chest and, yes, even his flat, male nipples. To her delight, he looked as if he might shoot up off the bed, too.

And he grew even larger against her.

And flexed.

And then Maggie flexed back.

There were so many hormones flying about that Maggie feared an explosion. In fact, an explosion was guaranteed if they continued on this course.

But wait. Wait, wait, wait. Maggie realized that she hadn't spoken the cautionary word aloud. "Wait!" she practically shouted now. She didn't know if she was trying to be heard over the roaring of blood in her ears or his . . . probably both, because the heightened color on his face as he stared down at her, not to mention his ragged breathing, proved he was as turned on as she was.

"Wait?" he inquired in a strangled voice. "*Now* you tell me to wait? What is amiss?"

"I can't make love with you here . . . now . . . not with my daughters in the house."

"*Now* you gainsay me?" His eyes darkened angrily to a steely gray. "Why not?"

"Because it wouldn't be right," she insisted. "I have to set an example for them. I'm a single mother . . . an unmarried woman. My girls can't ever think of me as being promiscuous."

"In my land, children respect their elders' privacy. They know that lust and marriage do not necessarily go hand in hand."

"Yeah, well, you're not in Oz now, Toto," she said snidely, then immediately regretted her words. "It doesn't matter what the morality is in your land—or my land. It matters what *I* think." She put a palm over her heart for emphasis. "And I want my children to grow up believing that lust or love, or whatever you want to call it, do go hand in hand with marriage. Or at the least, a committed relationship."

He made a rude sound of disgust. "Like all women, you want something for your favors, then. Whether it be coin or the bindings of marriage, females are ever out to snare men with their wiles."

"You don't know me at all if you think that."

She saw the stiffening of his jaw and the accusatory gleam in his eyes. She knew exactly what he was thinking.

"I wasn't teasing you, Joe."

"It felt like teasing. Are you one of those women who enjoy the chase, and get your pleasure from making a man grovel?"

"*No!*" she asserted forcefully. "And I doubt whether you've groveled a day in your life."

"Then why come to me in your siren robe, giving me those come-take-me looks?"

Now he was getting insulting. She tried to push

him away, or squirm out from under him, but he wouldn't release her.

"I came because I wanted you, you big lout. Because I wanted you so much, I forgot that I have responsibilities." She turned her face to the side, hating the fact that her eyes were misting over.

He tipped her chin back with a forefinger so that she was staring up at him as he propped himself on one elbow above her. His anger had melted away, replaced by a rueful acceptance. "A big lout, hmmm?" he remarked with a self-deprecating grin as he fingered the ends of her hair, still damp from her recent bath, then sniffed her. He nodded, as if pleased with the scent of her shampoo. Lilacs . . . the same as her bath salts had been.

"The biggest," she answered with a small sob.

"And you wanted me a great deal?" He was leaning so close that his breath fanned her lips as he spoke. When she declined to answer, he nipped her bottom lip with his teeth and rubbed his erection against her at the same time.

She jerked back at the exquisite sensations those brief caresses engendered. If that wasn't bad enough, he nudged her legs farther apart with his knees, then cupped her bottom and rocked her hips against him.

She squealed. She actually squealed. Then she admitted, "A great deal."

"And still do?" he persisted.

Now he was alternately wetting the inner whorls of her ear with the tip of his tongue and blowing it dry. It was as if a thin, erotic thread connected her ears to her breasts and genital

213

area, because each flick of his tongue was causing her to swell and throb in delicious agony.

"Still do," she whimpered. "But, I repeat, we can't make love."

To her surprise, he nodded. "Well, a kiss then. Surely it would be no great shock to your daughters' sensibilities to see a man kissing their mother."

She laughed softly at his too-obvious ploy. "You don't even like kisses."

"Oh, m'lady, you have sung that song too many times already. I have told you more than once that I have changed my mind on that issue."

"A kiss? That would be all?"

"Well, a little touching, too."

"A little touching? Aha! Men have been saying that throughout the ages. A little touching leads to a lot more, and before you know it, well, you can guess where it all leads."

"The injustice of your remark wounds me, m'lady," he said. "If I promise to give you only kisses and little touches, then that is what I will do. My word is my bond."

She nodded, because she really did want–no, need—a little bit of his loving tonight . . . something to seal this change in their relationship.

"To be fair, I must advise you that I have been told I have clever hands."

Clever hands? What does that mean? I don't want to know. Yes, I do. Oh, boy!

"Mayhap it is the calluses on my palms from wielding a long sword for so many years. Or mayhap it is the flexibility of my fingers, which must needs thrust a spear or pull on the reins of a blood-maddened warhorse with equal dexterity. Or mayhap it is the things learned in the Eastern harems that—"

She put her hands on either side of his neck, pulling him down for a kiss.

He drew back a hairbreadth from her lips and said, "I may be willing to accept your terms, but be forewarned: there are things I want to do to you that no man has ever done afore. . . ."

Maggie's heart skittered wildly at his words, and a hot dampness pooled between her legs.

"Even so, I will keep my word, for now. Mere kisses and little touches . . . that is all."

Joe kept his promise then, but there was nothing mere or little about him.

And, as to clever hands . . . *Lordy, lordy!*

Jorund sat at the head table of Mag-he's great hall early the next afternoon, awaiting the Thanksgiving feast.

Actually, there was no great hall . . . not even a hall at all, for that matter. And only one table. But then, Mag-he's keep itself was not all that large; he could touch the ceiling in any of the chambers. It was not as humble as the longhouses of his Norse cotters, nor as grand as the wood castles he, his father, and his brothers had erected in his homeland, following the Saxon and Frankish styles.

But one thing in this land might prove better: the food set out on the table smelled delicious, though foreign to his palate. Not a salted fjord fish or a bowl of *skyr*, the soured cream favored by many in his country, was in sight. And there was no central hearth with a boar on the spit or an ever-present cauldron of the meat or vegetable of the day—usually rabbit and leeks. No loss to him were any of those things.

Instead Mag-he, without the aid of any house-carls, had prepared a roast turkey with sage stuffing, whipped potatoes, and candied sweet potatoes. Jorund had no idea what a potato was until Mag-he explained that it was a root vegetable, like a turnip. How one went about whipping a root, he could not even guess. There was also corn—another vegetable he'd never witnessed before—cranberry sauce—which caused his eyes to narrow and his belly to knot up because it had the same jiggly texture as that hated jail-low from the Rainbow hospitium—bread, butter, milk, and pumpkin pie.

Another thing he did not miss from his time was the often smelly, vermin-infested rushes on the floor. It was a constant struggle on the part of womenfolk to keep them fresh with juniper and dried herbs. Here there were luxurious carpets . . . thick as the plushest wool fleece. But then, hounds did not abound indoors here, grousing about for bones and relieving themselves hither and yon. Just an irksome cat that had its own privy box. The insufferable Rita had taken to following him about, giving him the evil eye. He would consider cleaving the bothersome beast from its hissing mouth to its twitching tail if he did not recognize the misplaced affection these three females held for the fat cat.

He started to reach for a piece of bread, then pulled his hand back abruptly when Beth made a cautionary tug on his sleeve. Beth was the name of one twin, he had learned; Sue-zee was the other. Jorund was not devoid of social graces, but he felt so awkward in this strange country whose customs he was yet learning. Even the use of a fork still came clumsily to him.

"We have to say grace first," Beth informed him as she took his hand.

Grace? Who is Grace? Jorund glanced behind him to see if another person had come in, or worse yet, another bothersome cat.

Sue-zee took his hand on the other side. Then both girls joined hands with their mother at the other end of the table.

Jorund closed his eyes briefly at the wave of poignant memory that swept over him at the feel of two tiny hands engulfed by his. The entire hand of each of them barely covered his palm. And the skin . . . ah, the skin was softer than the film on his mother's thick cream.

Dismayed, he opened his eyes to see the girls gazing at him with what could only be described as . . . adoration. *Adoration!* That caused him to be even more dismayed. What had he done to earn such adoration? Nothing. He did not deserve—nor did he want—such sentiments. Really, they were pathetic little creatures in their need for a father figure, he concluded. Any man would have suited. At least, that was what he told himself. But deep down, he suspected the only pathetic one in this picture was a Viking who was quaking in his boots . . . or rather, his cloth running shoes.

"Dear God, bless this food we are about to eat. . . ." Mag-he began.

Oh. Grace must be a prayer.

"And let us give thanks for all the bounty you have given us this year."

"Amen," the three of them said at once.

The only bounty I've been given is a kick in the arse through time to a land of lackwits, he thought ungraciously, and tried to tug free of the girls' hands, but the little imps held on tenaciously. Now that they had him, they were not about to let him go.

"Now let's begin our annual ritual," Mag-he told her daughters. They nodded, but first Mag-he elaborated to him: "Each Thanksgiving we list the things we are most thankful for from the past year."

Holy bloody hell!

"I'm thankful that no more killer whales were captured last year," Beth, the gentle twin, said.

Huh? What an odd sentiment! I would think a child her age would be thankful for a new pair of slippers, or a riband. But a whale's noncapture?

"I'm thankful that I passed math this quarter," Sue-zee proclaimed with a brash smile at her mother.

"What is this math?" Jorund asked.

"Numbers. Adding, subtracting, multiplying, dividing. Yuck!" Sue-zee explained with disgust.

"Ah," he said with understanding. "I know exactly how you feel. Ever did I have trouble with my numbers as a child. Likewise, my brother Magnus of the Big Ears. The priest who was hired to tutor us nigh pulled his hair out with frustration . . . what little there was on his bald tonsured pate. My brother Rolf the Shipbuilder was the scholar . . . he fostered in the Saxon court, but I was destined for the battlefield, even as a youthling, and . . ." His words trailed off as he realized that everyone was gaping at him . . . and that he'd interrupted the thanking ritual.

Mag-he spoke next. "I'm thankful that I got my doctorate degree finally, and that I'm now a full-fledged psychologist."

Jorund thought her efforts might have been better directed toward more traditional female tasks . . . like begetting more children, especially boys—there was always a need for more young men to go off to battle or build ships or plow fields. With a grin, he decided not to share those sentiments with her. She would no doubt call him a male show-vein-is pig, just as Reva had called Josh one day a few weeks ago. Or perchance she would clout him on the side of the head, as his mother was wont to do with his father when he pronounced what she called "male blather" or "ale talk."

Sue-zee spoke again. "I'm thankful Joe came home."

"Me, too," Beth said.

Oh, no! No, no, no, no! Do not be thankful for me. And do not call this my home. I am just a wayfarer passing through. The only reason Jorund kept these sentiments to himself was that he'd promised Mag-he not to hurt her daughters. He looked at her for help.

Mag-he just nodded her head, seemingly at a loss for words, too. Why didn't she correct her daughters? It was her job to steer the children's thinking toward the right path.

On the other hand, Mag-he might also be thankful that he had "come home." More likely, she was thanking her One-God that she had peaked three times the night before under Jorund's expert fingers. She should be thanking her One-God that Jorund was going to bring her even more pleasure at the first opportunity. He knew that he was thanking the gods that she was a woman with enthusiasm for bed sport. He could not wait till he showed her the renowned Viking S-spot. She would be more thankful than she'd ever been in all her life, he would warrant.

"Actually," Beth began, "it was really the Vikings who discovered America. So we should probably be thankful today for the Vikings."

"Funny you should mention that. I had forgotten. You know, that Leif Eriksson was a barmy fellow . . . just like his father Erik the Red. I remember one time he . . ." Jorund's words trailed off as he realized that Mag-he was staring at him with dismay. He assumed he was not supposed to be speaking of his ancient past around her children.

"What are you thankful for, Joe?" Sue-zee asked.

Caught was his first thought. He'd been caught having lewd thoughts in the midst of a family event. His mother really would have clouted him now, having an intuition concerning her boys' lustful fantasies, even when they were no longer boys. His eyes went involuntarily to Mag-he's *shert* front—made of another of those stretchy materials that he loved—which clearly delineated her nipples.

She blushed, sensing his wayward thoughts, then frowned in warning.

"I'm thankful I'm alive," he blurted out, grasping at the first thing he could think of. When he saw the expression of disappointment on their faces, he added, "I thank the gods that they have given me a family with whom to share this special day."

Jorund wished he were dead.

He was strapped into a metal box, with Beth and Sue-zee on either side of him, and they were in the midst of riding a metal monster called 'the Comet,' or 'the Vomit,' depending on which child was speaking. Sue-zee was laughing gaily. Beth was tapping her fingers with boredom, much preferring another trip to the orca park, where there had been not one single message from Thora. And Jorund was holding on to the front bar with white knuckles, his Thanksgiving turkey in his throat, along with the candy apple and cotton candy and root-beer Slurpee he'd just consumed. If his brother, Magnus, ever heard that he'd consumed a beverage called a Slurpee he would roll on the rush floor with laughter.

Mag-he—the coward, or the wise woman, depending on one's perspective—was standing down below, waving up at them. He was going to wave something at her, like a birch rod, if he ever survived this ordeal. She should have warned him about the danger of this amusement ride, which he thought was ill-named. There was nothing amusing about putting oneself into a metal box that rode up one hill, then down another, higher and higher into the sky, sometimes upside down, then hurled the passengers straight down at excessive speed till their stomachs lurched and rose to their bulging eyeballs. Then the procedure was repeated over and over again. It was insanity, pure and simple. They ought to establish a Rainbow Hospitium right in the midst of this chaos.

If Mag-he ever again dared to refer to him as a type-tea personality, he intended to set her crooked mind straight. There might very well be men—or women, or children for that matter—who enjoyed great thrills by making their hearts nigh stop beating, but he was not one of them. In truth, a Saracen horse soldier had once put a scimitar to his throat while dangling him off the side of a cliff, and Jorund had not felt such fright as on this rolling hell-ride.

Why could they not have stayed at Mag-he's home and watched football—a brutal game more to his liking, where grown men tried to beat each other's brains out—on the tee-vee box? It was the custom of most Americans in this land on this day. But no, these three lackbrains had to make one last trip to the Orcaland park before it closed for the winter.

Soon—though not soon enough for Jorund's satisfaction—they emerged from the demented ride. He staggered on weak legs over to a bench, where he plopped down and put his face between his outspread knees. Sue-zee sat down beside him and exclaimed happily, "Wow! That was so cool. Can we do it again?"

He raised his head slightly and slanted her a look that he hoped conveyed his feelings on the subject. He was afraid that, if he spoke aloud, foul words would spew from his mouth.

"Can we go on the Ferris wheel now?" Beth asked her mother, who sat down on his other side and stared at him with concern.

"What's a fair-ass wheel? Is it a fright machine, like the rolling coaster?"

"No," Mag-he said with a short laugh. "Even I am not afraid of the Ferris wheel."

So they walked over to another area, where the girls quickly jumped into another metal box. He and Mag-he followed in the next box. If Jorund hadn't been so disoriented by the effects of the rolling coaster, he would have paid more attention to his surroundings. It was only as the fair-ass wheel began to move, backward and upward, that he let his gaze roam skyward and saw just how high this fair-ass wheel was. Enormous. Then he glanced down at the fence that enclosed the fair-ass wheel arena where a sign clearly proclaimed, *World's Largest Ferris Wheel.*

That was all Jorund needed to learn. "You people are barmy," he declared, unbuckling his seat belt. He began to climb out of his metal box, which was already high up in the air.

"Joe! You can't do that," Mag-he cried out. "Come back here."

"Way to go!" Sue-zee, the bloodthirsty little type-tea, was cheering.

"Be careful," Beth shouted down to where he was dangling from the slow-rising box. Despite her concern, it was obvious she was enjoying his wild antics, too.

"Joe, you have to stay on the Ferris wheel till it stops," Mag-he informed him with chagrin.

"Not bloody likely," he said, equally chagrined, swinging an arm out to grasp at a metal supporting pole, which he used to shinny down to the ground.

"You crazy son of a bitch!" the machine operator was screaming, practically frothing at the mouth. He had a front tooth missing and a bulge in his cheek.

"You are fortunate I do not have my sword with me," Jorund retorted as he landed on his feet with a thud.

"Well, sword this, buddy," the fellow hollered recklessly, meanwhile sticking a middle finger in the air.

Normally Jorund would have ignored the scrawny know-nothing, but he had learned from his friend Steve just what this gesture meant. He could not let the insult pass.

"Nay, I prefer to do *this*." Jorund said, shooting him a sharp punch in the mouth, thus loosening another tooth.

Needless to say, they were soon evicted from the amusement park. But Jorund did not care . . . he had had enough amusement for one day.

That night Joe was in the den, buffing his sword with a soft cloth and a jar of her silver cream. He claimed that fresh blood—as in battlefield blood—was the finest polish for "a warrior's best friend," but Maggie didn't know if he was kidding or not. She certainly wasn't about to open a vein to find out.

"Are the girls abed?" he asked, without glancing up from his task. She had been standing in

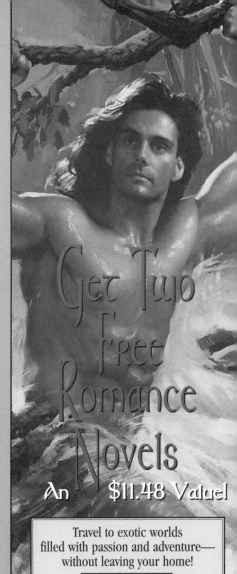

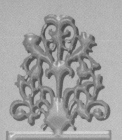
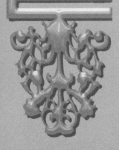

Thrill to the most sensual, adventure-filled Romances on the market today...

FROM 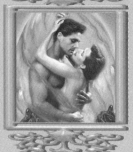 LOVE SPELL BOOKS

As a home subscriber to the Love Spell Romance Book Club, you'll enjoy the best in today's BRAND-NEW Time Travel, Futuristic, Legendary Lovers, Perfect Heroes and other genre romance fiction. For five years, Love Spell has brought you the award-winning, high-quality authors you know and love to read. Each Love Spell romance will sweep you away to a world of high adventure...and intimate romance. Discover for yourself all the passion and excitement millions of readers thrill to each and every month.

Save $5.00 Each Time You Buy!

Every other month, the Love Spell Romance Book Club brings you four brand-new titles from Love Spell Books. EACH PACKAGE WILL SAVE YOU AT LEAST $5.00 FROM THE BOOK-STORE PRICE! And you'll never miss a new title with our convenient home delivery service.

Here's how we do it: Each package will carry a FREE 10-DAY EXAMINATION privilege. At the end of that time, if you decide to keep your books, simply pay the low invoice price of $17.96, no shipping or handling charges added. HOME DELIVERY IS ALWAYS FREE. With today's top romance novels selling for $5.99 and higher, our price SAVES YOU AT LEAST $5.00 with each shipment.

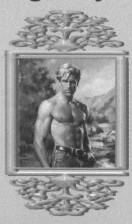

AND YOUR FIRST TWO-BOOK SHIP-MENT IS TOTALLY FREE!

IT'S A BARGAIN YOU CAN'T BEAT! A SUPER $11.48 Value!

Love Spell ✦ A Division of Dorchester Publishing Co., Inc.

GET YOUR 2 FREE BOOKS NOW–AN $11.48 VALUE!

Mail the Free Book Certificate Today!

Free Books Certificate

YES! I want to subscribe to the Love Spell Romance Book Club. Please send me my 2 FREE BOOKS. Then every other month I'll receive the four newest Love Spell selections to Preview FREE for 10 days. If I decide to keep them, I will pay the Special Member's Only discounted price of just $4.49 each, a total of $17.96. This is a SAVINGS of at least $5.00 off the bookstore price. There are no shipping, handling, or other charges. There is no minimum number of books I must buy and I may cancel the program at any time. In any case, the 2 FREE BOOKS are mine to keep—A BIG $11.48 Value!

Offer valid only in the U.S.A.

Name_____

Address_____

City_____

State _____ Zip _____

Telephone_____

Signature_____

A $11.48 VALUE

Get Two Books Totally
F R E E —
An $11.48 Value!

▼ Tear Here and Mail Your FREE Book Card Today! ▼

the doorway and hadn't realized he'd been aware of her presence. She stepped into the room now and wished he'd put the sword aside. The fact that he felt the need to keep the weapon in tip-top shape bespoke a time when he would be leaving them.

"Yes, but they're still so overexcited by their day with you that I doubt they'll be asleep anytime soon."

She saw the muscles in his jaw go rigid.

"Thank you for being so kind to them. I know they were a pain in the neck, clinging to you, and . . . well, I appreciate your . . . uh, tolerance."

"They were just being youthlings, no different from . . . from other children their age."

She knew that he had been about to say they were no different from his own daughters. Why wouldn't he talk about his girls? Greta and Girta, he'd told her reluctantly, but he almost never mentioned them by name. The psychologist in Maggie recognized that Joe would never heal until he faced his loss head-on. It was a necessary part of the grieving process. And how about his wife? It was even stranger that he shut her out of his mind. He must have loved her very much.

"Do you know what your daughters said to me when I went up to look at their wishing star tonight?"

"What?" Maggie braced herself for the worst.

" 'I wish you were my daddy.' That is what they said, Mag-he."

Yep. The worst. "I told them not to say stuff like that to you, but I guess . . . well, I guess they can't help themselves. Don't get bent out of shape over

225

it. Hey, next week they'll be hoping that whale trainer at Orcaland is their father, or some hot-shot movie star, or . . ." Her words trailed off at the disbelieving look Joe leveled at her. They both knew this was not a passing fancy on her girls' part. "So what did you say to them?"

"I told them that, by necessity, I could stay in this land only for a short time."

"And?" she prodded.

He released a long-breath. "And then Beth asked if I would be their daddy just while I am in this land . . . at least till after the yule season."

"Oh, Joe! And what did you say to that?"

"Naught . . . I said naught. I was saved by Sue-zee asking me if I could chop down a Christmas tree for them. I said that I could indeed chop down a tree, though why they would want me to do so is beyond my understanding."

Maggie laughed then and sat down next to Joe on the couch. Briefly she explained the tradition of Christmas trees. "You're lucky they didn't ask you for firewood and snow, as well."

"You bring dead evergreen trees into your homes to celebrate Christ's birth?" His eyes were wide with amazement.

"Yes, and we adorn them with bright lights and glittery balls and homemade decorations."

"Now see, that is the strange thing about your land, Mag-he. You deem a man demented because he rides atop a whale naked, but you see naught wrong with people voluntarily putting their lives at risk on rolling coasters and fair-ass wheels, or worshiping dead trees. I ask you, who is truly insane?"

She smiled and put a hand on his arm, about to squeeze it in playful remonstrance when she felt the heat emanating from him. It was only then that she noticed the flush on his face as well. Was it a sunburn? She put a hand to his forehead and gasped. He was burning up. This was no mere sunburn.

"Joe, why didn't you tell me you're not feeling well?"

"Dost have a hearing problem, m'lady? I told you after eating all those sweets at the amusement park that my stomach was rebelling. Riding that metal monster just churned it up more. Of course I am unwell."

She left and came back with a thermometer. "Lift your tongue and let this rest in your mouth for a minute or so. I need to check your temperature."

"Temperature?"

"Body heat."

"Oh, I can assure you that I am hot. For you." He waggled his eyebrows at her with a half-hearted attempt at humor.

"Not that kind of heat. Open your mouth."

"No."

"If you don't want to do it that way, I'll take you to a hospital, where they can take your temperature in another orifice. It's what they do with babies—and stubborn adults."

"You would not dare."

"Try me."

Reluctantly he opened his mouth for the thermometer, but the whole time he held it under his tongue, he glowered at her.

She soon discovered that he had a fever—one

227

hundred and four. Forcing him to take two Tylenol, she helped him into the sofa bed and declined his request that she join him. The silly man wouldn't have been able to do anything in his condition anyway. Well, maybe he would, but she doubted he'd be up to his par.

Ridiculous thoughts.

She slept restlessly that night. When she awakened the next morning, she realized that she had reason for concern. Joe was almost delirious with a raging fever . . . now a whopping one hundred and five. She rushed him to the emergency clinic at a nearby medical center.

And there she discovered something even more alarming about Joe . . . something that would change her world forever.

Chapter Twelve

The Bayside Medical Center released Joe the same day with a stash of antibiotics and extra-strength painkillers.

Maggie suspected that the only thing keeping them from admitting him to the hospital was his lack of medical insurance. Despite her being part of the medical establishment, she had to agree with the majority of people in this country: the health-care industry and its concern with the bottom line was deplorable.

She had a hard time keeping the girls away from him in the den, which had been transformed into a sickroom. Finally Maggie sent them to a Saturday movie matinee with a girlfriend and her mother. By the time they returned at dinnertime and went upstairs to listen to tapes,

Joe was sleeping restlessly. He was still extremely sick, though his temperature had gone down.

Then the telephone rang. "Joe Rand, please," a male voice on the other end of the line said.

"He's not available right now. Who's calling?"

"This is Dr. Zalvanchic from Bayside Medical Center."

"Joe is asleep right now. In fact, he's been sleeping since we left your office this morning. Is that OK? I mean, I assumed that sleep was the best thing for him. He still seems to have a fever, but his temperature has gone down a bit." She had stopped at a pharmacy that morning and bought one of those high-priced thermometers that were placed in the ear, thus allowing her to check his temperature even while he slept.

"That's good. That's good. It means the antibiotic is working," the doctor said, but there was a note of worry in his voice.

"What are you keeping from me?" she demanded.

"Ms. McBride, what's your relationship to this man?"

She bristled. "Friend."

"Does he have any family nearby? Wife? Parents? Siblings?"

"No," she answered hesitantly. Why would he ask such questions? Was it a privacy issue? Or something more?

"Where's he from?"

Oh, God! How should she answer that? "Norway, I think."

"Hmmm."

"What's the problem, Doctor?"

"Well, you see, we've got a puzzle on our hands

here. The lab work came back, and the blood tests show a rare strain of virus that I haven't seen *ever*, and I've been in practice for forty-odd years."

"It's not the flu?"

"It's most definitely not the flu."

An alarming thought occurred to her, something she should have considered immediately with two daughters in the house. "Is it contagious?"

"Not at this stage. Nothing to worry about there."

"Is it a serious virus?" Her throat closed over as she choked out, "Terminal?"

The doctor laughed softly. "No, nothing like that. It's just that this particular virus hasn't been around for hundreds of years . . . maybe even a thousand years."

"Huh? Hey, even I know that there were no blood tests back then."

"I realize that, but there were specific symptoms mentioned in some of the Anglo-Saxon medical journals for a disease called Seafarers' Lament. Mr. Rand's unusual symptoms fit that disease to a tee. And they don't fit any modern virus we have on record."

"Unusual symptoms? Like what?"

"Swelling in the armpit and groin areas. Distinctive blotches on the skin . . . pink patches with white dots. Tremors in the thighs. Excruciating headaches at the base of the skull. Shrinkage of the tongue. Dilation of the pupils with a purplish shading to the cornea. A red tint in the urine sample. In those days, the malady was most often fatal, but today . . . well, modern treatments should work. You say that he already appears to

Sandra Hill

be improving? Well, it's pure luck that we hit on the right drug for his virus so quickly."

"Yes, but now I'm really worried."

"I think we should admit him to the hospital, if only for observation. I have colleagues at Johns Hopkins University who would love to study this chap."

Suddenly, in the midst of the information the physician was relaying, one thought came through loud and clear: Joe really was from the tenth century. No, she amended, *Jorund* really was who he had told her he was, though she'd have a hard time thinking of him as anything but Joe. The man was a time traveler from a thousand years ago.

How was that possible?

And, of more immediate importance, how could she subject him to the public scrutiny that would surely ensue if she allowed them to admit him to a hospital? He would be like a freak on display.

But how could she not admit him if his life was in danger?

"Doctor, would it be possible for me to treat him here at home? I have some medical training, and as I told you, he already seems to be improving. Besides, he has no insurance and no money to pay for an expensive hospital stay."

"Well, I suppose. As long as you follow my instructions carefully, and call me, or my service, the minute you notice any changes for the worse, I suppose it would be all right. To tell you the truth, we're understaffed here with the holiday weekend. Yes, I think your suggestion would be satisfactory ... for now. I want to see him first thing Monday morning, though."

Maggie agreed, but what she thought was, No way! She would not go back to that hospital unless there were a medical emergency. After getting detailed directions from the doctor, Maggie went down the hall to the den once again. For a long time she sat on the edge of the bed, bathing Joe's face and chest and bare arms with cool cloths. The whole time, Maggie's mind reeled with the enormity of what she'd just discovered.

Joe really was a Viking.

Two weeks later ...

"Can we stop at McDonald's?" Joe asked from the passenger seat as her car zoomed by the popular fast-food restaurant.

Maggie had come home from work today to find Joe dressed and ready for a ride to Orcaland, which was closed for the season. He had wanted to stand by the fence and try to commune with some invisible whale off in the distance. Apparently the whale was out of range, or ignoring him.

Maggie had trouble accepting the fact that the man had telepathic talks with a whale. But then, she'd had trouble accepting him as a time traveler, too. That was an issue she hadn't yet discussed with him. She told herself she was avoiding the conversation till Joe was well, but deep inside, she was afraid that, if she spoke the words aloud, she would have to accept that they were really true.

"Did you hear me? Stop at McDonald's."

"No!" she exclaimed much too loudly. The man

233

was driving her batty with his constant requests . . . and questions—oh, yes, especially the questions. He was like a toddler who'd just learned to talk and couldn't stop jabbering.

His monologues usually went like this: "Drive me to the bay. Buy me some beer. What's a condom? Oh. Well, buy me some of those . . . several dozen, at least. No? Then sell my arm ring so I can have money of my own; I'll buy the damn condoms myself. Where's the *TV Guide?* Why can't I watch you shave your legs? What's wrong with practicing my swordplay in the living room . . . with Rita? Now, if I were practicing the trick my uncle, King Olaf, taught me, where I play with three swords at once, with one of them always being in the air . . . *then* you might have cause for concern. What's a thong? No, I did not lock Rita in the bathing room . . . really. Sit down and watch TV with me. It does not make you braindead. Is oral sex what I think it is? How do they get toilet paper on the roll? I'm randier than a goat. When are you going to make love with me?"

The last had become a continuing refrain, ever since he'd started to feel better. Most ridiculous of all his statements had been, "I would probably recuperate more quickly with a good swiving or two."

"You're too sick," she had told him.

"Then oral-sex me." The man was impossible.

But that was then. Now his fixation was on food. "Why can't we stop at McDonald's? The girls would be happy to have such provender." During the past two weeks of Joe's recuperation, he had somehow discovered Big Macs and french fries, for which he'd developed a passion. Even Beth, who was not normally a meat eater, had become addicted to the junk food, especially chicken nuggets.

"We're going to have dinner at home. It's important that my girls and I sit down at the table together for a home-cooked meal . . . at least occasionally."

He groaned. "We're not going to have that tough-you again, are we? It makes my stomach cramp. I do not want to hurt your feelings, dearling, but that stuff is worse than jail-low." Maggie could feel herself go dreamy-eyed every time he used the term *dearling*, and she suspected that he tossed it into conversations fairly often for just that purpose.

"It's tofu, and it's good for you."

"Bedplay is good for me, too, and I don't see you passing any of that about. I don't suppose"— he flashed her one of his devastating grins, the kind that he probably knew made her insides melt—"that you would come to my bed tonight and demonstrate thongs for me?" So, he had known what thongs were, after all. *The lout!*

"Not a chance!"

He made a low sound of disgust and sank down in his seat so his head was resting on the seat back and his knees were raised in the cramped space.

"Besides, I need to talk with you, seriously," she said, further explaining her refusal to stop at the restaurant. "Since the girls will be late tonight— they have choir practice—I wanted some time alone with you."

"Alone?" He straightened and his face brightened with hope.

She shook her head at his persistence. "To talk."

He slumped again. "*Serious* talk?"

"Very serious."

"I'm not going to give you my sword."

"It's not that."

"I won't marry you."

She stiffened with insult, and the brute didn't even have the sense to know he'd offended her. "Who asked you?"

"Females need forewarning about such things."

Oooh! The man could make her go from happy to mad in two seconds flat. She clenched the steering wheel and refused to rise to his bait.

Then he turned his head to the side, still resting on the headrest, and winked at her.

Maggie's hormones kicked up a notch with just that wink. She pulled her car into the driveway and turned off the ignition. Only then did she tell him, "You are too good-looking for your own good, do you know that?"

"I know," he said, and dazzled her with another of his grins. They both unbuckled their seat belts but had yet to open their car doors. Out of the blue, he stated flatly, "You want me."

"Yep."

"But you are going to continue restraining those base impulses?"

"Yep."

" 'Tis not good for the temperament to—"

"Don't even bother with that line," she advised with a soft laugh. "It's as old as the hills, and as ineffective as a butter knife cutting an ice cube."

"I presume I would be the knife and you the ice?"

"Uh-huh," she replied hesitantly.

"Ah, but sometimes the knife is hot enough to melt the ice," he announced with a sweeping gesture of one hand toward his genital area.

"That was so bad." She wagged a finger at him reprovingly.

"I apologize for my crudity, m'lady. I can only attribute it to an overabundance of male need."

She laughed. "That line's as old as the hills, too. 'Testosterone made me do it.'"

"Kiss me," he commanded, leaning closer. All humor had left his face.

And God help her . . . despite the seriousness of all she needed to discuss with him, Maggie yielded to the demand. He angled his head over hers and put a hand to her throat, just where a slow pulse beat her erotic response to his nearness. She pressed her lips to his, and let him master her into wet, clinging compliancy. Then he forced her lips open with his thrusting tongue.

The kiss was short . . . just long enough for him to prove his point: this Viking was hot.

"You *are* a Viking," she accused.

They were sitting at her kitchen table. Mag-he was sipping a cup of herb tea in a delicate porcelain cup . . . raspberry, he would guess by the fruity scent. He was sipping a beer, straight from the can.

"Of course I am a Viking. Have I not been telling you such since I first landed in this godforsaken country?" Then the implications of her words sank in. "Do you now believe that I have time traveled here?"

"Yes . . . no . . . I don't know what to believe." She released a long sigh. "Actually, I do accept now that you are who you claim to be. The logical side of my brain says it can't be true, but I do believe in miracles. So that's the explanation I choose to give for it."

"You consider me a miracle?"

"In a way."

He laughed. "See, wench, we really should engage in bed sport. We would no doubt make miraculous love."

She laughed, too. "While I'm thinking of it, Joe . . . You don't mind my calling you Joe, do you? I've referred to you that way for so long that Jorund would come hard to my tongue."

"I rather like the idea of coming hard to your tongue."

"Tsk, tsk, tsk," she said.

"In any case, it matters not whether you call me Joe or Jorund."

"What I started to say was that you really shouldn't refer to a woman as a wench. It's sexist . . . comparable to the word *babe*."

"Babe, wench . . . I prefer to think of those as endearments of a sort . . . like *heartling*." If she believed that, he had a sunny beach on a northern fjord he would like to show her. "But tell me why you now believe my story, but would not afore."

She explained . . . a complicated tale involving the physician who had healed him and Seafarers' Lament. It was a malady he was already familiar with: his cousin and two of his brother Rolf's sailors had died of it three years past. No doubt he'd contracted the disease from that bloody whale, Thora, who'd made him ride atop her back in the cold, disease-ridden seas.

"Tell me about yourself," she urged all of a sudden.

"What do you wish to know?"

"Everything."

"I already told you everything afore."

"I wasn't listening closely then."

He gave her an exaggerated glower. "There is not much to say, to my mind. I am one of four living children born to Eric Tryggvason, a high jarl of Norway, and Lady Asgar, a Christian of Saxon birth who has adopted the northern ways these many years."

Mag-he stared at him, transfixed, her chin propped in the cup of two hands, her elbows resting on the table, her tea forgotten. "You've already mentioned your older brother Magnus, the farmer. He's the one with the big ears and an overabundance of women and children, right?"

"The selfsame once." He missed his brother, just speaking of him. Had Magnus returned to Norway by now? Jorund hoped he had not stayed at sea searching for him.

"And you've also talked of your younger brother, Rolf . . . the one you were searching for. A shipbuilder, you said. But who was the fourth sibling?"

"My sister, Katla. She was married a dozen or more years ago, at age thirteen, to a Viking prince from Normandy. I have not seen her in many a year, though I hear that she fares well."

"Thirteen! Your sister was married at age thirteen?"

239

He shrugged. "Women wed young in my land. Their lives are not usually as long as those of women in your country. Mostly they die of childbirth fever. 'Tis the reason why my ancestors first began the practice of *more danico*, I warrant."

"*More danico* meaning polygamy, I presume?"

"True, but let us not argue that issue again. Suffice it to say, the countries and the times are different."

"Tell me about your wife."

He stiffened.

"Did you love her hopelessly? Do you miss her still?"

He put a hand to his chin and rubbed thoughtfully. "I do not wish to speak ill of the dead, but Inga was a conniving witch. She and her brothers decided that I would make a suitable husband, based on my wealth and that of my father. So they invited me to a feast and showered me with mead. The next morn, I found myself with a big head and a naked woman in my bed . . . no longer a virgin. Inga, that is . . . not me. Soon after, I was forced to announce the wedding banns when Inga's monthly flow stopped and she was breeding."

"Surely you can't lay all the blame on her."

"I did then, but I mellowed toward her later. After all, most marriages are arranged in my time. And woe to the party who will not comply. I recall the time King Olaf wanted his sister, Astrid, to wed Erling Skjalgson, a man of good lineage and fine looks. But Astrid refused since Erling was not a prince, of equal station to her. The next day, so wroth was Olaf that he had Astrid's pet hawk taken from her, and he returned it to her that eventide with all the feathers plucked off. Need-less to say, Astrid soon agreed to the marriage."

Mag-he was staring at him in horror. "That's awful."

"Nay. That is life in my land."

"Back to your own marriage—did you ever for-give Inga?"

"Yea. In time. She was young. I was old enough to know better. And besides, she gave me a great gift."

"Your twin daughters," she guessed.

"Yea, that she did." He did not want to speak of them. It was too painful. But Mag-he was like a puppy tugging on a man's boot. She would not let up. "I was there at the birthing . . . which is not the usual practice in my land. I saw them first, as they emerged from the womb, wrinkled and blue and more beautiful than anything I had ever seen afore, or since."

"You loved them from the start then?"

He nodded. For the first time in a long time, he allowed his memories to spill forth. "In many ways, Greta and Girta are similar to your twins. Girta was a daredevil, as you say in modern lan-guage . . . outspoken and adventuresome. Greta was the gentler soul, but willing to try anything her sister dared her to. They loved me uncondi-tionally. I loved them madly."

Mag-he reached out a hand and squeezed one of his. There were tears in her eyes . . . and his as well, he realized with mortification. Vikings were not supposed to cry. He wiped at the tears. "I let them die. For that I will be eternally guilty. 'Tis probably the reason for my punishment . . . being

241

banished into another time. I am not even welcome in Valhalla."

"That's the most ridiculous thing I've ever heard," she said ferociously, in that husky voice he so appreciated. "Don't you dare blame yourself. Bad things happen. It's no one's fault."

He would like to believe her. He really would. But enough of his spewing forth his confidences. " 'Tis your turn. Now that you have opened a hole in my chest and let my heart hang out, tell me about yourself. What are your secrets? Why have you never married?"

"Well, the reason I never married is because Suzy and Beth's father didn't have marriage in his plans. When I told him I was pregnant, he suggested that I abort the babies."

"Kill them in the womb?" It was not unheard-of in his time, but a deplorable practice, nonetheless . . . especially to Vikings, who prized children above all else.

"Yes. Oh, I try to be tolerant of him, but it's hard for me to look at my girls and accept that he never wanted them."

"Perchance he would have changed his mind on seeing them birthed, as I did."

"Maybe, but I don't think so. He had all these things he wanted to do with his life. Children—and me, for that matter—wouldn't have fit in. He wanted to become a famous, wealthy surgeon. Set a record for skydiving. Climb the highest mountains. Race cars. Scuba dive. Whatever. Always a new challenge."

"And were you a challenge to him?"

Her eyes went wide with surprise. "How perceptive of you! Yes, I think I was. I was a virgin when I met Judd . . . a twenty-one-year-old virgin. You have to understand my background to see why I was ripe for the kill. I developed earlier than most girls my age. Breasts and curves at age twelve were not welcome, believe me."

"I like your breasts . . . and your curves . . . especially your fine arse."

She flashed him a glare of reprimand for interrupting her . . . and for liking her breasts and arse, no doubt.

"Kids can be cruel, and some boys started calling me a slut. And other girls made assumptions that, if I had the visible manifestations of a sexpot, then that's what I must be."

A sexpot? Oh, that must be a woman who spreads her favors hither and yon. Like Rosalyn.

"Today it would be called sexual harassment. But then, teachers and my parents just put it down to harmless teasing. Well, it wasn't harmless."

"You never mention your parents. Where are they now?"

"They died when I was fifteen. That didn't help, either . . . having no one to confide in, except the elderly aunt I went to live with. She has since died, too. The only family I have is my girls; so you can see why I am so grateful for them."

He nodded. "Go on."

"I got a severe throat infection when I was thirteen, which changed the tenor of my voice. A sexvoice, you called it. My classmates did, too. I started wearing clothes that hid my body, and I rarely spoke, unless spoken to, but by then it was too late. I got a reputation without ever having any of the fun . . . not that I would have consid-

243

ered sex fun at that early stage. All of these repressions lasted through high school."

"Where did you meet this Mud person?"

"Not Mud . . . Judd," she corrected with a little laugh.

"My mistake," he said, stone-faced.

But she could tell it had been deliberate. "In college. During my senior year. Oh, he was smooth. I give him credit for one thing, though: he brought me out of my shell and made me see that my sensuality belonged to me, and no one else . . . that I shouldn't care what anyone else thought of my body or my voice. So I started to dress differently and act the way my personality dictated."

"He took advantage of you," Jorund observed with disgust.

"I suppose he did, but he did help me in some ways, too. I can't believe that I never thought of it that way before. And for all his bad traits, he gave me Suzy and Beth, and for that I have to be thankful."

"And did you love him hopelessly?" He was throwing back at her the same question she had asked of him earlier.

She shook her head. "No. I thought I loved him then, of course. I wouldn't have opened myself to him unless I did. But, in the end, I wasn't all that upset when he didn't want to marry me . . . except for the girls' sakes. And fortunately I had a trust fund from my parents and a small inheritance from my aunt, which allowed me to finish grad school and take care of my children. Lots of single parents aren't so lucky." She gazed off into the air, tucking away some memory or other, he supposed. Then she concluded, "So that's my story."

"Can we go to bed now?"

She laughed, no longer somber with remembrance. "Stop teasing me."

Jorund hadn't been teasing. After all they had disclosed to each other, he really would have liked to hold her in his arms. And swive her a time or two, he supposed. The time was not right, she had told him on more than one occasion, and he did not know if that right time would ever come. *Bloody hell!*

"Now that we've gotten that out of the way, Joe, let's get down to what I really wanted to talk with you about."

"More talking?"

"More talking."

The woman talks entirely too much. He groaned.

"Joe, we have to discuss the implications of this time-travel stuff. I've been thinking. . . ."

The woman thinks entirely too much.

"I don't believe this was a random time traveling."

"Random time traveling? What the hell is that?"

"It's a phrase I came up with myself," she admitted sheepishly. "If it was random, it would mean that it could have happened to anyone who happened to be in the right place at the right time. Like your brother Magnus, for example, who stood right next to you. Also, it would mean that the time traveler could have ended up anywhere and in any time, not necessarily in Galveston, and not necessarily in the year two thousand. Do you see what I mean?"

"I'm beginning to," he answered. *And that is not a good sign.* "In other words, there must have been a specific reason why I was sent, and where I was sent."

"Right."

"So, what's that reason?"

"I haven't a clue. Do you?"

He pondered the puzzle for a few moments. "All I can think of is that it's too much of a coincidence that I lost twin girls and that I came to a place where there were twin girls."

She tapped her fingers on the table pensively. "I agree. The girls' wishing on a star, or praying, or whatever, must have brought you here."

He nodded. "They seem to have great need of me."

He saw that she would have liked to argue that point. But then her shoulders slumped.

"Of course, you have great need of me, too. Did you perchance wish for me upon a star, too?"

"I did not!" she declared vehemently, but her words were belied by the blush on her fair cheeks. "The most important thing to me isn't why you came, but what will happen to the girls when you leave . . . as you most assuredly will."

Jorund wasn't as certain of that as she was. "I suspect I will not be returned to my time to complete my father's mission until I have accomplished some mission here. It will not happen of a sudden, without forewarning; I am convinced of that."

"I just don't want my girls to be hurt."

"Methinks you are overly protective."

Her chin shot up in the air, as if he had struck her.

"Mag-he, all your life you have tried to control life, which is an impossibility. You tried to control your sensuality as a youthling. You thought you could control a man in your first relationship. I wouldn't be surprised if you avoid men today for fear of not being in control. And you try to control your daughters too much. Part of growing up is being hurt and learning to handle the pain."

Her eyes were welling over at his harsh assessment.

"I do not mean to offend you, m'lady."

"You aren't," she said with a little sob. "Much of what you say I already knew, deep down."

"The bottom line, as you people say in this land, is that you must ask yourself this question: Would your daughters be better off not knowing me at all? Or would it be better for them to have had me in their lives, even for a short time?"

Jorund couldn't believe he was actually speaking of playing a part in those little girls' lives. If ever there was a disaster waiting to happen to his already broken heart, it was Sue-zee and Beth.

"How did you get to be so smart?" she asked, dabbing at her eyes with a tish-you.

"I'm a Viking."

Chapter Thirteen

"I don't believe it!"

It was a Saturday afternoon, two weeks later, when Maggie arrived home from a half-day mental-health conference in Dallas. She'd known that Joe was bored, staying home, with no job. There wasn't a big call for Viking warriors in the work force. But never in a million years had she expected this.

There was a hole in the side of her house. A huge hole. And Joe, dressed in jeans and a sweaty T-shirt, despite the mid-December chill, was wielding the sledgehammer that has caused the damage.

No, that wasn't quite true. Steve was there, too, driving a small backhoe. What was he doing here . . . out in public? The press had been hounding him for weeks, ever since that reporter had recognized him at the Moving Wall. He'd even moved into the hospital temporarily, to protect his much-wanted privacy.

Maggie glanced around her yard. It wasn't just Steve who was there. There were Suzy and Beth, too, along with several other outpatients from Rainbow, including Natalie, Rosalyn, Harvey, Chuck, and Fred. They were all helping to remove the debris—debris that was actually the side of her house—and putting it in a Dumpster. *A Dumpster? Where did that Dumpster come from?*

Fred, dressed as a Village People version of a carpenter, was looking full of himself in a hard hat and tool belt as he followed Joe's orders. Harvey was off to the side counting the number of two-by-fours in one pile and round rocks in another pile, then tabulating his results on an official job-site clipboard. Chuck was being an elephant today, swinging his loose arms forward like a trunk as he carried large pieces of siding to the Dumpster; Maggie, who still had not diagnosed Chuck's real problem, was not surprised to see the words on the bright young man's shirt: *It is as bad as you think, and they are out to get you.* Natalie was singing, of course, as she fetched and carried, and Rosalyn looked surprisingly fetching in tight jeans and a T-shirt that proclaimed, *Librarians Do It by the Book.*

And, oh, good Lord, was that Nurse Hatcher in coveralls and workman's boots, appearing for all the world as if she could take down Maggie's entire house with just a huff and a puff? She was avidly listening to something Fred the Carpenter was telling her. *Oh, no!* It wasn't possible. Was it? A love connection between Gladys and Fred?

"What do you think you're doing?" Maggie gritted her teeth as she stomped over and confronted Joe.

His head jerked up with surprise. "Mag-he! I thought you weren't going to be home till dinnertime."

"My meetings ended early."

"We wanted to surprise you," he complained in a little-boy voice.

She felt like spanking his behind, like a little boy deserved. What did one do to a misbehaving big boy? Whack him on the butt with a two-by-four? There were plenty of them lying around.

"Surprise!" everyone yelled at once, belatedly.

Maggie turned around to see the entire motley crew, including her two grimy daughters, gazing at her expectantly, as if they expected her to congratulate them.

As if! "What is this mess?" she asked, turning back to Joe, who set his sledgehammer aside and was wiping his brow with the back of a forearm. She was trying hard to stifle her fury, for the sake of her daughters, who'd never seen their mother lose her cool. Yet.

"A fireplace," Joe announced. "I'm building your daughters a fireplace."

"Huh?" *A fireplace?* "What next? Igloos in Florida?"

"Tsk-tsk! Dost think sarcasm is called for, Mag-he?"

Maggie gave her daughters her full attention now, and they had the good sense to step back a pace, sensing her disapproval.

"We just mentioned to Joe that we've never had a fireplace," Suzy explained in the whimpery voice that usually meant tears were about to flow.

"And we told him how every Christmas we have to hang our stockings on the living room archway, 'cause we don't have a fireplace," Beth added. Her voice was small and weepy, too.

"Where did you get the money for all this?" she demanded of Joe. There had to be hundreds of dollars' worth of building materials scattered about her lawn, not to mention the rental of the backhoe.

"I sold one of my arm rings to Martie."

She looked at his upper arms. Sure enough, one of the bracelets was gone. "Martie?"

"Yea. Martie Wilson. Remember, you told me one day that Dock-whore Sea-bold's lover—"

She inhaled sharply with distress. "I never told you they were lovers."

He waved a hand dismissively. "You told me that Dock-whore Sea-bold's woman-friend was a trader in antiquities. I called her shop, and she came over to make me an offer yestereve when you took the girls to choir practice. She wanted my sword, but I could not sell her that. A warrior's weapon is his boon companion."

A headache the size of his boon companion hit Maggie like . . . like his sledgehammer.

"Besides, in my world, jewelry is treated the same as coin. Why else would I be wearing arm rings? Do you think I am so vain I adorn myself when going into battle, or on a seafaring voyage to rescue my brother?"

Maggie didn't know what to think. "You shouldn't have sold the arm ring, Joe. It was a prized possession."

"Pfff! A mere object! 'Tis not as if I sold a limb, or anything so dire."

"How much did she give you? Are you sure you got a fair price?"

"Seventy-five thousand dollars."

"S-seventy-five thousand dollars!" she said in a squeal.

"Yea, and you are not to worry. Methinks Martie is an honest woman. Sometimes 'tis necessary to trust, don't you think?" His words obviously had a double meaning. "Are you not surprised?" he inquired then, proud of himself as he waved a hand in a wide sweep to encompass the horrendous hole in her house.

The man is clueless.

Then he plastered a slow grin on his face for good measure...the one he knew made her insides turn to mush.

Well, maybe not so clueless.

"*Surprised* doesn't begin to describe how I feel." She put a hand to her forehead and counted to ten. "Do you even know how to build a fireplace, Joe?"

"Of course." He then ducked his head sheepishly. "Well, actually, I have ne'er built one afore, but how hard could it be? Besides, Steve said he helped his brother-by-marriage construct one twenty years ago."

"Twenty years ago!"

"And the man at the Home Station—"

"Home Depot," Steve corrected.

"The man at the Home Deep-oh," Joe amended, "gave us detailed diagrams."

"I used to be a construction foreman," Fred added, puffing his chest out importantly.

"You were?" they all exclaimed as one.

His face turned bright red, even his balding head under the hard hat.

"Well, why did you not say so afore?" Joe exhaled with disgust, and handed his sledgehammer to Fred, who almost dropped the heavy object, apparently not prepared for its excessive weight.

So, by Sunday night, Maggie McBride and her two daughters had a stone fireplace in their den. And, though she hated to admit it to Joe, it was really pretty nice.

Even though Christmas was still two weeks off, stockings had already been hung with care . . . *four* of them. Suzy and Beth had insisted that Maggie go down to the craft store and have one made with Joe's name on it, identical to the three they had already. Of course, there was a paw-shaped stocking for Rita, too.

She was still going to kill Joe the minute she caught him alone. He had been avoiding her like the plague. *Smart man*. But now she'd cornered him. He was alone in the den, basking in the glow of the fire and his newfound family.

"Uh-oh," he said when he saw her. He pretended to cringe with fright. "Despite the warmth of my surroundings, I can feel the very coolness emanating from you, Mag-he."

"You've been avoiding me all day," she accused.

To her surprise, he nodded. "I am not a Viking for naught. I know when to stay out of a woman's path. Only a fool could fail to see the murderous gleam in your eyes. You would like naught more than to put a blood ring 'round my neck."

"I couldn't have said it better myself. The fireplace was a nice gesture, Joe, but you are never, ever to do anything like that again without my permission."

"My brother Rolf advocated never asking for permission first. He said 'tis better to do the act, then apologize later, but he was probably talking about something involving sex."

Maggie wagged a forefinger with exasperation. "Don't try to change the subject on me. Give me your word that this won't happen again."

He gave her an amused, level stare, then agreed. "Whatever you say, dearling." But Maggie wasn't fooled, not one bit.

Joe had other plans.

Joe had a job.

The takeover of the Rainbow Hospital by Medic-All had been finalized the week before. Thus far there were no visible changes in staff or policy, but Maggie knew they were sure to come after the New Year.

Whether she would stay or not depended on how the experimental programs she'd initiated were handled. If they went, she went. Unlike some employees, she was fortunate to have a sizable nest egg that would allow her to live for an extended period without a paycheck, if need be. She hoped it wouldn't come to that.

But the most surprising thing was that Jerome Johnson, president and CEO of Medic-All, had remembered Joe the Viking in a positive way. When he'd learned, last week, that Joe was no longer a patient, he had urged Rainbow to hire him to restructure its physical-fitness program. Apparently, when Jerome urged, everyone followed his wishes. So now Joe was about to start running the program three days a week, beginning today. And he was ordering everyone about as if he were a . . . well, a military leader.

"Why can't we give fencing lessons?" he was asking Harry in the Monday-afternoon staff meeting.

"Because this is a mental hospital, damnit," Harry snapped. "We don't give lethal weapons to patients. And that's final." Her boss usually didn't lose his temper, but Joe had already demanded new rowing machines, a running track, and bowling balls, which he referred to as catapult balls, and bowling lanes, which he referred to as hurling tracks. Amazingly, Harry had agreed, having been given a slightly higher budget from Medic-All for this purpose.

When the meeting was over, Harry gave her a meaningful glare, which she interpreted as, "Keep that man out of my way."

"Hurry up, Mag-he," Joe urged as they walked down the corridor. "We have to pick up Sue-zee and Beth after school soon. You know that I promised the girls we would go out in the woods and chop down a Christmas tree today."

She groaned, having forgotten. "I still say my artificial tree would serve just fine."

The expression on his face said the issue was settled.

"I don't suppose you will be angry if I tell you that I bought you a little gift." He spoke hesitantly as they approached the parking lot.

"Joe, I already told you that I disapprove of your selling your arm ring. And I certainly don't want you buying me stuff with that money. Furthermore—Oh, no!" Maggie gawked, practically bug-eyed, at the parking lot. "You didn't. Please tell me you didn't."

He smiled brightly at her. "How could we go yule-tree chopping with your piddling vehicle?"

He had.

Sitting next to her Volvo was a brand-new red pickup truck.

It was going to be the best Christmas ever.

Maggie was sitting beside Joe on the sofa in the den, where their newly decorated, wonderfully pungent, way-too-big Christmas tree held center stage, with the crackling fire in the new fireplace providing just the right ambience. Of course, the windows were open to offset the heat. She couldn't stay mad at the brazen brute when he'd given her—and her girls—such wonderful gifts for the season. Just the shine in Suzy's and Beth's eyes when she'd tucked them in a few moments ago . . . well, it made up for all the aggravation Joe gave her. And he could be aggravating, no doubt about that.

"Thank you," she said.

"You are welcome," he answered, not even bothering to ask what for. Putting an arm across the back of the couch, he snagged her by the shoulders and pulled her into the cradle of his arm. Nuzzling her hair, with a soft murmur of, "Lilacs, mmmmm," he added, "I expect you will give me thanks with more than words . . . in time."

"In time," she emphasized. She didn't need to repeat to him her concern over Suzy and Beth.

She'd told him enough times in the past few weeks that she wouldn't engage in an affair in the same house with her daughters.

"I wonder if that time will ever come," he whispered against her ear.

She bristled and tried to pull away–not because of his words, but because of what he knew how to do with her oversensitive ears. Lordy, lordy, the man could set her afire with just a few breaths and some whispered words of wicked things he'd like to do with her.

"Will you take off your undergarments for me?" he suggested all of a sudden.

"Wh-what?"

"Now, do not go all atwitter on me. I am not suggesting we make love, precisely. I just want you to go into the bathing room and take off your undergarments. You said we could not make love with the girls in the house, and being a creative fellow, I have come up with a plan for having sex-less sex."

"That's some creativity." Her nervous giggle betrayed her interest.

"Yea."

"It sounds a little . . . perverted."

"Yea," he concurred with a little smile.

"Joe," she protested.

"Now, sweetling, you can put your *braies* and sweat-her back on. But when you return, and sit here chattering about this and that, I will know you are naked for me beneath. You will be aware of me, and I of you. Perchance it will satisfy my baser instincts, for now. Do it."

Maggie had never heard of such a thing before.

Certainly no man had ever suggested anything so . . . well, erotic.

To her surprise, she did as he asked, blushing even as she complied, alone, in the bathroom.

When she returned, Joe was sitting in one of the wing-back chairs beside the fireplace. He motioned for her to sit in the chair opposite him.

"Sit as I do," he directed in a husky voice. He moved his hands so that they clutched the wings at the top of the chair, and he spread his legs wide.

She followed suit.

Then he just stared at her for a long, long time.

Under his intense, carnal scrutiny, the fine hairs rose to attention all over her body. Her nipples became hard, aching points, pressing against the suddenly heavy weight of her sweater. Between her legs, hot liquid pooled in the swelling folds.

With just a look, Joe made her want him . . . more than she'd ever wanted any other man.

A moan escaped her parted lips.

He moaned, too, in reaction, a low, male sound of pure temptation.

She thought he would smile then, his ego appeased that he had reduced her to this pathetic state with a mere stare . . . but he did not. Instead he held her gaze, communicating some seemingly serious message. Then he said, "I have wanted you from first time I set eyes on you."

"Oh," was the only response she could come up with. What a perfect thing for him to say! Had he sensed her need to hear those words . . . to justify her hair-trigger arousal?

"When I look at you, I want to make fierce love with you . . . to teach you with my callused hands and hard staff not to tease a fighting man."

Merciful heavens! She was picturing all the wonderful things those rough palms could do to her soft skin . . . how his hardness would feel inside her. A thrum of stimulation rippled through her and lodged between her legs like a sweet burn. "I never teased—" she started to say.

He shook his head to stop her protests. "At the same time that I yearn for savage bedplay with you, I yearn as well for gentler things. Your head upon my chest. Our fingers laced. Soft kisses. Whispered words."

Maggie's heart felt as if it were ballooning inside her, and would surely burst with the pure joy of his declaration. Did he realize just what he was saying?

"These things frighten me, Mag-he," he confessed. "I am much more at ease with lust, you know."

She nodded, understanding perfectly.

"Arch your chest for me, Mag-he," he entreated.

She did. Without glancing down, she knew that her nipples were hard pebbles, clearly delineated by the thin knit of her sweater. And she did not care. For once in her life she was glad—very glad—that these overt signs of her sensuality were there for his enjoyment.

"Oh, Mag-he," he said with a long sigh. "Do you know how much I want to suckle you? I would take your breasts deep into my mouth and draw on your nipples till you cried out for release. I would worship your breasts for a long, long time."

She moaned aloud and gripped the chair wings tighter, arching her breasts out even farther so that the throbbing tips were caressed by the coarse threads of her sweater.

"Let us put an end to this delicious agony," he said in a voice choked with emotion. Maggie could see that he was as excited as she was.

Joe took one hand off the back of his chair and laid it over the ridge in his pants. With a jerk of his head, he indicated that he wanted her to do the same. "Find the bud of your woman-pleasure and stroke it so," he instructed as he ran his fingertips up and down his erection.

To her amazement, she did just as he wanted, and experienced no shame—just a glorious, spasming orgasm as she writhed on her chair under her own touch. As much satisfaction as she received, though, the greatest thing was watching Joe rear his head back, the cords in his neck standing out, and squeeze the chair arms with white knuckles as he rode his climax.

As Maggie's senses floated back to earth, she discovered something new: it *was* possible to have sex without physical contact from a lover.

And she could only wonder about something else: if this man could melt her bones and heat her blood and make her hormones hum with just this, what would it be like to actually make love with him?

Love with a Viking was getting harder and harder to resist.

* * *

On Friday night, Maggie had taken a bubble bath and donned her red silk robe. Barefooted, she rushed downstairs to turn off the warming oven. She'd prepared a nice dinner, which she didn't want to dry out.

Joe still wasn't home. After working in the Rainbow facilities all afternoon, he had gone to a gym with Steve to experience something new to him: working out. Joe claimed that everyday work for a Viking soldier was "working out." Still, he'd accepted Steve's invitation.

Just then she heard a car pull up outside, then leave, followed by the sound of a key in the door. She went into the hallway, waiting.

He entered and gazed at her for a long moment. As he hung his jacket in the closet, his movements slowed. He was clearly perplexed. "Where are the girls? I do not hear the Em-tee-vee blaring."

"Their grandparents arrived suddenly this afternoon . . . Judd's mother and father. Since the girls won't be staying with them over Christmas this year, Jack and Martha wanted them to come back to the farm for a visit."

"A visit?" he asked. "How long a visit?"

"The weekend."

"The weekend," he repeated. It took only an instant for understanding to dawn. "And you left me sitting in a gym, bi-sigh-cling myself to mind-numbing boredom? Are you daft, lady?" Then the slow grin she loved so much began to creep across his lips. "What are you wearing under that wicked garment, wench?"

"A belly-button ring."

"And?"

261

Then it was she who gave him a slow grin.

She saw his Adam's apple move . . . once, twice, three times, as if he tried and was unable to swallow. Finally he said, "No."

"No?" she gasped out.

"No, you are not going to control this situation, as you have all others in your life." He continued to stare at her casually, as if she hadn't just offered herself to him, with a huge dollop of sexual promise.

"You don't want . . . I thought you wanted to make love with me." *Oh, how humiliating!* She wished the slate tiles of the foyer would just open up and swallow her whole.

With a *tsk-tsk* of disgust, he pulled his T-shirt out of his low-slung sweatpants, and over his hair, which hung in a single braid down his back, still damp from a shower at the gym. Then he tossed the shirt to the floor, slicing her with a disbelieving look. "Are you serious, wench? Of course I want you. I want you so much my teeth ache and my loins tremble. Thor's toenails! I can scarce breathe."

She saw then that his chest was indeed heaving with some great stress. And what a great chest it was, too. And broad shoulders, a washboard abdomen, well-delineated muscles everywhere, all leading down to narrow hips and waist and a deliciously flat stomach. There were blond hairs covering his chest and arms, a darker shade of blond than on his head, but straight and fine as gold silk. How would it feel to the touch?

And, oh, it was humbling to admit, but the man was in much better physical shape than she was.

She was a slug compared to him . . . all soft and squishy in places he was hard as steel. He was narrow and trim, while she was all curves—way too many curves, she thought, as all her insecurities came back. She should have jogged more lately. She should have spent every spare moment on the StairMaster. She should have done crunches till the cows came home . . . or at least till the Viking came home.

He was the exact picture of a Norse god. Better, even.

She, on the other hand, was no Norse goddess . . . not by any stretch of the imagination.

"You came to the door like a siren, prepared to lure me into your game," he accused.

"I did not," she protested, knowing full well it was a lie, or at least a half-truth. Subconsciously she had recognized the significance of her daughters' absence, but her skimpy attire hadn't been a deliberate attempt to lead him . . . to control their lovemaking. Had it?

"Ne'er once did you think of calling me at the gym and informing me of these events, I warrant. Ne'er once did you contemplate that I might like to be the man in this process. Tell me true: were you or were you not trying to seduce me?"

"You are really beginning to sound like a male chauvinist." Her chin shot up defensively. "Do women never seduce men in your time? Is it so wrong for a woman to take the first step?"

"You know it is not. That is not the issue here."

"And what would that issue be?"

"Me. The man you know me to be. I am Jorund the Warrior. The first time we make love must be

263

on my terms. We will make love—of that there is no doubt—but it will be my way."

"A Viking kind of love?" She was attempting to inject some humor into their conversation, but there was no masking her nervousness.

"Precisely."

Precisely? Precisely? What does that mean?

Do Vikings make love differently from other men?

Oh, boy.

I mean, oh, man . . . oh, man, oh, man!

"The only question in my mind is whether, this first time, I should woo you or conquer you."

What an arrogant, sexist thing to say. But both possibilities sounded good to Maggie. In fact, his hoarsely rasped-out words caused her knees to go weak. She backed up a pace and grabbed for the upstairs banister with one hand, for support.

"You have made me wait too long for wooing, Mag-he," Joe told her, as if they were discussing the weather and not some erotic activity that would no doubt blow her mind. He was bent over, untying the laces on his athletic shoes. "What think you on the matter?"

Maggie thought she was already too aroused to think, let alone speak.

Joe stood and in one sleek movement pushed off his sweatpants and Jockey underwear, together. Stepping out of them one foot at a time, he then gave her his full attention.

"Mercy!" was the only thing she could think of to say.

His stomach muscles lurched, as did another part of him.

She repeated, "Mercy!" Obviously Joe did want her, as he'd said. A lot. *Mercy, mercy, mercy!*

Joe Rand . . . or Jorund—was a big man. All over. And while Maggie had never been one to yearn for great size in that department, she wasn't about to deny its merits, either.

"I have made my decision," he announced, stepping slowly and purposefully toward her.

A decision? About what? Did I miss something here? Oh, he must mean his question about the format of our first lovemaking. His next words confirmed her conclusion.

"Methinks a conquering is in order."

Chapter Fourteen

Jorund was almost embarrassed by the hugeness of his erection. Almost.

Really, he could not remember a time in his life when he'd ever wanted a woman so much. Had she ensorcelled him? He knew that he was treating her unfairly, accusing her of trying to be a leader in the sexplay. But—*blessed Odin!*—he had to do something to slow down his catapulting excitement.

He glanced down at his *excitement* and snorted with disgust. *For the love of Freyja!* Instead of lessening, his engorged member had become even more painfully erect.

Rita waddled in, probably figuring it was time to bedevil him again. Instead she took one look at his *excitement,* then appeared to do a feline double lock before raising her fat head with disdain and ambling off. Obviously she was not impressed.

But Mag-he was. Truly, did she not have the least bit of sense to be staring at him so, gape-mouthed with wonder? Did she not know that a maiden's eyes on a man's most prized instrument caused it to react on its own? As his brother Magnus always said, "A man's cock can be his best friend, or his worst enemy." And his other brother, Rolf, always said, "A manroot has no brain." He agreed with both sentiments.

"Are all Vikings like you?" She was still ogling his staff.

"I'm the only one," he lied.

She giggled. She actually giggled. He considered crossing his legs and covering himself with his hands, but that was so out of character for him, who was usually proud of his endowments . . . except that his endowments had never been quite this endowed. In truth, he wished the slate floor would open up and swallow him whole. Instead his other brain—the one between his legs—decided to take over.

"Take it off." His statement came out more like a growled order than a sweet request.

"Take what off?" The wench was holding on to the stair post, white-knuckled, as if she might fold bonelessly to the floor without its support. He was of the same mind.

She should know perfectly well what he'd meant, but then her eyes did seem dazed. Perhaps she was a bit disoriented. So he told her, "The siren robe." If he was going to be standing

267

naked as a plucked chicken with a bull-size erection, he was bloody well going to have company.

"Oh." Her skin was flaming, from her face right down to the edge of the deep neckline.

He liked her blush ever so much. Usually Jorund sought out women well experienced in bedplay . . . ones who could teach him new tricks. But he had to admit he was anticipating the joys of teaching Mag-he a thing or two . . . or twenty.

She untied the cloth belt at her waist, then stopped. "Joe, I'm not as beautiful as you are, or in nearly as good shape as you are." Shyly she parted the sides over her shoulders and let the fabric slither to the floor in a crimson pool.

His heart stopped beating for a second, then exploded inside his chest into a thundering beat. "Oh, Mag-he, you are beautiful to me. And your form is shapely, just the way I like."

Actually her form was more than fine to him: it was perfect. She was taller than the average female, more like the statuesque women of his race, though there was naught Nordic about her appearance. Her hair was raven black, cut far too short to be feminine, but attractive nonetheless. Her lips were full and red and kissable beyond all bounds of sensuality. Her eyes gazed at him through misty blue pools of passion.

But it was her body that drew him now . . . a body that was curvaceous . . . made for love. Her breasts were large and full and rose-nippled. They were not excessively large, except in relation to her small-boned frame, and they were uplifted, not sagging with their heaviness. He intended to pay great homage to those breasts; that was a promise he made himself.

He knew that Mag-he thought she carried too much weight, but she was wrong. Men did not like skin-and-bone females, as was the fashion of her time. That was one thing he knew had not changed through the centuries. On that issue, men were men.

He let his eyes roam lower. Her creamy torso tapered in at the waist, but then flared out at the hips . . . hips perfect for bearing a man's babe, or a man's lustful body. The navel ring sparkled in its place, midbelly. He could not wait to taste it with his tongue. Was it cool? Or hot?

The thatch of dark hair below was curly and already glistening with woman-dew, he would wager. Her legs were long and comely, and her feet high-arched and narrow. He intended to investigate every part of her thoroughly before morning. Bloody hell, it would be before midnight, he amended in his head, if he kept going at this rate.

"So beautiful," he repeated in a voice raw with passion. Then he reached for her.

Maggie did feel beautiful at that moment. Under Joe's appreciative scrutiny, her womanliness was suddenly something to glory in, instead of repress. She wanted him to find her sexy, and he apparently did.

When he opened his arms to her, reaching as he strode toward her, Maggie was filled with such joy that she hurled herself into his embrace. He caught her with a surprised laugh and lifted her high. But when she wrapped her legs around his hips and her arms around his shoulders, she must have startled him, because he gasped and exclaimed, "Mag-he!" just before his knees gave way. He lurched forward, landing on his knees on the first rung of the carpeted stairs. Then, still pitching forward, he pressed Maggie backward, and she found herself sprawled on the steps, legs wide, and Joe on top of her.

He blinked at her, wide-eyed with shock. Maggie wasn't sure if he was about to laugh or cry. Despite the carpet that had broken his fall, Joe's knees must pain him dreadfully. "Are you hurt?"

"Beyond belief," he choked out, and insinuated his erection more tightly against her. "Too late, too late, too late," he moaned as his lips took hers hungrily and he thrust himself inside her slickness. Well, not quite inside. Halfway. He was so big, and Maggie had not done this for a long time.

With his eyes closed and his head reared back, he pulled himself out, then thrust again. Three times he repeated this exercise before imbedding himself to the hilt.

To Maggie's mortification, she began to spasm around him. Her eyes were probably rolled back in her head, with only the whites exposed, so intense was the pleasure he gave her. She shut her eyes. And she continued to spasm. It was much too soon. How pathetic she was. She began to cry and tried to squirm out from under him, but he would not allow that.

"Shhh," he said, "you feel so good. Like a supple glove of warm, oiled leather." Then he rolled so he was on his back on the steps and she sat on his lap, impaled and filled. "Peak again for me, sweetling," he urged in a voice smoky with sex, putting his hands on her hips to hold her still. Her first instinct was to undulate on him. But no, he took her hand and made her touch herself at that place where they were joined. She glanced down. The base of his erection was barely visible where blond hair blended with black.

Just that sight made her go hot with liquid pleasure, *there*.

Does he feel the scorching heat as well?

His gray eyes appeared glazed, like misty silver, and from his parted lips came a soft moan.

He does.

His firm hands on her hips forced her to keep him inside her. He refused to let her seek her release through movement, only through her own sinfully erotic touch. Within seconds she came again in violent convulsions that grasped and released, grasped and released, grasped and released his still-engorged penis. In fact, she thought he might have elongated and thickened with the flexible accommodating of her inner muscles. She wanted desperately to move, to feel the friction of his penis, but he kept murmuring against her ear, "Not yet, not yet."

Maggie realized he was indeed playing the role of the conqueror. Didn't he realize that she'd already surrendered? But no, that wasn't quite true. There was a part of her that still fought these out-of-control passions. He must sense that.

And so she threw her head back and moaned and moaned and moaned as shudders rocked her body, and she came endlessly. "Oh, oh, oh, oh, oh, oh, ooooh!"

And still Joe had not climaxed.

But that did not mean he was unaffected. Hardly. He rolled them over so she was on the bottom again, and his stiffened arms were braced on the step, on either side of her head. From his lips came a panting noise, "Wfff, wfff, wfff, wfff," like an overheated horse. He was clearly trying to rein in his excitement. For what purpose?

Finally, when he had calmed down a bit—though he was still fully erect and imbedded inside her, like a permanent erotic fixture—he smiled down at her and gave her a brief kiss. "Where are those condoms we bought?" he whispered against her ear, at the same time he nipped at the lobe. Even his breath was a carnal caress at this stage of her seemingly endless arousal.

So that was why he was holding off. Birth control. He wanted condoms. "In my purse . . . in the hall closet."

In one lithe movement, he put a palm under each of her buttocks and stood, still planted inside her. Then he began to walk across the foyer.

With a little yelp, she wrapped her legs around his hips and her arms around his shoulders, as she had before. The slight jarring created by his stride reverberated into sensations inside her that were . . . interesting. Maggie was beginning to think she was either a wanton, or a woman who had been very sexually deprived for a long time. Maybe a little of both.

In a few moments, condoms in hand, Joe carried her through the archway into the living room, where he deposited her on an antique chaise lounge, which she'd inherited from her great-grandmother. It was upholstered in green velvet, backless, and had an arm at only one end. A useless piece of furniture, she'd always thought . . . till now.

With surprising expertise for a task he'd never performed before, Joe put on the condom, then made a great fuss over arranging her nude body just so on the chaise . . . half reclining, with her head against the armrest, her hands behind her head, and her legs spread with her feet resting on the floor.

The old Maggie would have been mortified beyond belief to be so exposed.

The new Maggie wondered what surprising, sinful things he would do next.

Kneeling on the floor at her side, he was studying her body from head to toe, like a connoisseur considering the purchase of a fine painting. Did he like what he saw? The answer she saw on his flushed face and parted lips was a glorious *Yes, yes, yes.*

"Let's just make love," she urged, and her voice came out even huskier than usual.

"We will, heartling. We will," he promised, still studying every curve and plane of her body.

When was he going to start touching her, and doing other things? *Oh, good Lord!* Was it possible that Vikings didn't make love the same way people did today? No, that was silly. Sex was sex. Wasn't it?

Aaarrgh! Can a person go crazy from hormone overload?

"When?" She arched her body involuntarily, like a purring cat in need of a good petting.

Her posture caused his eyes to go wide, and he clenched his fists at his sides, still restraining his impulses. *Darn him! He'd better unrestrain soon, or . . . or else.*

273

"When you are wild . . . with want."

Oh, boy! Maggie simultaneously felt a sharp throb between her legs and an ache in her breasts, and she thought, I am already wild.

Jorund could not believe his eyes. His Mag-he had gone wild for him. What a picture she made, reclining sensuously on the low sofa . . . a sofa that was, by the by, constructed perfectly for bed-sport. Jorund, kneeling on the floor at her side, could not get enough of gazing at her. But he'd best be careful, or he would explode before he ever entered her body. That was a shame he intended to avoid at all costs.

The ripeness of her mouth attracted him first. He let his touch trace the outline of her full lips, then dipped a finger inside and moistened them. A lamp on a nearby table provided just enough golden light for him to view the glistening wetness he had created. Then he tunneled his fingers in her short hair, and moved his lips over hers, back and forth, till they fitted together perfectly. He had been telling Mag-he the truth when he stated at one time that he had no particular fondness for kissing. But, oh, she had changed his mind. Now he could not imagine making love with her and not tasting her lips and tongue and teeth. With that in mind, he stroked her with his tongue, in and out, in and out, in and out, and she drew on him. He had never known a kiss could be so intimate, or so like sex itself.

When he finally tore his mouth away, her lips were swollen and even more kiss-some. Her breathing was as ragged as his. He saw the pleading in her luminous blue eyes. Her eagerness both excited and scared him at the same time. *Beware,* some inner voice warned, *this woman could be your downfall.*

But then another voice, accompanied by some whalelike clicking noises, countered, *Or your greatest achievement. Follow your heart, Viking. Follow your heart.*

But Jorund ignored the voices in his head. He had a beautiful, sensual woman begging for his erotic loveplay. "Soon, dearling, soon," he assured her as he moved his ministrations lower.

It was her breasts—her beautiful, beautiful breasts—that caught his attention now. For a long time, he played with them, pushing them up from underneath, tracing the dusty areolae, fingering the prominent nipples. She was a mewling, mindless creature by the time he was through with her, imploring him for release. That was the way he wanted her. In truth, he was a bit mindless himself.

"Tell me what you want, Mag-he," he entreated in a voice thick with male need. "Tell me your desires."

Her eyes went frenzied, and he knew she was fighting the part of her personality that wanted to be in control. She did not want to tell him her secrets, her wanton yearnings, because then he would have some power over her. *Foolish wench!* She did not yet realize that she was the one who had power over him.

He saw on her face the moment that she yielded to his mastery. Her hands were still folded behind her neck, where he had forced them to

275

stay, but now she pulled them out resolutely. She put her left hand on the nape of his neck, drawing him downward, and with her right hand placed under one breast and pushing upward, she gave him her breast to suckle. And—*oh, holy Thor!*—how sweet it was!

For a long time he stabbed her nipple with his tongue, and licked, and plucked, and bit, and sucked, and fluttered her. Then he did the same to her other breast. Such wonderful agony was this to her that she cried out her pleasure with little mewling moans and bucked her hips rhythmically on the sofa, trying to find her release against thin air. In the end, even as he continued to minister to her sensitive breasts, he put the heel of his hand on her mons, and she bucked against his callused flesh till she peaked in unbridled convulsions.

"Ne'er have I enjoyed anything so much in all my life as watching your pleasure," he told her.

When her breathing slowed down a bit, she opened her eyes and glared at him. "You'd better end this soon, Viking, or you'll be sorry."

He doubted that. Laughing softly because she was such a delight, Jorund moved to his knees at the foot of the sofa. Then, hooking her under the knees, he yanked her toward him till her buttocks rested on the edge of the sofa and her feet were planted on the floor, on either side of his legs.

He explored her abdomen then, her trim waist, her delicious navel with the warm metal ring, the crease where her buttocks met her thighs, but mostly the dark nest of curls and the parted cleft that was so very wet with her readiness for him.

He spread her legs even wider, to expose her more.

Then he tasted her, just a quick swipe of tongue over swollen nether lips and a bud that was turgid and prominent.

Mag-he screamed out his name, not that modern one, but his real one; "Jorund!"

He thought he would melt at how sweet his true name on her tongue sounded to his ears. But it was too soon for melting, though the scorching heat in his vitals did not bode well. Just a few more minutes, he promised himself.

Relying on all he'd learned over the years about bedplay, and a few surprising ideas he thought up now, Jorund then used his tongue and teeth and lips on Mag-he's slickness . . . and never in all his life had he brought a woman to such wetness. Like a nectar of the gods was her cream. He pushed his tongue inside her as far as he could go, trying to find her most erogenous zones—that was a term he'd learned from Dock-whore Ruth on the TV box—then decided to save those delights for later. When he sucked on her rigid bud—the center of female eroticism, or so he'd been taught—Mag-he let loose a continuous wail of "Yeeeeeessss," the whole time pounding on his back with her fists.

Needless to say, she peaked again. Perhaps it was even two times. It was hard to tell with all that continuous convulsing.

It was time.

Raising his head, Jorund saw that Mag-he was lying sprawled on the sofa like a limp doll, with her eyes closed. Well, not for long, he pledged

277

silently. Putting his hands on her waist, he lifted her bodily so that she lay farther up the sofa.

Her eyes shot open.

Yes, he wanted her wide-awake for this.

Bracing his arms on either side of her, he eased his erection into her hot depths. As before, she immediately started shattering around him, her inner muscles grasping and releasing him in welcome, not unlike that handshaking practice.

He tried to go slowly, with long, easy strokes, his fingers entwined with hers above her head, but he had prolonged his ecstasy too long.

"You stretch me," she commented in wonder.

"Yea, I do," he remarked pridefully. Was that not the way it was supposed to be with a man and a woman? "Should I stop?"

She laughed, a seductive, feminine trill. "Don't you dare." She drew her knees up, wrapping her legs about his hips as if to lock him in.

He needed no such encouragement. He was not able to let her go. This time he lunged so deep, he feared his penetration had reached her womb. He paused in question.

She blinked at him repeatedly. Then she said, "Goodness!"

He assumed that meant she was pleased at how well he filled her, so he continued. Caught in the throes of a hurricane, his sexplay became a raw act of possession as he drove into her, hard.

He was wild.

She was wild.

The power of their joining was a palpable thing swirling between them as they gazed in wonder at each other. His burning eyes held hers, but she did not look away. Had a coupling of man and woman ever been so staggering to the senses?

"I love you," she whispered as the pinnacle of their rapture approached, and he continued to hammer himself into her. Her words surprised him and did not surprise him at the same time. He could not say that he was displeased, but he did not repeat the words back to her. He could not.

Still, he gave her the greatest pleasure he could with his shaft and his expert fingers and mouth. At the height of her fierce undulations and his deep strokes, he slid his fingers between her legs from behind. At that one touch, her molten folds exploded around his shaft, which was now so engorged it pained him. Jorund reared his head back, released a harsh, masculine roar of victory, and came to pulsating satisfaction.

Then he fell heavily on top of her, sated to the point of bonelessness.

I love you, sweetling, he said inside his head. But he did not say the words aloud. In truth, he did not know where the sentiment came from. He did not really love this modern woman. Did he? He was no longer capable of love. Was he?

Cloudy thoughts swam in his brain as he eased himself off the too-small sofa, onto the carpeted floor. He took Mag-he with him, nestling her face in the crook of his neck, one of her arms over his chest, and one leg draped over his.

He wanted to say something to her, to thank her for the most incredible experience of his life, but "thank you" seemed so inadequate to express all he felt. Instead he hugged her tighter and kissed the top of her head.

* * *

Maggie must have swooned, or slept. All she knew was that some time must have passed since the most spectacular sexual marathon of her life—of anyone's life, she would bet—and Joe was sleeping soundly beside her.

Her face was resting against his shoulder, her palm over his chest, where his heart beat slowly in sleep, and a leg was thrown over his, with her knee pressed up against his genitals—genitals that were now semi-limp. Did the man never give up totally . . . even in sleep? Was he always half-ready to go?

Her body felt bruised and battered from Joe's lovemaking . . . and wonderfully satisfied, too. She was exhausted, no doubt due to her being out of shape. And more than anything, she was confused by the whirlwind that had overcome her in the form of a very sexy Viking. This was so much more than she'd ever expected. *He* was so much more than she'd ever expected.

A warm shower, that was what she needed. Then she was going to crawl into bed and sleep till noon. Only then would she feel rejuvenated enough to contemplate with a logical mind all that had happened to her tonight.

Carefully she eased herself off of Joe. He was in a deep sleep. She attempted to stand, but her legs gave way. She sank back to the floor, on her knees, and giggled. Then she clamped a hand over her mouth and glanced guiltily at Joe. He snored softly. *Well, good.* There was some small gratification in knowing she'd worn him out, too.

It was an ignominious posture, but Maggie

began to crawl from the room on her hands and knees. When she got to the hall she would stand, with the support of walls and stair rails.

"Going somewhere, wench?" a silky, male voice inquired. At the same time, an iron hand snaked out and grasped her ankle.

Maggie peeked over her shoulder and groaned. Joe was approaching her, on hands and knees, too, like a big, stalking cat. That image was only reinforced when he came up and over her from behind, covering her with his massive body, and purred into her ear. Already she could feel his erection against her leg.

"No, Joe, not again. Haven't you had enough for now?"

"Did I not say afore that my biggest talent was my stamina?" he boasted. She didn't look, but she suspected he was smiling.

"Is that like the Viking version of understatement?" she remarked dryly, and tried to crawl away.

He swatted her on the behind and yanked her back. She could feel the heat of his skin as he undulated over her, like a cat, though he barely touched her skin.

"It's too soon," she protested. "I couldn't. Really. Oh, my goodness!"

In one sleek, feline move, he lifted her hips and entered her from behind.

And Maggie soon discovered that, in fact, she could.

While his male member stroked her inside with long, leisurely plunges, his fingers and his whispered words praised her breasts . . . then the wet folds that she had thought were too sensitive to be touched again so soon. But—*oh . . . oh . . . oh*—they were not.

Maggie realized then, if she had not already, that this was not a modern man who did things according to politically correct rules. He was a Viking warrior with savage sexual appetites and barbarian ways of seduction. An uncivilized lover.

She would have him no other way.

This time a sated Maggie lay flat on her stomach on the floor, with Joe splayed top of her, laughing in her ear. "So what do you think of Viking lovemaking, m'lady?"

"I'm afraid to ask what you do for an encore," she said with a strangled laugh.

"Aaahhh, I am so glad you asked. Have I not told you about the famous Viking S-spot?"

It was midnight. They were lying nestled in each other's arms on the sofa bed in the den, watching a rerun of *The Andy Griffith Show*, which Joe adored, for some reason.

They were sated . . . for the moment, anyhow. One never knew about Joe. Just a little while ago, she had inquired of Mr. Hornier-than-Thou, "Do Viking women walk around bowlegged all the time?"

He'd tilted his head at her, baffled by her question. Then he'd laughed. "Nay, just the lucky ones."

There were no lights on now, but the Christmas tree in the corner was twinkling brightly, and Joe had built a fire in the fireplace, even though there was enough heat in the room to fire a nuclear station. Sexual heat, that was.

Joe had carried her here after they had taken a

shower together. Words didn't begin to describe that experience, involving hot water, liquid soap, and a loofah.

Afterward they had sat at the kitchen table in nothing but oversize bath towels, scarfing down beef Stroganoff over buttered noodles, and an entire half-gallon of orange juice. Joe had wanted a beer but she'd suggested o. j., as being more regenerative. *Hah!* Little did she know!

Then they had made love again, this time with her sitting on top of the vibrating dishwasher, and that was where she discovered the secret of the Viking S-spot. *Holy cow!* Joe could write a book about the phenomenon, if he stuck around this century long enough, and if he was unable to find a job as a warrior. It certainly put the G-spot to shame. She knew for darn sure he'd be a hot ticket on the talk-show circuit.

Then again, no. Maggie didn't want to share this man with anyone else. That was selfish of her, of course, but she regarded him as her special secret.

Joe had then carried her to the den. Now she wondered why he was so quiet.

"What are you thinking, Joe?"

He chuckled. "Already you are back to the sigh-colic-jest questions."

She slapped him playfully on the chest, and he playfully winced as if she'd hurt him. When she tried to shrug out of his arms, he tucked her more closely into the cradle formed by his arm looped over her shoulder.

"I was thinking that I must be more virile than I thought if I can make a woman peak twenty-five times in a matter of"—he glanced over to the mantel clock—"four hours."

"Oh! That is such a lie. I never climaxed twenty-five times."

He lifted an eyebrow at her.

"Were you counting?" she accused.

"Are you daft, wench? I was too busy trying to catch my breath."

She buried her hot face against his chest as all her old insecurities slam-dunked into her brain. Was she a slut at heart? Too sensuous? Too uninhibited? "Was I too . . . too . . . ?"

Her words were muffled, spoken as they were against the warm skin of his bare chest, but he heard her. Tipping her chin up with a forefinger so he could see her face, Joe finished for her, ". . . wanton?"

"Yes. Was I too wanton?"

"Oh, Mag-he! How can you ask such a question?" He threw his head back and laughed uproariously. When she sliced him a glare, he gave her lips a quick, smacking kiss. "Your woman-joy is my man-pleasure, silly lady. I was teasing you, but in essence I was puffing my chest out with pride at my good fortune."

"Really?"

"Really."

"So what were you thinking about so seriously then?"

"I was thinking that mayhap living in this godforsaken country and time might not be so bad. I was thinking that perchance my mother was right when she said home is where the heart is. She was answering my question at the time as to how she—a highborn Saxon lady—could adapt so easily to the harsh northern climate and a vastly different culture. And finally I was thinking—and this scared me mightily—that your home is becoming too much like home to me."

Tears welled in Maggie's eyes. "Oh, Joe, that's the nicest thing you could have said."

"So you think, but how will I ever be able to depart this land if my affections grow so strong? All this time, I have been heeding your cautions not to let your daughters get too close, for fear of the hurt they would suffer once I leave—which I must do inevitably—but not once did I realize that I was being pulled into this selfsame net."

My affections . . . Maggie homed in on those words of Joe's. What did he mean by that? Suddenly she recalled blurting out to Joe, in the midst of their lovemaking earlier tonight, that she loved him. Had he heard her? Did her words bother him? Was he trying to tell her, indirectly, that he returned her affection? She couldn't help herself. Maggie asked, "Are you in love with me, Joe?"

"Pfff! How would I know? I have never been in love afore."

"Some men claim that if you have to ask the question, then you're not."

"Ha! Most men don't know their manroot from a beet root." He sighed deeply. "All I know is that I go breathless just looking at you. Is that love? I could swive you till my cock falls off. Is that love? When you leave a chamber, even for a few minutes, I miss you. Is that love? My heart swells almost to bursting when I watch you with your daughters. Is that love? I want to do things to you that no man has ever done or contemplated. Is that love? I want to protect you with my shield from all harm. I want to stop all men from gazing at you. I want to see . . . I want to see you . . ." He was unable to finish his litany.

Maggie was weeping openly now. "You want to see me what?"

He reached beneath the covers and placed a hand over her belly. "I want to see my babe growing in your womb."

Chapter Fifteen

That afternoon, they decided to go yule shopping.

Mag-he claimed she needed to buy some last-minute gifts to put under the tree—*Odd practice, that*—but he suspected she wanted to get him out of her house, lest he try to teach her more tricks in bedplay. *Smart lady.*

He yielded to her wishes readily because he was thinking he should buy some gifts, as well. The Norse people did not celebrate Christmas, as such, though they welcomed any opportunity for feasting and gift giving. But mostly Jorund agreed to go shopping with Mag-he because he did not want her to become bowlegged—*Ha, ha, ha*, he thought. *A little Viking humor.* Quite frankly, he did not want his manpart to fall off from overuse—*Ha, ha, ha! A lot of Viking humor.*

She was driving her car, and he was sitting in

the passenger seat, strapped in. He was going to have to learn to drive if he stayed in this land much longer. Driving a car was a necessity here, much as riding a horse or a longship was in his time.

"Did you hear me?" she asked.

Oh, she must have been talking while he'd been humoring himself. Too much swiving must turn a man's brain to gruel. On the other hand, was there such a thing as too much swiving?

"I said, I think we'll skip the mall."

"Methinks we should skip the shopping and stop at McDonald's. My stomach is growling."

"Your stomach is always growling. We are not going to McDonald's again. If you eat many more Big Mac's and french fries, you're going to turn into a clown . . . a Ronald McDonald clown."

"Shopping is women's work," he grumbled.

"And a man's work would be . . . ?"

"War." Then he waggled his eyebrows at her. "And swiving."

"Why did I ask?" She shook her head at him, as if he were hopeless. "Anyhow, we're going to the Strand historical district. Besides, you already went shopping at the mall with Beth and Suzy the night I had a staff meeting at Rainbow."

"And ne'er did my feet hurt so much in all my life. Those girls must have stopped at every blessed trading stall in the entire mall. And I swear, if I hear 'Jingle Bells' one more time, I may just throw up the contents of my stomach."

"The girls told me you had a good time," she pointed out with a smile. "They said you even had a long conversation with Santa Claus."

"Santa Claus! Oh, I am glad you brought up the

subject. That fat, old, white-bearded fraud! You'd never catch me wearing a red suit, not even if I owned a set of flying reindeer. Do you really believe in the Santa Claus myth? Do you?"

"Well, I certainly believe in the spirit of Christmas."

"That is a nonanswer if I ever heard one," he scoffed.

"If time travel exists, why not Santa Claus?"

He saw the grin she was trying to stifle and realized that she jested with him. He made a harrumph of disgust.

"Anyhow, you won't have to worry about Santa Claus downtown. Oh, he'll be there, by the dozen, I'm sure, but the Strand is much more Christmasy in a traditional, old-fashioned sense."

"What is the Strand?" he asked, gazing at Maghe's lips, which were swollen from his numerous kisses. He rather liked the idea that she carried his mark in some way.

"The Strand is the district at the heart of Galveston. In its heyday, which was the late 1800s and early 1900s, Galveston was even called the New York of Texas."

Jorund thought about letting Mag-he blather on, but he had to refute that last preposterous statement of hers. "How could a city in Tax-us be the new York? Everyone knows that York—or Jorvik, as we Norse call it—is in England. Even I know they cannot move a city across the ocean."

Mag-he turned toward him, taking her eyes off the roadway for a brief second. "Not that York. I'm referring to New York City. Oh, never mind. It's not important."

She was correct: it was not important. What

was important was that his attention had snagged on her red Christmas sweat-her, which had a green tree on the front . . . a green tree with colored balls, two of which were stationed right about where her nipples were–nipples for which he had developed a particular fondness. He was also fond of what was beneath her black silk *braies* on the bottom.

"Are you wearing undergarments?" he asked all of a sudden.

"Joe! What a question to ask!"

"Are you?"

"What would make you think that I'm not?"

"A man can be hopeful, can he not? Methought you might have wanted to surprise me, since I must go celibate today."

"I think celibacy refers to a longer period than three or four hours."

" 'Tis a long time for me," he grumbled. Sighing with disappointment, he stared out the window on his side at the passing scenery.

"I'm not," she said softly, "wearing underwear."

His head swerved to the left. She was blushing profusely. Suddenly he decided shopping would not be as boring as he had contemplated.

Mag-he returned her attention to her driving, and went on talking, probably to cover her embarrassment. "Many of the spectacular buildings erected then are still in existence on the Strand, surviving even a devastating storm in 1900. I think you'll like it."

He thought he would like to go home and practice some more oral sexing, or mayhap he would just polish Mag-he's belly button ring for her . . . with his tongue. And he still wanted to try licking her toes, which he had discovered were very ticklish.

"What are you grinning about?" she asked.

"Toes," he said, and winked at her.

She blushed again. But she did not turn the car around. Apparently she was bound and determined to go shopping.

He slumped down into his seat, disgusted. Oh, it would be interesting to watch Mag-he today, knowing she was nude for him beneath, but there were dozens of sexual exercises he wanted to experiment with, and only a limited number of hours left till the girls came home tomorrow night. And what did the feckless wench propose? Shopping!

In truth, women were the same throughout the ages. It mattered not if it was a shopping mall in a city or a trading stall in a market town. He didn't doubt that the first Christian man, Adam, was as beleaguered by his woman, Eve, as all men were. It would not have mattered to Eve that she had everything she could possibly need, living in the Garden of Eden. She would have wanted to go shopping, he would warrant. For apples.

"Did you see that?" He sat up straight, undid his seat belt, rolled down the window, and leaned his head outside.

"What? What?" Mag-he asked, swerving her car over to the side of the roadway, then turning off the motor.

"Out there." Jorund pointed over the water. "I thought I saw a killer whale jumping into the air. Do you think . . . Yea, it must have been Thora."

The Strand area was located on the opposite side of the island from the Gulf near a thriving

Sandra Hill

commercial port. Surely a whale would not swim into those congested waters. But then, this was not a normal whale.

Much as he and Mag-he peered over the water, there was no sign of Thora. Perhaps he had been mistaken, but he did not think so. There had to be a reason for her showing herself now. What could it be? Was it a sign, or a warning?

"You're not going back to your time *now*, are you, Joe?" Mag-he asked him in a tear-filled, panicky voice.

He brought his head back inside the car and stared at her, horrified. That thought had never occurred to him. It was too soon. Oh, he had been complaining for weeks about not being able to go home. But now that the possibility loomed on the horizon, he realized that he did not want to go . . . not yet. Conflicting feelings battered him. He had to go, for his brother Rolf's sake. He had to stay, for Mag-he's and her daughters' sakes.

He could not think about all this now. Instead he made a *tsk*ing sound and put his arms around her, kissing her face and neck and lips. "I am not going anywhere, sweetling," he assured her.

But a whaley-like voice inside his head clicked and squealed in orca language, adding to his words an ominous *Yet*.

"Hey, Dr. McBride. How's your belly button?"

Maggie's head jerked upright with surprise, but then she noticed the young man with purple spiked hair. He was standing in the doorway of the tattoo parlor where she'd had her body piercing done earlier this year.

"Just great, Orvis," she answered. Orvis was the

son of the owner, Herbert Dupree, a long-haired, graying, sixties hippie who had never really grown up.

Before she could turn and introduce Joe, he set their overflowing shopping bags on the ground and stomped forward, grabbed Orvis by the front of his raggedy T-shirt, which read, *A Hangover Is the Wrath of Grapes*, and lifted him off his feet so that the young man was at eye level with him.

"Troll, do you dare speak of my lady's intimate body parts?"

The kid appeared as if he might pee his pants, so surprised and terrified was he. Even worse, they were garnering attention from the shoppers and tourists in the busy Strand district.

"Put him down. Right now," she ordered Joe as she tugged on his arm to pull him back. "He's just a college student who works in this shop, where I had my belly-button ring put in." In fact, as Maggie recalled, he was a prelaw student at UCLA.

"Oh." Joe looked from her to the dangling boy in his hands. "I thought perchance your *braies* had dropped down a bit, and he could tell you were not wearing undergarments." He snaked out a hand to palm her behind then, and squeezed. His other hand was still holding Orvis up in the air by his T-shirt.

She yelped and jumped away.

"I was just checking," he said, and smiled widely, apparently satisfied that she hadn't lied. Then he turned back to the boy, inquiring, "You meant no insult?" He was still not convinced the kid wasn't some dire threat to her reputation.

The kid just shook his head, speechless.

Joe dropped him unceremoniously to his feet.

"Apologize at once," Maggie told Joe in an undertone, "or else we're going to have police here, arresting you for assault."

"Assault? That was no assault." He blinked at her in incomprehension. "An assault would be a blood eagle to his back, or sword dew spilled. This youthling is unharmed." He turned his attention back to said youthling. "Is that not true?"

Orvis nodded his head like a dashboard doll.

Joe reached out a hand then and shook Orvis's hand vigorously. "I am Jorund Ericsson. How do you do?"

Orvis shook his hand back, but under his breath Maggie heard him mutter, "Holy shit!"

Joe glared at the ogling shoppers who still stood about, till they finally slunk away, figuring he might start on them next. Then he turned his gaze to the storefront. "Ah! A body-piercing market stall. Mayhap I should have one of my body parts pierced, too."

Maggie inhaled sharply, and the air went down the wrong tube. She began to cough uncontrollably.

Joe just blathered on: "I can think of one body part that deserves particular homage after all of last night's bedsport. What think you of—"

"No!" He barely had time to gather up the shopping bags before she grabbed his arm and dragged him away from the store and down the unique street, with its high curbs and overhanging canopies. Horse-drawn carriages passed by slowly, contributing to the Victorian ambience of the place. A Viking in Dickens's world, she thought with a shake of her head. But actually, anything went on the Strand. Even the occasional oddball shops, selling body piercing, kites, and army surplus gear, somehow seemed to fit in with those carrying fine antiques, gourmet chocolates, imported cigars, and designer clothing.

"I was jesting, Mag-he. Dost really think I would mar such perfection? Or sustain such pain for the sake of vanity?" He winced and pretended to cross his legs.

Where had this playfulness and sense of humor come from? Joe had been such a grim fellow when she'd first met him. *Hmmm.* Maybe she was a good influence on him. But she couldn't let his outlandish statement stand. "Perfection, huh? A little full of yourself today, aren't you?"

"With good cause, m'lady," he bragged, pointing out, "You would know that best of all."

Maggie couldn't stop her face from heating with embarrassment.

"Mayhap I should get a tattoo, then," Joe offered, stopping in his tracks and resisting her efforts to move him along the sidewalk.

"No!"

"I could purchase a tattoo of a killer whale," he suggested. "Mayhap that would be a good thing to do, Mag-he, like an offering to the gods to appease their wrath."

"The gods of orcas?" she inquired with raised eyebrows.

He shrugged. " 'Twould appear anything is possible." His forehead creased with thought. "Yea, I could put a drawing of a whale on my arse. Thora has a fondness for my arse, you know."

"You are impossible," she said with a laugh, shoving him into the Old Strand Emporium, where they soon ordered deli sandwiches and mugs of draft beer. From the back could be heard a cacophony of musical sounds coming from the Wurlitzer Band Organ, player pianos, and old-time banjo-player jukeboxes.

"Mayhap I will buy one of those music machines for Sue-zee for Christmas," Joe suggested as he took a long swallow of beer.

"Are you crazy?" she asked, then immediately ducked her head with shame. What a question for a psychologist to be asking . . . especially of a former patient. "I mean . . . do you know how much those jukeboxes cost? At least five thousand dollars."

He pulled out a wad of bills from his back pocket and laid them out on the table. "Don't I have five thousand dollars?" Joe hadn't yet mastered the currency system.

She motioned for him to put the money away before the bug-eyed diners at the other tables decided to help themselves. "Joe, you have sixty thousand dollars left. That's not the issue. You can't be buying such expensive gifts for people."

"Why not?"

"Because you already bought a laptop computer for Beth and a pricey video-game system with a dozen cartridges for Suzy, both against my protests."

"You wouldn't let me buy that word-*shert* that proclaimed, *I Love Cats. They Taste Just Like Chicken.*"

"Get real," she commented. "Rita would never forgive me."

He raised his chin stubbornly. "Viking people

love to give gifts, and to receive them, too." He was back to the subject of expensive gifts. "Why is it wrong to purchase items that might please someone?"

"Because sometimes your generosity goes too far."

"Mag-he," he said with a long sigh, "generosity is when a person gives something till it hurts. Spending a few thousand dollars on people I care about is not going to affect me at all. Furthermore—I do not care how much you resist—I intend to buy gifts for Steve, Hair-vee, Chuck, Fur-red, Rosalyn, Not-a-lie, and Norse Hatch-her, as well."

Maggie put her face in her hands. The man just would not listen to her. The hospital gave Christmas gifts—small items, to be sure—to all its patients. It wasn't a good idea to get too personal with the patients.

Or was it?

Maggie had seen on more than one occasion how Joe's relationship with the therapy group, even though he was no longer a patient, had helped everyone. Treating them as friends, rather than sick people, had raised their self-esteem, and jump-started some real mental-health progress.

"Okay," she agreed, "but we have to work together on this. You're not going to go off the deep end buying extravagant presents."

"Who? Me?" he asked. Then, out of the clear blue sky, he commented, "I am picturing you naked right now. Do you like that?"

The man had a one-track mind. And frankly, she did like it. A lot. But she couldn't tell him that.

He winked at her. *Oh, my.* Could he read her mind now? Then he stretched his long legs out, crossing them at the ankles. The whole time he sipped at his beer, which he continued to refer to as mead.

A lot of men and women in the restaurant took note of Joe with surreptitious glances his way, even a gray-haired lady with a sweatshirt saying, *Forget Youth. How about a Fountain of Smart?* And it was no wonder. He stood out in any crowd with his height, good looks, and the proud way he carried himself. Today he was dressed in a long-sleeved plaid shirt tucked into jeans. On his big feet he wore the same athletic shoes he'd been given at the hospital. His long blond hair was bound into a queue with a rubber band. But it wouldn't matter how he was dressed. Joe would draw stares even if he wore rags.

"Well, we could buy Natalie a Patsy Cline greatest-hits CD."

Joe nodded. He was familiar with CDs, since Suzy and Beth often forced him to listen to their music, especially Ricky Martin, for whom Joe had developed a particular aversion. And he had to recognize the name of Patsy Cline, because Natalie was always belting out her tunes.

"Maybe we could buy Suzy another Ricky Martin CD. Perhaps there's one she doesn't have."

"I want to go back to that military surplus store and purchase that Navy SEALs jacket for Steve."

Maggie bit her tongue to stop herself from pointing out that it was a hundred dollars . . . too much for a friendly gift, especially since he'd already bought a baseball card of Steve's at a memorabilia store earlier today for a whopping fifty dollars, and it wasn't even in mint condition.

"Ooh, I thought of something else. We should buy one of those hats we saw in the cow-man store for Dock-whore Sea-bold."

Maggie smiled. "You mean the cowboy store?"

"Is that not what I said?" Sometimes Joe got exasperated when she corrected his language mistakes. "We should buy him one of those big-ass black hats we saw in the window . . . that's a word Steve taught me, by the by. With a hat like that, Dock-whore Hairy wouldn't have to worry about his hair drape blowing in the wind."

"The Stetson?"

"Yea, that's the one. The stepson."

Oh, good Lord. What would Harry think of such a gift? Then she giggled, trying to picture her boss in the *big-ass* thing. Though cowboy hats were not uncommon on a Texas man—or woman—she had a hard time picturing Harry, noted psychiatrist, wearing a cowboy hat. But then, his hair comb-over was out of character, too.

A mischievous grin appeared on Joe's face then. "And I have thought of the perfect gift for Glad-ass Hatch-her," he announced. "A whip."

"That's not funny," she said. But it was, kind of. Once again Maggie was surprised by Joe's sense of humor. Maybe he was beginning to put his guilt over his children's death behind him.

"On the other hand, mayhap we will give Glad-ass some scented skin creams to soften her up."

Yep, he was developing a super sense of humor.

They discussed what to buy for the other members of his group, then went out to make their purchases. In addition, there were a few more impulse buys, like the kaleidoscope that Joe just had to buy for Suzy. Maggie would have thought the Viking man was a little boy as he oohed and aahed over all the objects in the kaleidoscope store, finally settling on a brass-plated scope of fine quality. He'd also found a cuddly stuffed Keiko to add to Beth's collection. And he'd picked out colorful kites for both of them.

This was going to be some spectacular Christmas for her daughters. While Maggie wasn't stingy, she had never gone overboard with Christmas gifts, not wanting her daughters to become spoiled, or to take away from the true meaning of the season. She didn't think it would matter if this year was a little excessive, though. Besides, it might be the only Christmas they had with Joe, and she couldn't begrudge his making it memorable for them.

It was late afternoon, and each of them were carrying two shopping bags, when Joe said, "Do you know what I really want?"

"A Big Mac and french fries."

He made a *tsk*ing noise at her. "No, I want to go home."

Maggie closed her eyes for a brief second, savoring the sound of *home* on his tongue. She suspected what he had in mind, and suddenly even the slight abrasion of her light clothing was like an erotic caress. "Your wish is my command, oh Viking leader."

He gave her a look that translated to, *Since when?*

They had almost reached her car when he

remarked, "Do you know what I want when we get home?"

The sultry lowering of his eyelids and the husky tone of his voice were certainly big clues. She felt her breasts peak and begin to ache. The man was turning her into a world-class bimbo. "Surprise, surprise!" she responded in a choked voice. *Am I really up to another marathon of sex?* she questioned, then immediately replied: *Absolutely.*

"Not *that,* Mag-he," he corrected. "I mean, of course I want to make love after this long day of deprivation." He flashed her a slow grin, then added, "Nay, it is something else I yearn for, and have ne'er done afore."

Uh-oh! Maggie couldn't imagine anything sensual Joe hadn't done, and that smoky look in his gray eyes certainly bespoke sex with a capital *S.* The ache in her breasts dropped lower. She waited for him to continue.

"A bubble bath."

It was Sunday night, Christmas Eve, and they were attending the choir recital in the church.

Maggie was wearing a new white silk pantsuit, trimmed with gold cording, over a glittery gold lamé shell, just right for the season. There was something about Christmas that called for a new outfit, or a special outfit pulled out only at this time each year to fit the occasion.

Tears filled her eyes as she watched her daughters in small gold choir robes, with wreaths of holly in their hair, singing in harmony with their peers. "Silent Night." "Hark, the Herald Angels Sing." "Oh, Holy Night." "It Came upon a Midnight Clear." "The First Noel." But actually, tears seemed to be the norm for Maggie the past few days as one poignant event after another took place.

Since Christmas fell on a Monday this year, they'd held the Christmas party at the hospital this afternoon, even though many staff members were off on Sunday and outpatients were not usually on the premises. The clinic's standardized gifts were doled out—chocolate Santas and rainbow plaques with motivational poems on them. Then Joe and Maggie distributed their individualized gifts, as well.

All of the patients from their group seemed stunned by the particular care taken in choosing their presents, but Steve . . . oh, the moment when Steve opened the gift wrap revealing his baseball card . . . well, Maggie would never forget it. And neither would anyone else who had been there. Steve had been overcome that Joe—and everyone knew, without being told, that Joe was at the bottom of these special gifts—cared enough about him to buy that particular memento. In the end, he had just stared at him hopelessly and said, "Oh, man. Oh, man. You're gonna force me to straighten out, aren't you?" He'd liked the SEALs jacket, too, and made a big deal of putting it on for everyone to see how it fit, but it was the card that had hit home hardest.

How had Joe known it would mean so much to his friend? She never would have thought of it herself.

The refreshments included homemade Christmas cookies made by the staff and sickeningly sweet cherry punch, which they enjoyed while watching tapes of all the Christmas episodes on the afternoon soap operas. It turned out that some of the nurses and attendants were hooked on the soaps, too. When the different shows brought out flashbacks to Christmas past as far back as twenty years ago, there were tears in some of the eyes watching.

After that, Joe had put Maggie in a most awkward position. He'd invited everyone to attend the church choir recital tonight. Since it was open to the public, Maggie couldn't very well object.

He was sitting beside her now in a blue oxford shirt, khaki pants, a navy blazer, and cowboy boots . . . yes, cowboy boots, of all things. They had been a gift from Steve, who had shown up at their house unexpectedly just before they'd left for the church. The boots had touched Joe almost as much as Joe's gift had touched Steve earlier that day. And he didn't even seem to mind that they pinched his toes and made him wobble a bit when he walked. "I'm a true Texan now," he'd boasted.

"The Lone Star Viking?" she'd quipped.

"Aw, shucks, darlin'," Joe had drawled in response.

Sitting on her other side were Harry and Martie. Harry's new hat, which he appeared to love, was sitting on the bench between them. Harry claimed that he would have to wear the hat, since it had been given to him by a former patient, but she could tell that he was delighted every time he plopped the thing on his head.

On Joe's other side was Steve Askey in a conservative gray suit and tie, with cowboy boots. He was staring with serious concentration at the altar where the choir was singing, as if the music was filling some important void in his life. But perhaps it was just being back in a church after so many years.

Natalie Blue was there with her parents, dressed in her usual cowgirl attire, but this time it was an outfit in the seasonal colors of red and green, with glittery tinsel taking the place of fringe. Her parents had wished Maggie a merry Christmas before the recital began, and whispered a quick thank-you in an aside for all of their daughter's recent progress. It was a sign of Natalie's improvement that she was even able to sit in a crowded church. Maggie hadn't said anything at the time, but she'd really thought it was Joe they should be thanking.

Chuck Belammy was looking very normal tonight in a Polo shirt and blue chinos, though his gaze kept drifting back to the Nativity scene. Maggie thought she heard an intermittent "baa-baa" come from his direction, though he kept it very low.

Harvey Lutz was straining his neck this way and that, obviously counting the stained-glass windows. He didn't count aloud, but his lips were moving.

Fred Bernstein came dressed as Santa, so for once he blended in with everyone else. The audience probably thought he'd just gotten off work at the mall. Sitting next to Fred was Gladys Hatcher, dressed in a bright flame-colored dress with a reindeer appliquéd on the front. There must have been a battery under the bodice, because every couple of seconds the reindeer's nose blinked bright red.

The biggest surprise was Rosalyn Harris, who'd arrived late in a burgundy sheath dress. Her hair was still pulled back straight off her face into a spinsterish bun, she wore no makeup, and the dress was not immodest by any means . . . high-necked, long-sleeved, and calf-length. *But holy cow!* Who knew she had such a wonderful figure? She was tall, svelte, and curved in just the right places. More than one male head turned in her direction during the recital, and not just those who knew of her sexual desires.

Christmas had always been a special time to Maggie. This year every little nuance and tradition and smell and sound seemed to resonate inside her soul. She was creating memories . . . memories that she feared would have to last her a lifetime.

Jorund surveyed the little church, took a deep whiff of the pungent scents of evergreen boughs and bayberry candles, flexed his fingers where they were twined with Mag-he's, and sighed. My mother would be so proud of me, he thought ruefully. All those years she'd tried to preach her Christian dogmas, while he went hither and yon, practicing his warrior skills. Oh, he, his father, his brothers, and his sister had all been baptized in the Christian rites to satisfy her wishes, but it was only a token action. They still practiced the old Norse religions, as well. But tonight, as the sounds of the Christian music flowed in his ears, Jorund felt a sense of peace with the One-God . . .

as if finally he were forgiven—that with the birth of the Christ child, he could be reborn, too. It was a heady thought.

"I'm glad I came," he whispered in Mag-he's ear. She smelled of some light floral scent—lilacs again, perhaps—and of her own distinctive woman essence.

"Me, too," she said and squeezed his hand.

There were tears in her eyes, and Jorund knew they were tears of pride for Sue-zee and Beth, who were performing at the church altar. It was one of the things he admired most about Mag-he—the ferocious devotion she showed her daughters. If he ever had children again, he would accept no less in a wife.

Oh, may God and all his angels weep! Where did that thought come from? I will never wed again. I will never breed babes again. Never, never, never! The joy of parenthood will ne'er be mine again.

Ironically, the recital ended then with a loud rendition of "Joy to the World," accompanied by the blare of trumpets. Was it a sign? And that clicking noise. . . . surely it was just a clock ticking somewhere in the church vestibule.

Afterward they were driving home—Jorund in the passenger seat, Sue-zee and Beth in the backseat. There was a warm feel to the comfortable silence that surrounded them. Forevermore, Jorund knew he would associate this kind of hushed tranquillity with Christmas. Perhaps this was what was meant by peace.

"Mom . . ." Sue-zee said.

"Hmmm?" she responded.

"This is the best Christmas ever."

Beth agreed, adding, "Like a dream come true."

Misty-eyed, Mag-he glanced over at him and murmured, "Thank you."

He looked at her, back at the girls, then at her once again. "Nay, heartling, I thank you."

Chapter Sixteen

Christmas was almost over in the Muck-bride household, and Jorund should have been at peace. He wasn't. Not anymore.

Oh, it had been one of the most wonderful days of his life. He could not deny that. Perhaps that was why his spirits had plummeted. Perhaps it was as simple as the fact that he did not want the day to end. No, he knew it was more than that. No matter what happened tomorrow, or some tomorrow down the road, this was a day he would never forget.

It was that inevitable tomorrow that was brewing unrest in him now.

First there had been the gift exchanging, followed by a special yule breakfast of bacon, "dippy" eggs, toasted bread, and pancakes shaped like Christmas trees, covered with butter and syrup, along with pitchers of milk and orange juice, and cups of black coffee, a bitter brew he could not like, no matter that it was a favorite beverage of adults in this time. Later they'd had a feast of baked ham with roasted potatoes, vegetables, and let-ass, a staple of practically every meal, but which was little more than grass, if you asked him.

After that, they had watched a move-he on the TV world box called *It's a Wonderful Life*. Mag-he and the girls had gone weepy-eyed at the end, to his dismay, but they had told him it was "good crying," whatever that was.

The gift exchanging had been the best part, with the girls exuberantly exclaiming over each gift, big or small, and Maggie breaking out in tears over the antique gold, heart-shaped pendant on a chain that he'd given her. The heavy gold was etched with writhing animals in the Viking style. Inside there was an inlay of amber and a somber photograph of himself, which Sue-zee and Beth had helped him make in a machine at the shopping mall.

The girls had given their mother numerous small gifts—bath oils, perfume, a leather carrying bag for her papers, a music box that played her favorite song from a move-he about a sinking ship. Mag-he in turn gave them clothes and wrist rings and music CDs and stuffed animals. Of course, they had pretended that the gifts came from Santa Claus, but they weren't fooling him. He knew Santa was a myth. He had closed the flue on the fireplace chimney last night, and when he'd checked this morning, it was still closed. Not that he'd been foolish enough to give that legend any credence.

Jorund loved to receive gifts—he would not deny that—and the girls had made him hand-crafted cards with poignant sentiments that shot straight to his already melted heart. In addition, they'd given him fun presents, like a miniature Ricky Martin doll, which they claimed resembled him, only younger; a sweatshirt that said, *Proud to be a Texan*; a scale model of a Viking longship; and a glass bowl of green Jell-O cubes that could be held in the hands and eaten that way. Good thing that last had been a jest, for Jorund did not think he would have been able to eat even one, especially after imbibing that horrible egg nog that Mag-he had claimed was a traditional yule drink. *What is wrong with good old mead as a yule drink, I ask you?*

Even the annoying Rita had not been left out of the gift giving. Mag-he had given her a feline foo-tawn bed, which was a type of comfortable couch. The damn cat was spoiled too much, in his opinion, and he didn't feel that way just because the beast had taken an extreme dislike to him at first sight. She shed her fur all over his garments. She hissed when he approached Mag-he. She coughed up hairballs into his running shoes.

In any case, aside from the ridiculous foo-tawn, Mag-he had also given Rita a Santa hat, which she deemed the latest in "cat coo-tour." Jorund had barely been able to stifle his chuckles of delight at how ludicrous the cat looked.

Sue-zee gave Rita blowing bubbles that had catnip in them, and Beth gave her a Christmas wreath made of tuna-flavored leaves to place above her new bed. The wreath played a meow-ing version of "Jingle Bells." To be sure, that smelly wreath was going to be lost before morn-ing. "Jingle Bells" was bad enough. A meowing "Jingle Bells"? Never.

Not wanting to be considered a cat hater, which he no doubt was, Jorund had purchased a cat present, too: a feathery kitty wand, which had a heavy metal disc for a base that suctioned to the floor, and a tall, thin metal pole from which numerous bird feathers were suspended. Cats apparently took great pleasure in trying to catch the elusive, fluttery feathers. The good thing about this one was that every so often, when Rita batted at a feather, the wand would swat back, causing the cat to fall on her fat rump with a shriek.

Mag-he had eyed him suspiciously, obviously wondering if he'd deliberately bought a toy that would drive Rita half-mad.

He'd just smiled innocently at her.

Of course, there was no explaining away the sec-ond gift he'd bought for Rita: a food bowl with the words, *The Cat from Hell*, emblazoned on the side.

Mag-he's gift to him had been a tooled leather belt to hold the scabbard for his sword and a set of books about Vikings, with fine gold-edged bindings. He could not easily read the books yet. But every day he was getting more proficient at recognizing written words and phrases. He was deeply touched that she'd given the books to him. It was as if she expected him to be here long enough to learn to read English well. And that was what was causing his low spirits.

He had not expected to care so deeply ever again. It had happened so quickly, as if predestined. That scared him mightily, because he sensed that he was soon going to have to make a decision: to save his brother and leave this land and those he had come to care for; or to stay and see how these affections might develop, and thus abandon his brother and his father's mission.

"Joe, you're not paying attention," Sue-zee complained.

He was sitting cross-legged on the floor, playing her new video game with her. It was a gruesome battle of gremlins against giants. "And they say Vikings are bloodthirsty," he grumbled good-naturedly. "They ought to see a nine-year-old girl with a game clicker in her hand."

Sue-zee jabbed him in the ribs with an elbow and hooted. "You're not going to give up, are you?"

"Yea, I am."

"Chicken! Bock, bock, bock!"

"You win, sweetling." With a wink, he declined to rise to her bait, and instead stood and arched his back to remove the kinks.

"Joe, could you come over here?" Beth urged. "You, too, Mom." Beth was playing with the new laptop come-pewter he'd given her. Truly, it was a magic box. And he'd seen only a few of its marvels which Beth had demonstrated that morning. A-oh-ell. The Enter-net. Webbing sites. E-mail. Chatting rooms. Whale research sites.

Beth was a truly remarkable child, with her fierce protectiveness of the killer whales . . . especially one particular whale named Keiko. On her own, she had established her own Webbing site where she was garnering support among young people all over the world. He would bet a Viking king's booty that Thora would love this girl.

Mag-he put aside the book she had been reading in the comfortable chair next to the fire—one of the Viking books she had given him. It was the end of December, but in Tax-us the weather was still fairly warm . . . certainly not cold enough for a fire. But Mag-he and the girls had insisted that it wouldn't be Christmas without a fire, now that they actually had a fireplace; so they'd put on the air conditioner, a device that magically cooled the house, and had him make a fire.

It struck him as odd that people would want a fireplace in their homes when fire was not used for heat or cooking. But then, this was a country that encouraged cutting down live trees and bringing them indoors to shed their pine needles.

The girls also yearned to have snow for Christmas—another strange tradition in this country—which was almost impossible in this part of Texas. He had told them with a laugh, "A fireplace I could produce for you, but not snow. I am not a god."

"I think you're a god," Mag-he had whispered in that husky sex-voice of hers.

She made him feel like a god.

Now she came up to stand beside him, behind her daughter, who was sitting on a chair in front of a piece of furniture called a desk. She was staring at the colored screen of the laptop, which showed words and colored pictures.

He put his arm around Mag-he's waist, then let

313

his hand sidle lower to palm her buttock. It seemed like forever since he'd last had the freedom to touch Mag-he, even though it had been only a week.

She gave him a startled sideways look, slapped his hand away, then let her gaze wander till she took in the fact that neither Sue-zee nor Beth had noticed. Only then did she reach over and pinch his buttock. "Behave," she ordered in an undertone.

"What did you say, Mom?" Beth asked. She was doing some complicated maneuvers on her laptop. Sue-zee had started another game by herself, and the sounds of *zing-zing-zap* could be heard in the background.

"Nothing," Mag-he replied innocently. "What did you want to show us, sweetie?"

"Vikings."

"Vikings?" he and Mag-he said at the same time.

"Yeah, I know how interested Joe is in Vikings . . . coming from Norway and all that," Beth explained. He and Mag-he had agreed not to tell the twins about his having time traveled, but instead to let them think he was a man of Norse heritage with a special interest in the tenth century. "Well, I did a search on Yahoo—that's a search engine—and came up with a zillion sites on the Internet. Then I narrowed my search to tenth-century Vikings, and you won't believe what I found. Are you interested?"

Jorund looked at Mag-he, and she looked back at him. Was he interested? *Bloody hell, yes.* He pulled an extra chair over next to Beth.

"Lots of the stuff you've told us about King Olaf is true."

"Of course it's true. Did you think I would lie?"

"Well, sometimes the things you say are pretty off-the-wall."

"Name one thing."

"That your father is—was—a Viking king."

"Well, he is—was—not really a king . . . rather a minor king. Actually, his title is jarl, which is similar to the English earl."

Beth skipped from one site to the next, showing him histories of tenth-century Vikings, along with pictures of their longships, jewelry, clothing, and native fjords. Jorund was fascinated. And he was also homesick, just seeing the images of his homeland.

He didn't realize that Mag-he had placed a hand on his shoulder, but she was just as captivated as he was, leaning over him. "Honey, do a search under the Viking histories for Vestfold. And then for Jarl Eric Tryggvason." She squeezed his shoulder. "Isn't that where you said you come . . . I mean, where your people come from? The southeastern section of Norway?"

He nodded.

Soon Beth had even more detailed information, though she declared that the tenth century was practically the Dark Ages and not much data had been collected in written form. The person who owned this particular Web site, a member of some group called the ess-see-a, claimed there was a man called Jarl Eric Trygvasson, brother to King Olaf Trygvasson. Apparently there was a grave mound in modern-day Norway with his father's name on it in runic symbols, dated the year 999. Beside it on one side was a smaller grave mound commemorating the death of Eric's daughter-by-marriage, Inga, and his two grand-daughters, Greta and Girta. Jorund had already seen the latter, but the former . . . well, it must mean that his father had died one year after he'd last seen him in 998. Had there been an accident, or had his father fallen in battle?

If that wasn't heartbreaking enough for Jorund, the next screen showed a large stone with runic symbols on it. Before Beth had a chance to read the text for him, Jorund began translating aloud the inscription, " 'This stone is dedicated in the year 998 to the memory of my sons, Karl Geirolf Ericsson and Karl Jorund Ericsson. They died at sea, brave of heart. May I join them one day in Valhalla.' "

More important, there was a picture there of Jorund's sword, Bloodletter, which had been buried in the grave. Surely that was a sign that he had returned home, for there was no duplicate of this specially crafted weapon.

Jorund was staggered by this news, and he could tell that Mag-he was, too, by the way she squeezed both his shoulders. Did this mean that he would never return home to his time? Or would he return after his father's death? Wouldn't he have removed the fallacious gravestone, if he had? On the other hand, mayhap he'd been too grief-stricken to care. No, the most damning evidence was his sword. He would be returning to his time.

Mag-he leaned down and whispered in his ear, "We'll talk about this later."

"Oooh, oooh, oooh!" Beth exclaimed. "Look at

what I found." She'd moved to another Webbing site. " 'Rosestead: A Viking Village.' See. Some guy and his wife built an authentic Viking village in Maine. And it's a working village, too."

Picture after picture was shown of the inhabitants at work . . . building longships, operating farms, caring for livestock, weaving textiles, making soaps, crafting jewelry, brewing mead, pattern-welding swords. It was like gazing back in time, and yet all of this was apparently taking place today somewhere in this country. *Amazing.*

" 'Tis odd," he commented tentatively, "but the icon marking each of these pages is identical to my family crest—writhing dragons wrapped around a cross. It represents the Vikings of my father and the Christians of my mother."

"It's probably just a coincidence," Mag-he observed.

"And that longship shown there. 'Tis called *Fierce Raven*. The ships my brother Rolf built all had the name *Fierce* in them, like *Fierce Destiny, Fierce Pride, Fierce Dragon.*"

"That's probably a coincidence, too."

"Yea," he agreed finally. "If people have no compunction about robbing graves, they would not hesitate to steal a family crest or a ship name, as well."

Beth read some more and told them that the village was originally started to preserve the Viking culture, since there was no true Viking country today . . . Iceland being more Viking in nature than Norway was. Because Vikings were assimilated into the countries where they conquered or settled, they had no real homeland of their own. In addition, Beth read that Rosestead also served as an orphanage for inner-city home-less kids.

"Wouldn't it be nice to have a place like that for mental patients, like the ones at Rainbow?" Sue-zee suggested from behind them, where she was still playing her game. She must have been listen-ing to them and playing at the same time.

Everyone turned with surprise.

She shrugged. "It was just an idea. Lots of the people at Rainbow aren't dangerous or anything, and look how well some of them are doing, just being around Joe, who's kind of a Viking."

"Who's *kind of* a Viking?" he protested. "I am most definitely a real Viking."

"Yeah, yeah," Sue-zee said, and went back to concentrating on her game.

"It's an interesting thought," Jorund remarked to Mag-he.

She nodded and appeared to be considering all the possibilities. Not that it was really possible. He would be long gone before any such project could be undertaken. Wouldn't he?

"They even have a visitors' program six months of the year, when outsiders can come in and tour the place. They're closed November through April," Beth went on. "Maybe we could go there for vacation next year, huh, Mom?"

"Maybe," Mag-he conceded, but her mind still seemed to be elsewhere.

For some reason the computer shut down on them momentarily, and when it came back on, they had lost the Rosestead Web site. But Jorund had seen enough.

"I must needs tell you something that I have just now decided. Methinks it will be glad tidings for you all." Jorund could scarce contain his excitement in making this announcement.

They all stopped what they were doing and stared at him expectantly. Mag-he tilted her head; she was a little suspicious.

He didn't know where the notion had come from, or why he was so convinced that it was the right thing to do. It just felt right.

"We're going to Maine."

Pandemonium broke loose. Joe was jabbering away excitedly. The girls were jumping up and down, thrilled at the prospect of a road trip with their beloved father figure. And Maggie was seething with fury.

"No!" she finally screamed to get their attention. When everyone calmed down enough to listen, she softened her voice. "We are not going to Maine." And she gave Joe a meaningful glower to indicate that it was cruel for him to have made the suggestion without consulting her first.

He just lifted his stubborn chin in defiance. The dunce didn't have the sense to realize his blunder.

"Mom!" Suzy and Beth whined.

"No!" she repeated, more firmly this time. "It's out of the question."

Then to Joe, she said, "Number one, it's too far away. Number two, we have to be here on New Year's Eve—remember, we promised to be at the talent show at Boot Scootin' Cowboy to support Natalie. Number three, that Rosestead place isn't even open in the winter. Number four, the girls have to be back in school the day after New Year's Day—that's only nine days from now. Number five, it's cold—very cold—in Maine this time of the year."

"We could get a couple days off of school," Beth argued. "They're allowed for educational purposes. And this would be educational, I bet."

"You never let us do anything," Suzy added.

"Girls, I want you to go upstairs and take your baths."

"It's Christmas. Why do we have to go up so early?" Suzy protested, tears welling in her eyes.

"I thought we were going to watch *A Christmas Story* on TV tonight," Beth added. "You said we could, Mom. Remember, that's the movie about the kid who wanted a BB gun for Christmas? It was so funny when he got those footed bunny pajamas, and when that kid's tongue got stuck to the flagpole."

Maggie remembered. She didn't need Beth's nervous jabbering to jog her memory. Did Suzy and Beth really think she would be so harsh? She wasn't about to let their Christmas end on such a sour note. "You can come back down after your baths," she said gently, pushing some loose strands of hair off of Beth's face and behind her ears. "Joe and I need to talk . . . *alone.*"

Once the girls were gone, Jorund knew he was in big trouble. But before he let that trouble hit him smack in the face, he had something important to do. Walking resolutely to the door leading from the den to the hallway, he shoved Rita out with a whisk of his foot, closed the door with a loud bang, then turned the key in the lock.

"What are you doing, Joe?" Mag-he asked, backing up slightly. She was wearing tight black *braies*, which were appropriately called tights, and a big, loose black tunic, caught in at the waist with a twisted rope belt of red and green. He hoped to hell she was wearing no undergarments, because he didn't have that much time before the girls returned.

"What am I doing?" he repeated, already yanking his *Proud to Be a Viking* T-shirt over his head. "I'm about to give you the best Christmas present you've ever had."

"No."

"Yea."

"We can't. I told you that I wouldn't do this with the girls in the house."

"Surely there must be an exception for Christmas."

She wavered. He could see it in her eyes. He would warrant she'd missed their lovemaking almost as much as he had.

"Mag-he, you are killing me with all these new . . . emotions. Not just our lovemaking, or being amongst twin girls again, but the whole Christmas season. I need . . . I need . . ."

She waited for him to finish, but he could not. In truth, he had closed the door to the den chamber in hopes of a quick swiving. He had not intended to spout such nonsense—at least, that was what he would have called it at one time— but the words just came out. Perhaps it was not just a quick swiving he was after . . . or not the *only* thing he was after.

Why does everything have to be so complicated in this land?

"You need what, Joe?" Mag-he asked softly.

He closed his eyes briefly, then opened them, staring at her bleakly. "I need to be touched," he confessed.

"Oh, Joe."

321

Sandra Hill

She was ripe for the plucking now, if he wanted to take advantage of her vulnerability. Somehow Jorund could not do that. He did not want to seduce her tonight. He wanted her to want him as much as he wanted her.

She bit her bottom lip with indecision and reached a hand out, cupping his jaw.

That touch—that mere touch—was almost his undoing. He moaned and turned his mouth to her palm, kissing it gently.

She moaned, too, a soft, feminine sound of capitulation. "I need your touch, too," she admitted. "I have missed you so much this week."

He nodded, waiting for her word to proceed. Jorund was a warrior. He knew when to advance and when to delay. Now his instincts said to wait for her cue.

"They'll be back too soon for us to do anything."

"Not for what I have in mind."

She arched an eyebrow. Yes, she was interested, despite herself.

"Something I heard about on the TV world box," he answered, backing her up against the closet door, beside the glittering Christmas tree. Even as he brushed his mouth over hers, restraining himself from deepening the kiss, he was already at work, loosening her belt. "A wall-bang-her."

Maggie gasped with surprise. He wasn't sure if it was because of what he intended to do, or because he'd already lifted her off the floor, shoved her tights down to her thighs—and yes, he had been right . . . thank the Lord . . . she was not wearing undergarments—and pulled his *braies* down far enough to release his erection . . . which was immense again. *Oh, for the tears of Thor! I resemble a tree limb. What is happening to my male parts in this land? I ne'er thought I would say this about my virility, but 'tis embarrassing.* Before she could blink, or raise some objection, he adjusted her legs to hug his hips, and plunged inside. Luckily, Mag-he had gone back on something called birth-control pills, and the condoms were no longer necessary.

"We can't." Maggie was already wrapping her arms around his shoulders and adjusting her legs more tightly about his hips, locking them at the ankles behind his back.

"We can," he said, then beseeched her in a raw voice, "Touch me, Mag-he. Touch me, touch me, touch me."

She undid the rub-her band holding his hair back and ran her fingers through the long strands lovingly. She traced the line of his jaw and his eyebrows with a forefinger. She rubbed his shoulders and caressed his back. Everywhere her hands and fingers could reach, she touched him.

Only then did he begin the long, slow strokes that he knew she enjoyed so much. The friction of her inner walls tugging at his staff on each backward stroke was sweet agony to him.

With one hand under her buttocks to hold her up, Jorund reached his other hand under her *shert* and began to massage one breast. He lifted its fullness from underneath, then palmed the whole, rubbing in a circular fashion till the tight bud in the center stabbed at his flesh. Mag-he had the most sensitive breasts, and it was only seconds before she was moaning aloud, and peaking around his pounding erection.

He wanted her to continue peaking for him till

he came to his own release. So, even before she stopped her erotic spasms, he was fluttering his thumb against her sex-bud . . . a continuous, rapid, back-and-forth motion that prompted another orgasm from Mag-he. The whole time, he continued his long strokes, which were becoming shorter and faster as he approached his own imminent exploding point.

"I love you," she cried out in the midst of her ecstasy, still alternately clutching and caressing his shoulders. Then, "Tell me, tell me, tell me," she begged.

He knew exactly what she wanted to hear, and perhaps it was the sex, or perhaps it was the Christmas spirit in the air, or perhaps he was finally surrendering to the inevitable, but Jorund couldn't help himself then. "I love you, heartling. I love you, I love you, I love you." He said all this to her as his seed burst into her body.

And for that moment, at least, Jorund's life seemed to have come full circle. He was complete.

"I said no, and I mean it," Maggie said, straightening out her clothes.

There was no afterglow period to their lovemaking this time, as much as she cherished Joe's words of love. She didn't blame him for the wild sexual interlude. She had needed his touch as much as he'd apparently needed hers. It had been as beautiful in its spontaneity as some of his long, drawn-out loveplay often was. But now Maggie felt awful, unable to savor what should be such a special moment. She couldn't seem to help herself. The girls would be back soon, and she had to settle the absurd question of their taking off across the country to some tourist attraction that wasn't even open to the public during the winter.

Joe stared at her, his eyes desolate and pleading. "Why is it so important to you?"

"I don't know. It just is." He'd already adjusted his clothing. Now he went over to unlock the door. When Rita rushed in, he made a disgusted sound. Turning back to Maggie, he reached out and took one of her hands in both of his. "My instincts tell me that this is something I must do."

Maggie pulled her hand from his clasp. She couldn't think when he touched her in any way. Besides that, her skin was still extrasensitive from their lovemaking. Pacing the room, she tried to get her emotions under control. "You want us—me and my two daughters—to take a fruitless, two-thousand-mile trip, all based on an instinct?"

"Yea, I do."

She noticed a familiar expression on his face. "Oh, don't you dare throw that trust business in my face again. This isn't about trust. It's about a whim."

"Mayhap it's about control, Mag-he. Mayhap you just can't bear to give up some of your precious control. I admit that I should have discussed this with you first, but I did not do it to usurp your authority. I was so excited over the idea that I blurted it out."

She took a deep breath. "Listen, Joe, we can go next summer when the girls are on vacation—"

"Next summer! What makes you think I will be here next summer?" His words were angry and bleak at the same time.

Maggie felt as if a vise were squeezing her heart.

"I'll go myself then. I will reserve a seat for myself on a gray dog."

"Gray dog?" Maggie laughed briefly. "You mean Greyhound . . . like a Greyhound bus?"

He waved a hand dismissively. "That is what I said, is it not?"

The idea of a tenth-century Viking boarding a modern bus and traveling a great distance to a place where he knew no one was so outlandish that Maggie hurried to convince him he was being unreasonable. "I can't let you do that."

His eyes threw flinty sparks at her, as if to say, *Try to stop me.*

"Joe, try to understand. I'm the only one who drives. Even if I could drive nonstop, it would be two days going and two days coming back. With at least one overnight stay in a motel, we're talking three days each way of driving alone. Were you planning that we would go, examine the closed-to-the-public village from the outside, then turn around and come right back?"

"You know I have made no specific plans. It's just something I want to do–nay, something I *need* to do."

As he needed my touch? No, don't think. You're softening, Maggie. Whatever you do, don't soften. "Don't you think you're being selfish?"

He seemed to give her question serious thought. "Nay . . . yea . . . it does not matter."

"And there's another thing: do you think it's wise to go so far away from the point of your time travel entry? There's a chance you'd cut yourself off forever from returning to your time."

"On the other hand, Thora may have traveled

north to colder waters. Mayhap she awaits me there. Mayhap that is why it is so important to me."

That prospect staggered Maggie. "You think that this might be a sign from Thora?"

"Mayhap."

"And you would abandon me and Suzy and Beth in Maine?" Maggie hated the pathetic tone of her voice.

"Not willingly." He drew himself up resolutely. "Heed me well on this, m'lady: I am going to this Rosestead village, but your arguments make good sense. So I will offer this compromise, though it vexes me no end to think of doing it."

He had her full attention now.

"We could go on one of those flying longships."

Flying longships? Flying longships? Oh. "By airplane?"

"Yea." His face was pale as a ghost at the possibility.

He plopped down on the sofa, pulling her down next to him. "I cannot credit that this love we have just discovered is destined to end here. Come with me, heartling. Please."

The girls burst through the door then, smelling of shampoo and lilac bubble bath. "Well?" they both asked expectantly.

Maggie barely hesitated a moment before informing them with forced brightness, "Looks like we're going to see snow this Christmas, after all."

327

Chapter Seventeen

"If ever I make it back to my time, I am going to have some fantastic stories to give to the skalds," Jorund grumbled.

Sitting next to the window—*in an actual flying machine, for the love of Freyja*—he was as rigid as a Saxon soldier with a Norse blade at his private parts, and twice as frightened. The only thing different was the lack of piss running down his legs . . . so far.

The airplane had the whimsical name of United. He supposed that was not so unusual, considering the names some Vikings gave their longships and favorite weapons.

Mag-he sat totally at ease in the seat next to him, trying to assure him of their safety with such ludicrous words as, "Only one plane in about a million ever crashes." As if that were any comfort to him. This metal container could very likely be the millionth one.

Once the craft was airborne, he released a long breath and continued his complaints. "Truly, my sagas will be retold through the centuries: how Jorund the Lackwit Warrior not only rode naked on the back of a killer whale, but landed in a madhouse, then willingly flew through the skies in a magic machine called an airplane, thus proving his madness."

Steve had loaned him his new SEALs jacket in anticipation of the low temperatures they would find in Maine. Mag-he and the girls, who sat in the seats behind them, wore layers of sweat-hers under their jackets.

While the girls were excited about the trip, he was tense, waiting for something—he knew not what—to happen next. Not an airplane crash. No, it was something else, he was certain. Mag-he, bless her trusting soul, was simply resigned.

For the next hour or so, he was able to relax, even though the airplane was traveling at an excessive rate of speed. When he turned to glance over the back of the headrest, he saw that the girls were napping. He had thought Mag-he was dozing, too, till she asked softly, "Do you still feel this trip has some importance?"

Clearly she was worried that their time together was nearing an end. He could give her no assurances to the contrary. Reaching over to lace his fingers with hers, he tugged her closer, then put an arm around her shoulders and rested her face in the crook of his neck. He would try to lighten her spirits, he decided. "Steve told me about a remarkable feat that some couples attempt while in an air machine."

She laughed—a choked, wobbly sound. "Stop trying to make me laugh." Her words were light, but her eyes remained melancholy.

" 'Tis called the Mile-high Association," he went on. "I believe it has something to do with sex in the clouds. That sounds interesting, do you not think?" Jorund was just jesting, of course. He might have been foolhardy enough to try flying in a metal box, but never would he dare fornicate on a cloud.

"Oh, no, you don't, buster." She punched him lightly on the upper arm. "Last night you might have been able to talk me into . . . into—"

"A wall-bang-her?" he offered with a grin.

"Yes. You might have been able to seduce me into vertical sex . . ."

Well, that's an interesting name for it.

". . . but no way are you sweet-talking me into sex in an airplane bathroom. Uh-uh."

Oh, so that is what the Mile-high Association is.

They both sat in silence then, but Jorund had some things that needed to be said, and Mag-he apparently did, too.

She spoke first. "You very cleverly evaded my question, Joe. Why are you so serious, aside from being scared to death of flying? What's bothering you?"

"If I should depart suddenly . . ." he blurted out.

Her body stiffened with alarm. "Oh, no! Do you really think you might—"

"Shhh." He squeezed her shoulder and held her

face with his other hand. "I don't know that I would be sent back without warning, but I must needs be ready."

"Tell me the truth. You sense that something is about to happen, don't you?"

He hesitated to tell her, but she had to be prepared. Finally he nodded.

She gasped.

He tried to explain. "I cannot tell you how many times over how many years I have prepared myself to go into battle. Each time, at the last moment, there is a rush of blood in the body, a humming in the ears, an excitement of sorts."

"It's called adrenaline."

Why was he not surprised that she would have a name for it? They had a name for every other bloody thing in this strange land ... including mouth sex, the bad temper women were in before their monthly flux, the perfectly natural inclination of males of middle years to swive younger women, and—

"Is that how you feel now? All hyped up?" she asked, tears misting her beautiful blue eyes. "As if you are about to fight?"

"Hmmm. Not exactly. More like something immense is about to happen."

They were both silent then. What could be more immense than his being hurtled back through time? What could be more immense than their permanent separation?

"You're strong, Mag-he," he remarked in a strangled voice. "You can handle anything."

He was not so sure about himself, though.

"No matter what happens, Joe, I can't be sorry that I met you, or that we made love."

He nodded, unable to express just how much his short relationship with her meant to him. In the end, he told her, "I will never forget you."

They were both too overcome to speak more, and Jorund turned away to stare out the window. The airplane was now traveling over an expanse of water. He narrowed his eyes and pressed his nose to the glass. *Aha!* He didn't even bother to tell Mag-he when he saw a killer whale spyhopping merrily down below. She would only tell him that it was impossible to see that far. But he knew. It was Thora; he was certain of that.

And her words to him, accompanied by the usual clicks and groans, came up the great distance from the water to the plane, loud and clear, for his ears only.

Soon, Viking. Soon you will know.

They arrived at Rosestead the next morning, and the Viking village was beautiful as a postcard . . . a perfect Hallmark holiday image.

"Wow!" Suzy and Beth exclaimed. They were practically jumping up and down with glee in the backseat of the rental car—not just at their initial view of an authentic Norse settlement, but at seeing real snow for the first time. Luckily this wasn't gray, slushy snow, but crisp, new-fallen flakes, like the snow globes found in gift stores.

"It was well worth the trip just to see this charming scene," she told Joe as they exited the vehicle. She was trying to make up for her earlier resistance to the trip, but her sentiments were honest.

He nodded distractedly. He was no longer hyped-up, but also somber with some odd anticipation . . . something she could neither fathom nor alleviate.

"Are you all right?" she asked, putting a hand on his arm. His face was pale, his lips pinched.

Giving her a sideways glance, he grimaced. "Bloody damn a-drain-a-line! My heart's pumping faster than a youthling's legs in his first wolf race."

At first Maggie had been alarmed by Joe's belief that something monumental was about to happen, but now it was more as if they were all on a slow-moving roller coaster. It was sure to be a rocky ride, but there was no getting off. What would be, would be.

She did say a silent prayer, though: *Please, God, if it be your will, let everything work out for me and Joe and my daughters. We love him so much.*

They'd gotten into the Bangor airport the night before, but Maggie had insisted that they get a motel room before heading for the village. If Joe and the girls had had their way, they would have come upon this scene in the dark, and that would have been a shame, she realized now.

With snow flurries coming down steadily, their first view of Rosestead was seen through a filter of the white flakes. Suzy and Beth were so excited as they emerged from the rental car, they were oblivious to the freezing cold.

Rosestead was located at a secluded site in northern Maine, accessed by a half-mile roadway leading off the interstate. A giant archway over the entrance read: ROSESTEAD: A VIKING VILLAGE. A smaller sign on the side listed its schedule. A banner over the sign proclaimed, CLOSED TILL APRIL. And there was a wooden gate across the entrance barring car traffic. It couldn't be any clearer than that. *Closed to the public.*

They emerged from the car, and Joe walked right around the gate. She and the girls had no choice but to follow.

A small, rolling mountainscape provided the backdrop to Rosestead on the left side. Several dozen thatch-roofed Viking longhouses—some large, some small; some clearly private residences, some workshops and businesses—were scattered about a private lake on the opposite side from the wooded hillside. She assumed that the lake led out to the ocean, because there were several beached longships, which would be of no use on a mere lake. In the middle of these longhouses, set back and elevated somewhat, was a larger dwelling that could only be described as a wooden, fortlike castle.

"That structure doesn't seem to fit in with the Viking ones," Maggie remarked to Joe, having to practically skip to keep up with his long strides.

"You are right. It is more in the Saxon and Frankish manner of building, but, if my eyes tell me true, 'tis identical to my father's home in Vestfold," he observed. "Some of the kings and jarls of Norway in the late tenth century were building castles of wood, just so. Longhouses were becoming too small for their extended families and housecarls and *hird*s of soldiers."

She nodded. If she hadn't already accepted that Joe had somehow come to her from another time, his ease in discussing the everyday life of the Dark Ages would have impressed her now.

"Look, Mom, look!" Suzy was gazing at the

lake, where a group of young people had begun ice-skating.

"Can we go, too? Please. Please. Please," Beth added.

"Maybe later," Maggie said, though why she would make even that tentative promise when they were already trespassing was beyond her.

A young, thirtyish man in a crew cut, jeans, and a sweatshirt that read, *U.S. Army* came out of one of the first buildings and yelled at them, "Hey, you guys. You can't come in here. The place is closed for . . ." He was striding quickly toward them when his steps faltered and his words trailed off. "Holy cow!" he muttered. At first Maggie thought he was awestruck because he thought Joe was a Navy SEAL, as evidenced by his jacket; many people were dazzled by the prestigious military unit. And he was apparently an ex-army man. But then she noticed that he was staring fixedly at Joe's face. He looked as if he'd seen a ghost.

"Who are you?" Joe demanded of the young man. His tone was so imperious, he sounded like some visiting warlord.

"Mike Johnson. The curator," he replied, not even questioning Joe's authority to grill him. "Who are *you*?"

"Jorund Ericsson."

Mike Johnson nodded. Then, with a disbelieving shake of his head, he repeated, "Holy freakin' cow!"

A young woman with blond hair and a little boy of five or so came out of the longhouse where Mike Johnson had originally emerged. Maggie assumed it was his wife and child. The woman watched Joe, wide-eyed, then exchanged a look with her husband.

"Where is your chieftain?" Joe asked. "The jarl of Rosestead?"

Mike inclined his head toward the wood castle, and Joe immediately stomped off in that direction. Maggie took Suzy's and Beth's hands and followed after him.

As they walked along, people were coming out of the longhouses, some in Viking attire, which they all probably wore during the regular tourist season, but most of them in jeans or sweatpants. There seemed to be a large number of young people. Hadn't Beth told them, when surfing the Web site, that there was a residential program for homeless inner-city kids here?

Interestingly, although this was a Viking village, there were Christmas decorations on many of the longhouses, a light-up Santa and a reindeer panorama in the front yard of another, and lots of illuminated pine trees. So it was a modern-day Viking village, she supposed.

No one tried to halt their progress, though they were clearly outsiders, trespassing. Little by little, the people following in Joe's wake grew into a murmuring crowd.

"Mommy, I'm scared," Beth said.

"Everyone's acting weird," Suzy added. "Even Joe."

"Don't worry, kiddos. It's just that Joe looks like a Viking, and this is a Viking village. They've probably never seen a *real* Viking before." That sounded like a good explanation. Too bad Suzy and Beth weren't buying it any more than she was.

Maggie wished Joe would take her hand. Instead he seemed to be oblivious to her presence. Soon his longer stride caused them to be left behind . . . at first only a few paces, then a greater and greater distance. To Maggie's dismay, she realized that he didn't even care whether she was there anymore, so intent was he on this . . . this thing that was drawing him.

Was this the beginning of the end?

Rosestead felt like home to Jorund.

There were differences, of course. Cold as it was here, winter in his country was frigid. A man's mustache and nose hairs developed icicles with just a brief visit to the garderobe. Some men claimed it was so cold their piss froze the second it left their bodies. In addition, the light coating of snow on the ground would have been eaves-high at his homestead by now, and would stay that way or pile higher till the spring thaw. The landscape itself was different, too. The northern fields were mostly rocky and untillable, unless they were farmed by skilled farmers like his brother, Magnus. But here, he could see, there would be thriving wheat fields and vegetable patches by midsummer.

Despite the differences, Jorund reveled in his first glimpse of the familiar wattle-and-daub longhouses with their thatch and sod roofs, the wooden keep so like his father's, and the dragon-ships. His throat constricted as he walked swiftly into the village. He had not realized how home-sick he was till now.

He passed the dragonships, which were propped on wooden cradles. Then he did a double take.

Holy Thor! There was a colorful figurehead on one of the prows that appeared identical to the one he'd given Rolf as a coarse jest years ago—a figure of a buxom blond woman with cherry-red nipples. They'd dubbed the wooden wench Ingrid, as he recalled. *How odd!* Had a copy of this figurehead been made in his country by the craftsman who'd chiseled the first? Or had this figurehead gone down with Rolf's ship a thousand years ago, and ended up on some beach as flotsam?

Well, that was of little import now. He needed to speak with the leader of this village. There were some significant questions he wanted to ask, like, How did his family crest get on Rosestead's Webbing site? Why did this keep so resemble his father's? What was the Ingrid figurehead doing here?

A man wearing standard Viking attire of a belted leather tunic over black *braies* and cross-gartered half boots, stepped out of the giant double doors of the keep. He walked across the small wooden bridge that traversed a narrow dry moat. Beside him on one side was a small boy of about two winters, clinging to his hand. On the other was a woman with long, auburn hair and green eyes. In her arms was a warmly bundled babe of perhaps a few months.

As the man came closer, Jorund got his first good view of him, then said with a gasp, *"Guð minn góður!"* Stopping in his tracks, he repeated in English, "My God!"

The man did likewise, muttering, *"Bld hel!"* He released the child's grasp to put both hands to his face, rubbing his eyes in disbelief. Except for the darker blond color of his hair, the resemblance between him and Jorund was remarkable. That

338

was why all the inhabitants of this village had been gawking at him so, he realized now.

It was his brother, Rolf.

"Jorund!" Rolf shouted joyously, now that his initial shock had passed.

"Rolf!" Jorund exclaimed, and rushed forward to grasp his younger brother, who was the same massive height as he, and lift him high in the hair, swinging him around as his father used to do with his mother when he came home after a long voyage a-Viking.

Once Jorund released his brother, they embraced tightly, choked with emotion. Then they stood, simply staring at each other with stupid delight. They both had tears in their eyes, which they wiped away surreptitiously.

"How did you get here?" Rolf asked.

"On a flying machine. An airplane," he informed him with disgust.

"From Vestfold? And the tenth century?" Rolf's mouth dropped open with surprise.

"Nay, you lackbrain, not from Vestfold. From Tax-us."

Rolf shook his head briskly from side to side, like a wet dog who had fallen into a fjord. "How the bloody hell did you get to Texas?"

"Ha! Funny you should ask! On the back of a killer whale. Do you believe it?"

"A . . . a killer whale?"

He nodded. "Her name is Thora."

"A whale with a name?"

"And Joe was buck-naked, too," Sue-zee offered with a little giggle, coming up behind them.

"Oh, I do not believe this," Rolf said, reaching down to lift both Suzy and Beth into his arms and give each of them a hug and a kiss. When he put them down, the girls scurried back to their mother, a little bit frightened by this exuberant stranger. "You brought Greta and Girta here? On the back of a whale? Was that not foolhardy of you?"

At first Jorund did not understand. Then he realized that Rolf thought these twins were his twins. "No, brother, these girls do not belong to me," he explained.

The expression of hurt on Suzy's and Beth's faces cut him to the quick. So he quickly added, "But they are the daughters of my heart."

The girls beamed.

"I will tell you of Inga and Greta and Girta later. Suffice it to say, they died in the famine."

"Oh, Jorund!" Rolf commiserated sadly and gave him another bear hug.

Jorund noticed Mag-he standing there silently, as well as the woman with the babe and child next to Rolf. He had been rude in ignoring them all, especially Mag-he, who had brought him, reluctantly, to this joyous homecoming. Tucking an arm around her shoulder, he drew her closer, and introduced everyone all around. "Rolf, this is my . . . uh, friend, Dock-whore Mag-he Muck-bride." He had been about to say "my leman," but suspected that Mag-he would not appreciate that title. Then, "Mag-he, this is my little brother, Rolf."

"Little?" Rolf scoffed.

"Younger, then."

"The brother you were searching for?" Mag-he asked.

"Yea, the very one. Isn't it wonderful?"

"More than wonderful," Mag-he said softly, and he knew they had much to discuss, later, about the implications of this reunion.

Then Rolf introduced his wife, Profess-whore Merry-death Ericsson, his son Foster, and his new daughter, Rose. *A wife? What an amazing happenstance! Methought Rolf would never wed again. Methought he liked his freedom too much.*

"A profess-whore?" Jorund asked with a grin.

"A dock-whore?" Rolf asked with a grin.

The two ladies shook their heads at each other, as if their men were hopeless youths.

"Seems to me there are way too many whores in this country," Jorund quipped, and Mag-he elbowed him in the ribs.

Despite his attempt at mirth, Jorund was puzzled. How could Rolf have left Norway one year ago, in 997, and already have two children? It was all so confusing. Perhaps the time portals where they had entered were just different . . . years could be gained or lost in the passing. Perhaps he could have even left after Rolf, but arrived before him.

It was enough to muddle the brain, if his weren't already muddled.

The women and children were all shivering in the cold. Rolf motioned for everyone behind them to go on home and invited the rest of them to come inside.

With his arm looped over Jorund's shoulder, Rolf said, "I have been praying for a sign from the past."

Jorund arched an eyebrow at him. "You? Praying?" Then, "Hell and Valhalla! I am your sign?"

341

"Yea." His brother nodded. "Finally, someone I can best in swordplay."

"Hah!" From the time they were children, Jorund had always triumphed over his brothers in the military arts.

"There will be no swordplay here." Rolf's wife spoke up for the first time. "Remember what happened the last time? Mike had to get fifteen stitches."

"Whate'er you say, dearling," Rolf replied, then rolled his eyes at Jorund, as if fifteen stitches were a mere child's wound.

It was.

"By the by," Rolf remarked then. "When did you arrive in this land?"

"Three months ago."

"Three months! What have you been doing all this time?"

"Well, of late, I have been teaching demented people."

Rolf stopped walking and stared at him, gape-mouthed, as if he were himself demented, which of course they had thought he was at one time.

Then, just to tease his brother, he added, "In a madhouse."

Rolf's jaw dropped a notch lower.

Leaning close to his brother's ear, he confided, "One of the pay-shuns is a sex addict. Another thinks he is Moses, on the days when he is not Charlemagne. Still another cannot get his cock to rise. One wench sings all day long. And there is a Norse there named Glad-ass. Is that not amazing, Rolf?"

Bursting out with a short laugh, Rolf punched him in the arm. "You are making all this up."

"Nay, I am not. 'Tis true. Really." He called up to Mag-he, who was walking beside Rolf's wife, Merry-death, conversing softly with her. "Mag-he, tell Rolf the truth. Do you and I not work in a madhouse?"

She cringed at his words. "We work in a *mental-health facility*," she said, making a point of the distinction in wording. "The word *madhouse* is not used anymore, Joe."

"Madhouse, mental-health facility . . . 'tis the same thing," he whispered to Rolf. But to Mag-he he said, "Whate'er you say, dearling," repeating his brother's response to his wife. A fine response it was, too. It was always best to let women *think* they had the upper hand.

"Why does she call you Joe?"

Jorund shrugged. " 'Tis a nicking name."

Rolf burst out with a chuckle. "Joe the Viking?"

Jorund rolled his shoulders in a gesture meant to convey, *What could I do?*

But then Rolf smiled at him, hooking an arm around his neck and yanking him close. " 'Twould seem that you and I have much to discuss, brother."

That was the Viking version of an understatement.

They were sitting at the high table in Rolf's great hall, the men sipping mead and the women tea. It was like stepping back in time, right down to the primitive weapons on the walls. During their tourist season, there were even rushes on the floor, which Meredith claimed were a pain in the neck to keep clean.

Lunch had been over an hour ago, but Maggie

was still in a state of shock. She'd sent Suzy and Beth out with some of the older kids, including a girl named Thea, who'd come up with extra ice skates for them, along with gloves, knit caps, and warmer jackets. Maggie had been assured the ice was very thick and completely safe.

She liked Rolf and his wife . . . a lot. Right now Meredith was discreetly nursing her three-month-old baby under a receiving blanket thrown over her shoulder. Maggie couldn't help noticing the way Rolf's loving gaze kept going back to his wife, even as he spoke with Joe. And Meredith was equally enamored of her husband, which was evident in the pleasure she displayed over her husband's joy in being reunited with his brother. Whatever made him happy made her happy; that was obvious.

"Besotted, are you?" Joe teased his brother. Apparently he had observed the same bond between Rolf and Meredith.

"For a certainty," Rolf admitted without hesitation, leaning over to kiss his wife loudly on the mouth, then to give an equally loud smack to his now-sleeping daughter's cheek.

Both brothers had been talking rapidly ever since they'd come inside, catching up on all their news. Joe told Rolf everything that had happened to him since he'd arrived in Texas, and it was interesting to hear the spin he put on everything. All agreed that Joe's method of time travel, atop a killer whale, naked, was much more dramatic than Rolf's simple shipwreck. And all agreed, as well, that not one, but two brothers being time travelers was a remarkable coincidence.

As Joe and Rolf continued to reminisce, Maggie asked Meredith, "Didn't you find it hard to accept the concept of time travel?"

"Absolutely," Meredith said. "I still do."

Maggie nodded. It was the same with her. She accepted and did not accept at the same time.

"I'm a professor of medieval studies at Oxley College. My parents are professors. My grandfather was, too. All my life I was trained to believe in scientific, scholarly methods of research. I think that the only way I was able to reconcile logic with such a fantastic notion as time travel was that it was a miracle."

"That's amazing. I came to the same conclusion."

"I can't believe in time travel as a scientific concept . . ." Meredith started to explain.

"But you can accept a God with the power to do anything," Maggie finished for her.

"Right," Meredith agreed with a smile. "I really, really needed Rolf at the time when he arrived. I didn't realize it at first, of course, but in the end the things he brought to me . . . well, I can only describe him as a miracle."

Suzy and Beth burst into the great hall then, along with the other excited children. Thea, who was Meredith's fifteen-year-old niece, wrapped her arms around Rolf's neck from behind, hugging him tightly. Her hair was purple, and she had five earrings in each ear and an eyebrow ring. Maggie imagined that she'd make an interesting Viking maiden during the tourist season. Her mother, Meredith's sister, was in London at the moment, trying to establish new markets for the reproduction Viking jewelry that was crafted at Rosestead.

345

Her daughters' faces were red. Snow dusted their bright caps and gloves. They were gloriously happy, as only children could be.

And where did they rush first? To Joe. Maggie wasn't offended, though. Instinctively she understood how important he'd become in their lives. He didn't supplant her; he supplemented her.

With both of them speaking at once, it was hard to decipher their words, but mostly they were talking about how exciting it had been to ice-skate, and wasn't snow the greatest invention in the world, and would he please, please, please be on their side in the upcoming snowball fight?

Joe listened attentively to all they said, seeming to be able to decipher who was saying what. He nodded and smiled, tugged playfully on Suzy's braids, and whisked some snowflakes off Beth's eyelashes. And Maggie's heart swelled and swelled and swelled.

She looked at Meredith, and Meredith looked back at her with understanding. Maggie had never realized just how much her daughters had needed a father figure in their lives—a man just like Joe. Was it really as simple as the fact that they had prayed on a wishing star, and God had sent them Joe?

Truly, she concluded, her Viking had been a miracle, too. A Christmas miracle.

Chapter Eighteen

Later that day, Jorund was still touring the Rose-stead village.

"I'm impressed," he told his brother. "Not just because you have built a thriving shipbuilding concern, and a world outlet for Norse crafts, and a tourist attraction, but you help troubled children as well. And look at how much you do to educate people in this land about Vikings."

"I *am* proud of my work," Rolf admitted with no token show of humility. It was the way of the men-folk in his family. 'Twas especially important to me that this enterprise succeed so that I could find a place for myself in this new world. I'm not sure what I could have done, if not for this."

Jorund understood. "A man needs to find work that suits his talents and feeds his soul."

"Yea, that is it exactly. Oh, I suppose I could

have gotten work as a carpenter, but I doubt I could have worked for someone else. I am too used to leading."

That sentiment Jorund agreed with, too. In truth, he was not sure he could fit in so well in this society.

"What will you do now?" Rolf asked. "Now that you have found me . . . does that not fulfill our father's wishes?"

"I am not sure," he answered truthfully. "One part of me is joyous and says I am finally free. . . ."

"Free to do what?"

"That is the problem. I'm not sure. Just free, I suppose. Another part of me argues that I must go back. Do you know—I probably shouldn't tell you this—but on one of the Enter-net history sites, it says that our father died in the year 999. That is only one year from the time I left. Mayhap if I go back I can forestall his passing on to Valhalla. And there was another thing, too. I saw my sword—the very sword I carry with me now—pictured on that Webbing site. It said that the sword was buried in my grave mound. Surely that means that I must go back."

"The Webbing site also mentioned that the grave mound was for me, too, and I am not returning. It must be a mistake." Rolf frowned with bafflement.

"I do not know," Jorund answered desolately. "Mayhap I died far from home. All I know is that our father cannot be left ignorant of your fate . . . before he dies." He added that last with a choked sound of pain. All of the Ericsson children were fond of their father.

Rolf put a hand on his shoulder. "Merry-death is an expert on ancient studies, and she tells me that the dates in the tenth-century histories are rarely accurate. Besides, it is not your responsibility."

"He is our father," Jorund cried out.

"Yea, he is, and though I expect ne'er to see him again in this life, it does not mean I love him any less because I choose to live my life here."

"But it's cruel not to let our father know that we—I mean, you—are well."

"I will say this, brother: you were ever the one to take on all the world's responsibilities."

Jorund bristled. "What mean you by that blather?"

" 'Tis not blather. Many a man would have refused to wed Inga if tricked into wedlock the way you were, but you felt responsible. Many a man has lost children and not felt the massive guilt that weighs you down, but you feel responsible. Many a man would have considered his father-duty ended when he completed his mission, but you feel a responsibility to tell our father in person. When does your responsibility to others end and your own happiness take precedence?"

He accepted that Rolf meant well, and much of what he said was true, but a strong sense of duty was in Jorund's nature. He could not change. Nor did he want to. At least, that was what he told himself. Inside he was not so sure.

"What of your Mag-he? Do you have a responsibility to her, as well?"

He shook his head. "Mag-he understands."

"Does she?"

He cocked his head to the side. "Do you doubt that?"

Rolf shrugged. "I don't know. I suspect you are confused right now, and I do not want you to make any hasty decisions."

"I won't," he promised. "In the meanwhile, I am obliged to attend a singing competition on New Year's Eve . . . involving one of the pay-shuns from the madhouse—I mean, mental-health facility." He grinned at his brother on making that correction. "Then, Sue-zee and Beth's birthing day is in February. I should probably stay till then. And Beth is planning a big protesting march at the orca park in April, and she asked specifically if I would be there for support, but—"

"More responsibilities?" Rolf was grinning at him knowingly.

"Then, too, I would really like to stay long enough to find out what happens to Josh and Reva." He ducked his head sheepishly.

"*The Guiding Light!* Do you watch that show, too? Ah, it is one of my favorites."

"Those two would make wonderful Vikings, do you not think?"

"I have said so on many an occasion to Merry-death. And Alan Spaulding, he would be a true Viking villain, if you ask me. Much like that Storr Grimmsson."

"Who is dead, by the by, thanks to our father's men. Be assured there was a long torture afore his passing to avenge what he did to cause your shipwreck."

Rolf nodded his approval. "And may he be swiving Hel, the queen of the dead, in her icy home in Niflheim, as we speak."

They smiled at each other, being reminded that they were of like minds.

"You know, Rolf, there is so much that is better in this land than what we had, but the excess bothers me."

"I cannot believe this. I had the same feelings when first I arrived. How can men be men if their hard work is not required to bring food to the table and shelter overhead?"

Jorund nodded. "And they take all this abundance for granted. When wealth comes too easily, it is not appreciated. And I'll tell you something else: this business of men and women being equal is sheer nonsense. Men are men, and women are women. Each have their given tasks. . . . Why are you grinning?"

"Because my wife would knock you over the head with an oar if she heard you talk so."

"Mag-he would no doubt do the same, but that does not make it less true." Jorund raised his chin defiantly.

They slapped their arms around each other's shoulders then and started to walk back toward the keep. Dusk was approaching early, and the snow was falling more heavily. Jorund inhaled deeply of the cold air. Just like home, he thought.

"I'll tell you one thing I favor about this country." Rolf wagged his eyebrows mischievously. "Drekking."

"Drekking? What in bloody hell is that?"

"Well, I have developed a fondness for this particular kind of hair soap called Breck, which is no longer sold in this country, but Merry-death and I bought boxloads of it from a remainder outlet. In any case, there is this most delicious activity that a man and woman can do together in the shower with Breck." He rolled his eyes meaningfully. "Drekking."

"Now, that is something I understand. You can do the same with liquid body soap."

Rolf's jaw dropped open. Apparently he hadn't expected his brother to adapt as well as he had.

"Why are you so surprised?"

"I am surprised because you were never so frivolous afore. In truth, from the time we were youthlings together you were always somber."

"Frivolous? Pfff. What is frivolous about sexplay? Did you think I was a monk just because I performed the somber work of war?"

Rolf grinned at him. Really, Jorund thought, his brother was doing a great amount of grinning today, at his expense.

"I will give this land credit for two things: Big Macs and french fries," Jorund remarked. "Ne'er have I eaten such delicacies, even in the courts of Byzantium."

"Hah! I think the greatest delicacy is Oreos."

"Too sweet!"

"Too greasy!"

They were about to argue the point further; then both shrugged.

"There is one remarkable thing I have noticed about this land—" Jorund started to say, then stopped himself. Why give his brother cause for more grinning?

"What?" Rolf prodded. "Do not be shy now, brother."

Jorund knew he would regret his hasty words, but . . . *What the hell!* That was a handy expression Steve had taught him. With his eyes at half-mast, he slowly divulged, "Well, have you noticed how much bigger your staff gets in this land?"

At first Rolf just stared at him blankly. Then his gaze moved lower, to his groin. "*That* staff?"

"Of course, *that* staff. How many other staffs are there?"

"And yours is bigger in this land?"

"Immense."

"You lie." Rolf hooted. Then, "Show me."

"I do not lie, and I will not show you. Besides, it only gets big when I am around Mag-he."

"You lackbrain. All men's man parts get big when they are aroused by their women."

"I know that," Jorund said with disgust. His brother was speaking to him as if he were an untried boy. "I am talking of huge. Not big, *huge.*"

"Methinks time travel has distorted your eyes."

"Methinks I will never tell you any secrets ever again."

"That is not a secret. That is news of great import. Viking men throughout the Old World will be seeking to travel to the future on the promise of that alone—big cocks."

Rolf and Jorund were laughing heartily when they reentered the keep.

"What's up?" Merry-death and Mag-he asked them both at the same time.

The women could not understand why that simple question caused the two brothers to burst into more hysterical laughter.

After three days, it was time to go home.

Suzy and Beth were already in the rental car, but they had the windows open and were waving and saying last-minute good-byes to all their new-

Sandra Hill

found friends. There were promises of e-mail letters to be exchanged and possible future visits.

Mike Johnson had been taking photographs the entire time during their visit, and now he was snapping last-minute shots . . . group pictures, individual ones, all different combinations. He was going to the one-hour processing center that afternoon and promised to send copies to them in Texas as soon as they were developed.

"Come back anytime," Meredith urged, hugging Maggie warmly. "It's especially beautiful here in the summer."

"Maybe." Maggie hugged her back.

It was odd, but she and the girls had been accepted by Rolf and Meredith like family. And yet they were not. Their only link with this Rosestead family was through Joe, whose connection with them was tenuous, to say the least.

She and Meredith glanced over to the side, where Rolf and Joe were talking seriously with each other. Whether Maggie and her daughters ever returned to Rosestead would depend on whether Joe stayed with her. And that was not a given, by any means.

Maggie had seen a different side of Joe here in the village. He was in his element, wearing Viking clothing, speaking Old Norse, teaching swordplay to the young men, playing Viking board games like *hnefatafl*, arm wrestling with his brother, engaging in footraces and horse races, drinking honeyed mead from a hand-carved horn, helping to chisel with an adz in Rolf's ship-building shop, chopping firewood like a demon, talking of his other life . . . a life Maggie could not understand, let alone share.

354

Deep down, Maggie sensed that Joe wanted to go back to his own time. Oh, his brother had managed to adapt to this modern life, but he had a skill—building ships—that was still valued today. What would Joe do if he stayed? Really, what kind of demand was there for a man who wielded a wicked sword? How long would it be before his self-esteem as a man began to slip? Would he become half a man . . . like his friend Steve?

And Maggie couldn't see his coming to work with his brother, either. This was Rolf's place . . . his small niche in modern society. Two strong, independent men like these two, would never be able to share leadership without eventually clashing.

"Don't expect too much too soon."

Maggie was jarred from her meandering thoughts by Meredith's admonition. "I wasn't—"

"Shhh," Meredith said, reaching over to wipe a tear from Maggie's cheek with a tissue.

Maggie hadn't even realized she'd begun weeping. "I thought that the only stumbling block to Joe's staying here in the future with me and my daughters was finding his brother," she confided. "Well, he's found his brother, but Joe hasn't said a word since we've been here. His silence is telling."

"It means that he's probably confused," Meredith said.

"Yes, it does. And I just don't understand why," Maggie cried.

Meredith thought carefully before she spoke. "These Viking men have to make the choice themselves. They do not think or act according to

355

our feminine whims. Did you know that Rolf left me for six weeks before we got back together? He let me think that he had died, or gone back to the past."

"No!" Maggie exclaimed. Then, "Did you whack him upside the head when you found out?"

"For sure," Meredith answered with a little laugh. "Rolf had to go back to present-day Norway, and then England, to get some answers before he made the decision to stay with me."

"Love wasn't enough?"

"Love wasn't enough."

Maggie let Meredith's comforting words sink in. "But Joe might be different. He might decide that the best thing would be to go back to his own time."

"He might," Meredith agreed. "That's something you have to prepare yourself for."

"I'm trying. In fact, I think I've been girding myself for that eventuality almost from the first time I met him. This relationship screamed *heartbreak* from the get-go."

"No," Meredith corrected. "I suspect it screamed 'the love of your life, baby' from the get-go. The fact that there might be some heartbreak as well was secondary."

"You're very wise. You should have been a psychologist," Maggie said, laughing.

"Come back," Meredith urged, repeating her earlier words. "No matter what . . . come back."

"I will," Maggie promised then, opening the driver's door of the car, but waiting for Joe before entering. "No matter what."

* * *

Jorund had said his farewells to his brother, and it was time to go.

"Will I see you again, Jorund? Ever?"

He shrugged. "You could come to Tax-us. Really, we could buy you a pair of cow-man boots. For you, I might even line dance."

Rolf smiled sadly, not at all taken in by his brother's teasing words or evasive response.

"I do not know," Jorund answered finally.

Rolf let out a whoosh of exasperation. "Why do you always make life so difficult? Really, it is an easy decision."

"Was it an easy decision for you?"

"Nay, but my situation was different."

"Hah! So you say now."

"Jorund, I thought I had to go back to complete our father's mission . . . a different one from yours, I concede, but his mission nonetheless. When I found out it was no longer necessary, I immediately returned to Merry-death. You thought the same thing—that you had to complete our father's mission—but your work is done."

"I am not sure of that."

Rolf pulled at his hair, which he had left loose today, the dark blond strands lying like a swath of gold on his shoulders. "You are so damn stubborn."

Jorund raised his brows sardonically. "Like you, mayhap?"

Rolf laughed and put an arm around his brother's shoulders, hugging him close as they began to walk toward the car.

"I am not like you, Rolf," he tried one last time to explain. "I need to have things settled one way

357

or another. I could not bear to stay here and know I had responsibilities elsewhere that I had neglected to satisfy my own whims. I could not bear to stay here knowing that at any minute that bloody whale might flip me back in time. I could not bear to stay and build strong bonds with Mag-he and her daughters, only to hurt them more by leaving later."

"Do you love the wench, Jorund?"

"Of course."

"Then you already know the answer, lackbrain."

He looked at Mag-he standing near the open door of the car, snowflakes powdering her too-short hair. She glanced in his direction, as if sensing his thoughts. There were tears in her misty blue eyes, and he knew the tears were for him . . . not for their departure from Rosestead.

Like a knife to his heart was Jorund's knowledge that he could hurt this woman so easily. Yes, he had his answer.

Better the small cut now than the open wound later.

It was New Year's Eve at the Boot Scootin' Cowboy.

Three whole tables of ten each were filled with friends of Natalie Blue, including her family, fellow group members, and some of the staff from Rainbow . . . even the new owner, Jerome Johnson and his lovely wife Freda, who loved country music. There was a festive air in the crowded club due to its being New Year's Eve, complete with glittery decorations, confetti, funny hats, and noisemakers.

But there was tension in the air, too, due to the

talent show, which was about to start. Judges
were already beginning to sit down at the long
folding tables set up in the center of the now-
empty dance floor. The judges were several radio
and TV country-music program hosts, a Nashville
record producer, a talent agent, and various other
local celebrities.

Tension wasn't just in the air, either. Maggie
looked at Joe, who was fidgeting in his chair.
Every couple of minutes, he would glance at the
doorway, as if he expected someone. In fact, he'd
insisted that a couple of chairs be left empty at
their table, on the other side of Steve, who sat
next to him, spiffily attired in a herringbone sport
coat with gray slacks and a white golf shirt, open
at the collar. He and Joe had taken up jogging the
last few days, since their return from Maine, as
part of Rainbow's physical-fitness program.
While Joe had always looked good to her, Steve's
appearance had taken a decided turn for the better. His skin was no longer pale, but tan and
healthy. He had always had an athlete's body, but
something about the way he carried himself had
changed. In an instant she realized that he carried himself just like Joe . . . with self-confidence.

"You've been a good influence on Steve," Maggie commented to Joe.

"Do you think so?" His lips turned up with genuine pleasure. God, he was a handsome man.
Tonight he wore his hair slicked back into its
usual queue and he'd shaved, so his face was
smooth. A trip to the mall yesterday had resulted
in her red sequined sheath and black high heels—
Joe's choice, accompanied by some hot looks and

a few winks—and his navy blue suit, white shirt, and tie. He wore the latter under protest, deeming it a torture device. It had seemed particularly important to Joe that tonight he fit what he considered the image of a modern man. Of course, he wore his cowboy boots—another torture device, in his opinion—so she guessed it was the image of the modern *Texas* man.

"Yes, I do think so. Steve's whole demeanor has changed, largely due to his association with you."

"That and getting a prescription for Viagra from that new doctor." Joe grinned at her as he spoke. More than once Joe had expressed amazement that there was a little blue pellet in modern times that could create such magic. More seriously he remarked, "You know, in the Norse culture, a man's worth is often measured by how well he fights. Valhalla, hall of the gods, is open only to warriors who die in battle. But I've been thinking that mayhap the true measure of a man should be how he has touched other people afore his death."

Maggie's heart constricted at such sensitivity coming from what, at the core, was a primitive man.

"I mean, think about it, Mag-he. What good is a man though he be the greatest soldier of all time, if he trod over those who surrounded him in everyday life? Believe me, I know many such men, and they are considered heroes."

"To me, you're the real hero." She said the words teasingly, but she meant them sincerely.

He put a hand to her nape and pulled her close for a quick kiss on the head. "Thank you, sweetling." Then he nuzzled her neck. "You smell so good. Years from now I do not think I will ever smell the scent of lilacs without thinking of you."

There was a drumroll then as the lights dimmed and a spotlight shone on the stage. The competition was about to begin. But Maggie's thoughts were centered on Joe's last, revealing words. He probably didn't realize what he had subconsciously let slip. The infuriating man was contemplating a future without her in it; she just knew it. They hadn't discussed the future since their return from Maine, though it loomed silently between them all the time. She hadn't pressed him for a decision, fearing what he would say. And he hadn't brought up the subject, she suspected, because he was still so confused.

Not a promising beginning for the New Year.

Six of the contestants had given their performances by the time a break was called and the lights were turned up. Natalie would be in the second round, and she was looking mighty nervous after hearing and seeing such talent in the first half—singing, guitar playing, comedy routines, clogging.

Everyone was ordering drinks or making quick runs to the rest rooms or conversing quietly when Joe stiffened and stared at the front door. The others at their table followed his gaze, noticing the strange intensity of his stare. Steve was the last to look because his back had been to the door, and he had to strain to look over his shoulder. Then he stood so suddenly that he knocked his chair over.

Steve stared at the doorway, then glared at Joe. "You interfering son of a bitch!" he said with a snarl. But his attention immediately returned to the doorway.

A woman in her mid-forties stood there, tall and thin and attractive in a natural, un-made-up way. Her blond hair hung straight to her shoulders. She wore a plain denim jumper under a heavy, fleece-lined winter jacket...unusual for Texas. In her hand was a small piece of carry-on luggage.

Steve put his hand to his mouth, where a small moan escaped. In his eyes, tears were already beginning to well into green pools.

"Shelley," he cried then, joyously, but he seemed frozen in place.

Even though it all happened in a flash, the scenario that followed was like a slow-motion film clip. She dropped the suitcase and ran toward him, a clear pathway being made by the curious spectators. "Steve," she practically screamed, and hurled herself into his arms.

Hugging each other tightly, as if they would never let go, he kept repeating, "Ah, Shelley. Ah, Shelley. Ah, Shelley."

And she kept saying, "You dumb jerk! How could you leave? How could you hide from me all these years? You dumb jerk!"

"I did it for you," he said.

"For me? You just about killed me. I kept expecting you to come back when you came to your senses. First it was one week. Then a month. Then years. You are dumber than Idaho dirt if you think you helped me by leaving." Still holding on tightly to his shoulders, she leaned her head back to look at him. "I could kill you."

He nodded, and kissed her with all the pent-up feeling that had been building in him over ten long years.

Finally she pushed him away gently and motioned for someone to come forward... someone who must have been standing behind her in the doorway. It was a boy.

"There's someone I want you to meet," Shelly said in a choked voice.

She took the hand of the boy—a boy of about nine years, with unique green eyes and a wiry, athletic body. On the shirt under his denim jacket could be read the words, *My Dad Was a Navy SEAL.*

Steve stared blankly at first, then put his face in both hands to hide the silent sobs that were racking him.

Shelly was merciless. "Steve, let me introduce you to Steven Askey, Jr."

Steve dropped his hands and murmured, "Sweet Jesus!"

"Dad?" The boy gazed up in adoration at a man he had never seen in person.

Only then did Steve reach for the boy and lift him high into his arms and give him a big bear hug.

"Hello, son."

An hour later Maggie finally got the chance to say to Joe, "Tell me how you found Steve's wife."

"Beth."

"*Beth?*"

"Yea, Beth told me you can find anyone on the Enter-net. And we did."

"I don't understand."

"The newspaper photographs of Steve at that warrior's wall apparently traveled across the country on some wiring service, whatever that is," he explained. "Shelley saw the picture in a newspaper in I-duh-hoe and has been trying to find Steve ever since. A fruitless search. She ne'er thought to look in a madhouse . . . I mean, mental-health facility. In any case, Beth and Sue-zee helped me phone Shelley in I-duh-hoe after we found her message on the Enter-net."

It took several minutes for everything he'd said to sink in. "Why, that little stinker! She kept a secret from her mother."

"Do not be angry with her. She—I—feared you would raise objections to my interfering in Steve's life that way."

"I would have."

"Yea, but look how well everything turned out."

"It did. I can't deny that," Maggie conceded, "but as a psychologist, I must say shock therapy is not standard procedure. By taking all the control safeguards out of the scenario—like having a private setting, removing the surprise element, asking for permission—this could just as easily have been a disaster."

Joe groaned. "We are back to the control thing again, are we not?"

She had to laugh. "Maybe you're right. Anyhow, everything worked out fine, but would you do me a favor? Consult me first in the future."

He nodded vigorously, which meant he would do whatever he damn well pleased, as always. "You look beautiful tonight, dearling," Joe observed then. He had a habit of changing the subject without warning, but sometimes in the most pleasant ways.

"You look pretty handsome yourself, fellow."

"Are you wearing undergarments under that skimpy apparel?"

"*Skimpy*? You picked it out."

"Yea, I did." He smiled at her, that slow, lazy smile that she loved.

"No, I'm not."

"Good thing that Sue-zee and Beth are staying with the sitting person tonight, then."

Maggie thought it was a good thing, too. It had been a week since she'd made love with Joe, and she needed that intimacy so much. Without the reinforcement of their loving, she feared that Joe would drift away from her. An irrational concern, she supposed, but when was love rational?

"How did you find out about Steve's son, by the way?"

"I did not know till I called Shelley on the telephone."

"How could Steve have a son when he's always claimed to be impotent?"

"Ah, but remember that he said it has been ten years since he last made love. Apparently 'twas a dismal effort on his part, which was what caused his abrupt departure. But 'twas not dismal enough that it did not result in his seed being planted in his wife's body."

She nodded. "Oh, look. It's almost Natalie's turn. I hope they come back soon." Steve and his newfound family were off in a private dining area, reacquainting themselves with each other. Natalie had just stepped onto the stage when they slipped into the empty seats. They seemed ecstatically happy. Steve's fingers were laced with Shelley's and his eyes kept going to his son.

Natalie was the eleventh of twelve performers scheduled. To say she was nervous was an understatement. All evening she had been going outside with her mother to get fresh air. Maggie only hoped she wasn't having agoraphobic attacks, as well as good old-fashioned stage fright.

"Ladies and gentlemen, our next contestant is Miss Natalie Blue," the announcer said in a deep Texas drawl. "She wanted me to tell y'all that this song is dedicated to the folks at Rainbow . . . but especially to the Viking who's responsible for her being here. Don't know what that means, but let's give a big Texas welcome to this sweet thang from Galveston . . . Miss Natalie Blue."

The stage went dark, and then a single spotlight shone on the young woman standing alone. Natalie looked so pretty in tight black denim jeans with a dress-up cowgirl shirt decorated with fancy fringe. The only problem was that she appeared to be shaking in her boots.

The backup band gave a slight strumming sound of chords . . . her cue to begin. Maggie held her breath. Would Natalie freeze, or bolt? It was an excruciating test to put anyone through, but especially someone with her background. Were they expecting too much of her?

Suddenly Natalie's voice burst forth, filling the entire club with a clear, twangy, poignant resonance. "I . . . fall . . . to pieeeeces . . ." she began the old Patsy Cline favorite, and by the end, she brought down the house. Patsy had never sung the classic as well as Natalie did. A standing ovation was Natalie's reward.

At the end of the evening, winning the free recording session in Nashville was almost superfluous. Natalie had won her greatest success that night in a Galveston night spot.

Maggie glanced at Joe and smiled. "This has been a wonderful night, hasn't it?"

He nodded. "Come, let us dance. It is almost midnight." Maggie had already explained the customs of this celebration.

"Don't you want some champagne?"

He shook his head. "I'd rather be intoxicated by you."

"You sweet talker, you." She laughed.

And suddenly it was midnight, and the band was playing "Auld Lang Syne," and noisemakers were going off, and she was in Joe's arms. The kiss they exchanged was warm and wonderful. Maggie couldn't help wondering then what the new year would bring for them, but she refused to let dismal thoughts ruin her evening.

"Happy New Year, Joe."

"Happy New Year, Mag-he."

As everyone sang the words to the song and came to the part about old acquaintances never being forgotten, Joe whispered in her ear, "I will never forget you, dearling. Never."

Instead of heartening Maggie, his words sounded like a death knell.

Chapter Nineteen

"I want to make slow love to you, heartling."

"Slow, fast . . . it doesn't matter to me," Mag-he said. "I just want to be with you tonight."

He nodded because he understood her need completely.

They were standing in her bedchamber in the wee dark hours of the morning of New Year's Day—nude, having made short work of removing their festive apparel. Thank the gods, Sue-zee and Beth would be gone till daybreak or later, since they were staying the night with the sitting person down the street.

Although he had examined her lush body from head to toe in detail on previous occasions, he could see that Mag-he was still shy with him. Women of his time were not so inhibited about their nudity. What was it about the females of this century? They worried about every little physical flaw: were they too fat? Or too thin? Were their breasts too small? Or too big? Their buttocks were of particular concern. Did they not know that most men favored a well-rounded backside on a woman? A lustful man needed something to grab onto in the bedsport. Besides, his Mag-he was perfect. So her modesty was out of place.

He strode across the small room and lifted her into his arms, causing a little squeal to erupt from her lips. He dumped her unceremoniously on the soft bed and followed after her. The lights were out, but the room was well lit from the full moon and star-filled skies, visible through the large double windows that were open to the cool night air.

She reached up her arms to him, but he shook his head. Instead he placed them above her on the pillows. "Let me do the work in this loveplay," he urged, his voice already raw with passion.

She laughed softly, a nervous, husky sound. "Do you plan on making me wild for you again?"

He had been brushing wisps of hair off her face and pressing butterfly kisses on her forehead and eyebrows and jawline, but he halted momentarily. "Nay . . . yea . . . well, of course I would like you to be wild, but that is not my objective. I just want to pay tribute to your body, which pleases me greatly."

"Oh, Joe."

He loved how his name sounded on her tongue . . . and yes, he had even come to like the shortened name she had given him.

Lying on his side, he kissed her . . . prolonged, deep, wet, drugging kisses that went on forever. "I cannot get enough of your sweet taste," he murmured.

"I feel the same," she whispered back against his lips.

He pulled back slightly. "I make a pledge to you, sweetling. Ne'er will I kiss another woman again . . . unless it be my lady mother or my sister. This delicious exercise that I have learned to savor belongs only to you."

Tears welled in her eyes, and he knew why. It was the unspoken message that he would be back in his own time, where he would have occasion to kiss his mother and sister. Well, so be it. It was a fact—or possible fact—that must be faced. But he could lighten her spirits. "I cannot promise that I will ne'er swive another female for the remainder of my days, though. The male urge is too strong. But I can deny myself the pleasure of kissing. In truth, I misdoubt it would even be a pleasure with another lady."

She gave him a weak punch in the arm. "You lout! Don't you dare think of making love with another woman."

He smiled at her ferociousness. They both knew she would be in no position to know what he did or to do anything about his transgressions.

But then he moved his ministrations lower, caressing her neck and shoulders, even her hairless armpits and the silken skin of her sides leading down to her waist. He grinned when he saw her navel ring glittering in the moonlight.

"Kiss it," she demanded.

Her words caused his groin to tighten and his male organ to swell. He gave the golden ornament and the enticing little cavity behind it a soft lick with his tongue.

She inhaled sharply.

That was a good sign. Viking men knew how to read erotic signals better than any others. At least, that was what Norse fathers had taught their sons.

Best I look for more signs now, he thought with a barely suppressed chuckle.

He worshiped her breasts then. Wetting them to sensitivity, he watched appreciatively as the rosy tips sprang to life under his expert fingers.

"Your mouth is so hot," she said, moaning as he suckled her deeply.

He considered that a compliment, and so did his engorging staff. *Another sign.* He took her nipple deeper, including the puffy areola. His tongue pressed up from the underside, and the roof of his mouth held her breast from the top. Then, and only then, did he show her things he would warrant no modern man ever had. She had taught him about kissing. Now he was showing her the best ways to pleasure a woman.

When he was through tasting her breasts, he reposed on one elbow and examined his work. She had peaked once already—*a definite sign*—and her nipples were wet, rigid pebbles, standing up on swollen breasts like rose-colored sentinels. If he knew what he was doing—and he did—even the air would feel like a caress on her hardened buds now. He would guess that she ached for him . . . not just in her breasts, but below. *Signs, one and all.*

Still leaning over her on a braced elbow, he let his fingers walk their way from breasts to abdomen, which she sucked in sharply, over the slight hillock of her belly, to the dark curls below. Without hesitation, he dipped into her womanly folds and came away with telltale slickness.

"You are ready," he informed her with a groan.

"Yes," she said, spreading her legs in welcome. "Come inside me. Now."

"Yea, I will." He gave her a quick kiss. "But not quite yet. There is something I need to do first."

She groaned. "I'm already wild for you, Joe. What else do you want?"

"This," he said, and rolled over atop her, kneeling betwixt her thighs. He could see by her widened eyes that she knew what he intended next.

She surprised him, though, by saying, "I want to do the same for you, Joe." And then she used wicked, deliciously wanton and explicit words to tell him exactly what she would do to him . . . later. Apparently she was not as timid as he'd thought.

He almost spilled his seed upon the sheets. *So much for signs!*

With adoration, he made love to that part of her body now. He felt almost possessive about the distended folds and sleek moisture, and especially the raised nub that was the seat of her woman-pleasure. The end result was that she lay writhing for satisfaction. The scent and taste and texture of her would remain with him forever.

There was probably a sign in there somewhere, but he'd stopped counting or caring.

Soon he eased himself into her hot sheath. She pulsed as inch by inch he slid into her depth till he was deeply seated, and they were one. Only then did he gaze into her eyes, which were wide and blue and staring directly back at him, reciprocating the adoration he had lavished on her. "I love you," he vowed then. The spoken sentiment came effortlessly to him now . . . straight from his breaking heart.

"I love you, too, Joe," she whispered, and the

words imbedded themselves in his soul . . . to be replayed over and over in some solitary future.

He made slow love to her then, as he had pledged. And from then on, till their simultaneous, crashing peaks, they murmured words of love to each other, poignant expressions of feelings so deep and eternal they seemed hard enough to last a lifetime, and so fragile that they could very well shatter at any moment.

As Mag-he lay, drowsily sated, he glanced through the wide windows and noticed a strange constellation of stars that resembled, of all things, a whale. He did not call the star shape to Mag-he's attention because he knew its significance. It was a time omen.

Jorund wanted to make promises to his beloved Mag-he, who wept silent tears now, but he could not. So he held her through the night, and as she slept, he kept saying over and over, in one form or another, "I may have to leave you, my love, but I also leave behind my heart, forevermore."

Two days later Joe was gone. And this time, Maggie feared, it was for good.

The girls had returned to school for the first time since holiday vacation, and Maggie had spent the morning and part of the afternoon at the hospital till some inner voice had told her to go home. This was not one of Joe's days for working out with the patients in the physical-fitness program, and he should have been at the house. Beth had conned him into helping her with her Keiko project. She was fascinated by what Joe had told her about whales and Viking sailors in the tenth century. Of course, Beth did not know that he knew of these legends firsthand. Beth had shown him how to speak into a tape player to record his tales, which she intended to incorporate into her Web site at a later date.

The house was empty, as she had somehow known it would be. Rita snoozed complacently on her window-seat cushion. If Joe were at home, she would have been off harassing him, with hissing, or shedding, or whatever. She wondered with hysterical irrelevance if Rita would miss him as much as she would.

Even before Maggie entered the den and saw the evidence of Joe's departure, tears were streaming down her face. On the sofa Joe had piled all of the clothing he'd been given or purchased while here, even the running shoes and the cowboy boots that he'd never gotten used to. He must have worn the Viking clothing that his brother Rolf had given him at Rosestead.

On the desk were two audiocassettes with childlike block lettering on them. One said SUE-ZEE AND BETH, and the other said MAG-HE. There was also a scattered pile of photographs . . . the ones they'd received in the mail from Rosestead yesterday. He must have taken some with him. A cursory examination showed that two were missing: the one of him, her, Suzy, and Beth standing in front of the Rosestead archway, and the one of him and his brother, smiling for the camera, just before they'd left for the airport.

With a sigh, Maggie first listened to the tape intended for her daughters, who were going to be devastated when they got home to the empty house. And it was empty without Joe in it. How had they survived without him before?

"Sue-zee and Beth, daughters of my heart, do not be upset that I have gone. I must go. My father needs me more than you do. Do not think that you have done aught to send me away. In truth, you made my leaving all the harder. Please be strong. Your mother will need your loving support now. Someday, if I am able, I will come back. But if I cannot, go visit my brother Rolf and his family often. I have told him to treat you as he would have my own precious daughters. I love you, dearlings."

Maggie was sobbing aloud by the time she finished the short message. Rewinding the tape, she turned to the other side of the desk. There was a huge pile of paper money. *The jerk! Leaving me money like some paid mistress, or something.* Then she listened to the tape intended for her.

"Ah, heartling, what can I say? The time has come, and I must go. Do not be bristling over the money, as I know you are, for I have no use for it where I am going. Deep down, I know this is the right decision for me . . . my destiny . . . but it is so hard, Mag-he. So very, very hard. I ne'er thought I would love a woman as I do you. You make me a better man, and in essence that is why I must go now. A better man heeds his responsibilities. I know how it feels to lose two children. I cannot let my father live out his life, never knowing that his two sons are safe and well. There is no other way. But, heart of my heart . . . my beloved . . . this is the hardest thing that I have ever done. Love me for all time, sweetling, as I will love you."

She noticed that Joe had made no promises to try to come back, as he had to her girls. And she knew why: he did not really think he would.

With a hand over her mouth, Maggie tried to stifle the silent sobs that were racking her. Soon she let loose and cried out her pain loudly.

The phone rang then and Maggie rushed for it, hoping beyond hope that it might be Joe, having second thoughts.

"Hello," she said, her voice cracking on even that one word.

"Mag-he? Is that you?" a male voice inquired. It wasn't Joe. "This is Rolf Ericsson."

"Yes."

"Is Jorund there?"

There was a long silence, and then she told him, "He's gone."

Rolf muttered a bunch of unintelligible words, which she assumed were Old Norse swear words. Finally he declared forcefully, "He'll be back."

"Did he tell you he would?" she asked hopefully.

"Nay, but I know him. He'll return when he comes to his senses. Should Merry-death and I come to be with you and your daughters?"

"No. We need to be strong, by ourselves. It's what Joe wanted."

She could hear Rolf talking to someone. Then Meredith got on the line. "You have to believe, Maggie," she advised. "He *will* come back."

Maggie wished with all her heart that she could believe. But Joe's words echoed in her head: *There is no other way.*

Despite all that, there were three McBride females, eyes red from crying, who refused to give up hope that night. Each, of her own volition, went to her bedroom window in hopes of seeing the wishing star. But the night was as black as eternity, and only hopelessness loomed on the horizon.

The next afternoon . . .

"Thora!" Jorund bellowed at the top of his lungs. His throat was sore from all his hollering, and he feared he might soon lose his voice altogether. "Get your bloody damn slimy carcass back here."

Nothing.

"You know, there are greedy men, even in these times, who would love to harpoon you, just for the sake of your skin and blubber. Methinks I should tell them of you."

Nothing.

Ever since he had left Mag-he's home the day before, Jorund had been sitting or standing on the land overlooking Galveston Bay, trying to make contact with his time-traveling orca. He'd been certain that the time was right now, but the stupid animal refused to connect with him.

"Thora!" he tried again. He refused to go back to Mag-he's, defeated, as he had the last time he'd left. In his breaking heart, he knew this was the right thing to do.

You don't have to scream, a clicking voice said to him in his head.

Finally! He peered outward, and sure enough, on the horizon he saw the infuriating killer whale leaping in the air, carefree, oblivious to the fact that she had ruined his life. Or was she oblivious?

"Where the hell have you been?"

Here and there.

Jorund rose to his full height, beat his fists against his chest in frustration, and made a low, rumbling sound in his throat, like a huge black bear he had once come upon in the forest.

Temper, temper, the whale chastised.

"I would like to show you my temper, you lack-brain whale. Come get me, and take me home."

The whale was swimming closer, going for long stretches underwater, then leaping high in the air. The bloody exhibitionist! Jorund thought. *But where is home, Viking?* the whale asked with its usual groans and clicks and squeals.

"What? Riddles now?" Jorund snarled, tearing at his hair in frustration. "Do you know how hard it was to make this decision? And now you question me?"

'Twas a good question. Where is home?

" 'Tis . . . 'tis . . ." Jorund sputtered.

Precisely. Now do you see?

"See? I see naught."

I have shown you your destiny, Jorund, and still you are blind.

"Do you mean Mag-he?"

That is for you to say.

The whale was closer now, several ship lengths away, but not close enough for him to lop off its irritating tongue . . . if whales did in fact have tongues. But, oh, the inclination to do the animal harm was strong.

"You brought me to this land, whale. Why?"

'Twas a gift, Jorund.

Those words made his eyes bulge. He was speechless with surprise.

Are Norsemen so thickheaded that they cannot see what hits them in the face?

"This one apparently is. Spit it out, whale."

You have a choice. It is for you to make, not me.

Enough of games and riddles! "Can you take me back to my time?"

Yes, I can. Actually, your brother Magnus is combing the seas near Iceland as we speak, searching for you still. And a dangerous enterprise it is, at this time of the year, as you well know.

"He is?" Jorund's breath hitched, but he was not sure why. Yes, he did know. In his heart of hearts, he had hoped that his departure from this time—and from Mag-he—was impossible. In that case, he would be unable to fulfill his responsibility. "Then I have no choice."

Have you heard a word I've said, Viking? You do have a choice.

"I cannot abandon my father. My mission will not be complete till he knows that Rolf and I are safe. And the only way for me to let him know is by returning to the past."

Oh? Really? The whale click-squealed, then went off into a series of spectacular leaping exercises. Sometimes the whale stood straight in the air for long moments. *Half-wit show-off!* Jorund thought. In the distance he could see some employees of Orcaland watching the exhibitionist whale through special eye devices called binoculars.

Frowning, he contemplated the whale's tantalizing question. Was there some other way to let his father know that Rolf was safe without

Sandra Hill

Jorund's delivering the message in person? *Please God*, he prayed to the Christian One-God, *if there is a way, show me*. Then he added a plea to Odin, as well: *Your wisdom is needed here, god of all the Norse gods*.

Suddenly tears filled his eyes, and he shouted with the sheer jubilation of his discovery. "There is a way; there is a way," he shouted excitedly to Thora, who swam close again. Jorund was practically jumping up and down with glee.

Of course there is, the whale replied smugly.

Jorund took his sword from its scabbard, the leather thong from his hair, and the zipper bag with the two photographs from his tunic flap. Carefully he wrapped the photographs around the sword till they were secure. *Where's duct tape when you need it?* His brother Rolf had taught him about that modern man's miracle.

Then, before he could think of the consequences, Jorund tossed the sword high in the air out over the water. End over end the sword sailed until the talented whale caught it by the hilt in its huge mouth.

"Can you deliver this to my brother, Magnus?"

I can.

"Will I see you again?"

I doubt it, Viking. My mission is complete.

"Who sent you?"

The whale just laughed. *Deep down, you know.*

"Good-bye then," Jorund called out.

The whale did an enormous backflip, creating a wave of huge proportions, the whole time holding the sword between its teeth so that it glittered in the bright Texas sun. The Orcaland people would soon be upon them.

One last thing, Thora told him before swimming off. *Tell Beth that Keiko sends his regards.*

"Keiko? You know Keiko?"

If whales could smirk, Thora did now. Then she flipped him a big splash of water with her tail fins and swam off. He thought he heard Thora mutter, *Can't wait to straighten out that Magnus and all his women!*

"Thank you," Jorund said then. Simple words, but they were from the heart.

You are welcome, Viking. Use your gift well.

Left alone then, Jorund glanced at his surroundings. So this would be his destiny. With a smile, he headed for home.

Maggie's first sign came from Rita. She was hissing in the front window, her back arched with outrage. Joe was the only one who brought that hostility out in her pet. Was this Rita's way of telling them that the man of the house had come back?

"Mom! Mom! It's Joe!" Beth shouted. She and Suzy were out the front door in a flash and running down the street toward the tall man who was walking purposefully along the sidewalk toward the house. He was wearing the usual Norse attire: a belted leather tunic over tight leggings and cross-gartered half boots. His blond hair was loose and blowing slightly in the breeze. He didn't look any the worse for wear, as he had the last time, but then he'd been gone only for a day. *A lifetime!*

By the time he reached her open front door, where she stood leaning against the frame for support, he had one girl in each arm, both of them chattering away and kissing his neck and face in welcome. But it was Maggie to whom he looked.

"Honey, I'm home," he said, mimicking the line he must have heard on the TV a hundred times. His tone was flip, but his eyes were dead serious, and vulnerable with question. He had to wonder if he was still welcome. After all, how many times could he leave and still be able to return?

"For how long?" she asked, trying to sound querulous, but failing because she was so happy to see the lout.

He set the girls on their feet and shooed them toward the house. Surprisingly, the twins scooted inside, giving them privacy. But the look they gave her as they passed was clear: *Don't screw this up, Mom.*

"Forever," he answered then, and opened his arms imploringly to her.

She hurled herself forward into his tight embrace. Against his neck she whispered, "Forever sounds just right to me."

Only later, when they all sat in the den, feeling very much like a true family, did Maggie ask Joe, "What will you do here?"

"I know not for certain. Build fireplaces? Teach demented people how to row a machine? Join the you-ess military as a warrior?" He shrugged. "Does it matter?"

She shook her head. "I just want you to be happy."

"I will be happy wherever you are. You are my destiny."

Epilogue

Two weeks later . . .

Everyone agreed it was the best Viking wedding ever held on the grounds of a Texas mental hospital.

Primitive at times.

Poignant at times.

Unconventional at all times.

Jorund's brother Geirolf wanted him to wait until summer and have a spectacular lakeside ceremony at Rosestead, following the ancient Viking rituals. Rosestead's famous rosebushes would be in bloom then. But Jorund was heard to exclaim, *"það kemur ekki komi til greina!"* That was the Old Norse version of "No way!" Jorund said his brother was living in another world— Viking soap opera humor—if he thought he was going to wait any longer than necessary to make

Maggie his bride, and he certainly wasn't waiting for a bloody rosebush to bloom before he broke the period of celibacy his fiancée was insisting upon during the betrothal period.

Rolf sighed in the end and said, *"Allt lagi."* That was Viking for "OK." He also said something about bullheaded Norsemen who made decisions with organs other than their brains.

It was important to Jorund and Maggie that all their friends from Rainbow be a part of their wedding. Of course, barricades had to be erected around the hospital grounds to hold off the news media and spectators who'd gotten wind of the unusual event.

The wedding was held on a Friday—or Friggs-day—to honor the goddess of marriage. It was an unseasonably warm and sunny day, even for Texas in January. Everyone took that as a sign that Jorund was in good favor with the gods, except for Maggie and her daughters, who claimed full credit, having made a wish upon a star to their One-God.

A small family-only wedding ceremony was held in church early that morning, to be followed by the traditional Norse nuptials on the hospital grounds that afternoon. Jorund claimed to be covering all his bases in tying the matrimonial knot.

The day started for both Jorund and Maggie with the ceremonial cleansings, which would normally take place in the castle bathhouse, similar to modern saunas. They compromised by having Maggie take a lilac bubble bath in her own home, with Jorund and his male attendants visiting a local athletic club, with boasted a Jacuzzi and sauna, as well. The symbolism behind these rituals had something to do with purification and the washing away of the virgin or single status. Jorund said the hot steam and cold rinse was more symbolic of his sexual state these past two sennights, which required many cold showers— hot, cold, hot, cold, hot, cold.

While these cleansing rituals were going on, the bride's and groom's attendants were supposed to be giving them advice. In Maggie's case, there was a lot of giggling going on. In Jorund's case, there was much scoffing and ribald jesting, especially concerning a certain body part of purportedly remarkable size.

Maggie wore the wedding outfit brought from Maine by her sister-by-marriage, Meredith Ericsson, which fit perfectly after a few adjustments. It included a long-sleeved, collarless chemise of gauzy white linen, ankle length in front and pleated and slightly longer in back. Metallic gold embroidered roses edged the wrists and circular neckline. A crimson silk overgown, open-sided in the Viking style, had matching bands of metallic embroidery at the neckline and hem.

The gold shoulder brooches and belt buckle were gifts from Jorund in the design of intertwined boars. The boar was the symbol of Freyja, goddess of fertility. Jorund and Maggie hoped to breed many children before she got too long in the tooth—Jorund's words—or he lost his virility—Maggie's words. In truth, there were rumors that Maggie already carried Jorund's seed.

Jorund wore his brother's wedding finery: a

Sandra Hill

black cashmere wool tunic with long sleeves, which hung to midthigh over slim trousers. At the waist was the leather belt Maggie had given him for Christmas, including his scabbard, minus his sword, Bloodletter. Rolf had presented him with a new sword that morning, Joy-bringer, which would play an integral part in the ceremony. A white silk–lined mantle, embroidered with roses matching the bridal attire, completed the outfit.

Rolf and Jorund, Meredith and Maggie had all agreed that they would be starting their own individualized Viking customs in this new world, including the passing on to each generation of these family bridal costumes.

Everyone who attended the wedding ceremony wore Viking attire, including the balding, middle-aged Fred Bernstein in furs . . . which in actuality were worn only on rare occasions and then only in the most frigid climate, but Jorund did not tell him that for fear of hurting his feelings. Fred was accompanied by Gladys Hatcher, who was heard to remark to some attendees that Fred was more than he seemed to be . . . that, in fact, with all the exercise he'd been getting lately, a person could crack coconuts on his butt. When said attendees had looked askance at Fred, who actually did look quite handsome as a balding Norseman, Gladys had added, "No kidding. His buns of steel would probably set off the metal detectors at the airport." Good-hearted laughter followed, as it did throughout the day.

Natalie Blue sang the processional and recessional song, "Sweet Dreams."

By the time the bridal party approached the trellis, decorated with imported lilacs, everyone

386

was in high spirits, especially Maggie's dual maids of honor, Suzy and Beth, who looked adorable in matching Viking gowns of robin's-egg blue, their hair in braids wound into coronets atop their head. Jorund had insisted that the girls wear in their braids ribands of all the colors of the rainbow, and soft-skinned, pastel-colored harem shoes on their feet. The girls kept gazing at Jorund with adoration, and on more than one occasion were heard to ask, "Can we call you Daddy yet?"

In some primitive Viking wedding rituals, an animal was sacrificed to the gods. It was not surprising which animal Jorund suggested: the fat white hairball sporting a robin's-egg blue bow, sitting big-as-you-please beside the refreshment table. After being jabbed in the ribs by a feminine elbow, Jorund compromised and sacrificed a Big Mac to the gods.

During the ceremony, Jorund handed his sword to Maggie, which was to be held in trust for their sons. The sword was a living symbol of the continuation of his bloodline. Jorund informed Maggie in an aside that, when their first son was born, a few grains of salt would be placed on the sword tip, which was in turn touched to the babe's lips. Thus would the newborn be given the courage of Viking chieftains throughout time, a contempt for danger, weapon skill, and even a facile tongue.

Instead of scoffing at this primitive ritual, the attendees listened raptly. And Maggie had tears in her eyes. "What if we have a daughter, and not a son?"

"Same thing," Jorund decided on the spot. "We are American Vikings, after all."

At that, Maggie gave the sword back to Jorund, thus marking the transfer of her guardianship and protection into his hands.

Finger rings were exchanged by both parties, each offered on the tip of the new sword. Once the rings were on their fingers, they joined hands upon the sword hilt and spoke their vows. Rolf and Steve stood as Jorund's witnesses. Meredith and Shelley were at Maggie's side.

When they were finally wed, the bride-run began, with Maggie being given a head start in her rush for the hospital door. Jorund chased after her, passed her by with a joyous laugh, and stood awaiting her when she arrived, breathless with excitement. Jorund blocked her way by setting his sword across the doorway. When he took her hand and led her inside, it represented the final transition from maid to wife.

The ancient rituals touched the heart, and made the attendees laugh out loud. On the whole, it was a rip-roaring, whooping event in the style of a true Norse celebration, combined with a little Texas low-down hoedown.

In fact, Jerome Johnson, new owner of Rainbow, gave one of the bridal toasts—honeyed non-alcoholic mead, of course—with these words: "Texans must be Vikings at heart, because both know how to have a damn good time."

Jerome had become a good friend and patron to Jorund. Not only was he lending them his yacht for a one-week honeymoon, he had even offered to help finance the health club that Jorund planned to open—a club that would cater not to perfect, already fit people—mentally and physically—but to those who needed to hone the talents that God—or the gods—had given them . . . to be the best that they could be. It was all about self-esteem, as Maggie, in her role of psychologist, had once told him.

"I want to make a difference in this world, like my brother Rolf does," he had told Maggie when first explaining this plan. "Too long I have been a warrior, taking lives. Now I want to build lives up."

Maggie's response had been a little sob and the words, "You already make a difference, Joe, just being you."

"And Texans and Vikings both think the universe revolves around them," Gladys Hatcher had yelled out, seconding Jerome's toast.

"And they're both the world's best lovers," Maggie had muttered under her breath, then ducked her head, just the tiniest bit tipsy from too many nonalcoholic mead toasts and the euphoria of this most special day.

But Jorund heard her and smiled. "Yea, that is the truth. Good loving. 'Tis a gift we Vikings give our women."

Author's Letter

Dear Reader:

Thank you so much for your wonderful response to *The Last Viking*. I hope you will like its sequel, *Truly, Madly Viking*, just as much.

In previous books, I have remarked on the fact that you've gotta love a Viking man. Then I went on in the other books to say that you've gotta love a Cajun man, too, and noted the similarities. Well, guess what? I think there are similarities between Vikings and Texans, too.

You've heard of long, tall Texans; well, surely there were long, tall Vikings as well. Both groups of men have wicked senses of humor and are a little bit thickheaded, proud, and loyal to the bone. And handsome? Lordy, lordy! If a Texas man tips his hat, hitches his hip, shuffles his cowboy boot in the dust, and winks at you, you'd better beware. If a Texas *Viking* does the same, run for the hills.

Please know that I take no credit for writing the T-shirt sayings in this book. They come from observation, word-of-mouth, and the Internet.

Please know, as well, that I am fully aware that there are no killer whales in Galveston. A little literary license, if you will. <grin>

Mental illness is no joking matter, of course, and I hope no one takes offense at my take on the mental-health industry and its workings. Keep in mind that this is a fantasy novel and was never intended to replicate the way in which actual psychologists or psychiatric facilities operate in real life. On the other hand, laughter—especially laughter at oneself—can be a marvelous balm, if not a cure, for any illness . . . mental or physical.

Please let me know what you think of my Viking, Jorund, in this book, and of my Vikings in general. I can promise you that there will be more Vikings in my future. At the very least, Adam and Rurik, from *The Bewitched Viking* are in the planning stages. And there might possibly be a sequel to *Frankly, My Dear* and *Sweeter Savage Love*.

Sandra Hill
P.O. Box 604
State College, PA 16804
email: <shill733@aol.com>
Web site:
<http://www.sff.net/people/shill>

THE OUTLAW VIKING

SANDRA HILL

As tall and striking as the Valkyries of legend, Dr. Rain Jordan is proud of her Norse ancestors despite their warlike ways. But she can't believe her eyes when a blow to the head transports her to a nightmarish battlefield and she has to save the barbarian of her dreams. If Selik isn't careful, the stunning siren is sure to capture his heart and make a warrior of love out of the outlaw Viking.

___52273-X $5.50 US/$6.50 CAN

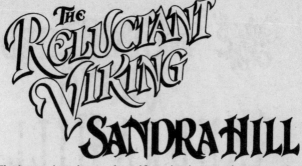

THE RELUCTANT VIKING

SANDRA HILL

The hypnotic voice on the self-motivation tape is supposed to help Ruby Jordan solve her problems, not create new ones. Instead, she is lulled from a life full of a demanding business, a neglected home, and a failing marriage—to an era of hard-bodied warriors and fair maidens, fierce fighting and fiercer wooing. But the world ten centuries in the past doesn't prove to be all mead and mirth. Even as Ruby tries to update medieval times, she has to deal with a Norseman whose view of women is stuck in the Dark Ages. And what is worse, brawny Thork has her husband's face, habits, and desire to avoid Ruby. Determined not to lose the same man twice, Ruby plans a bold seduction that will conquer the reluctant Viking—and make him an eager captive of her love.

___52297-7 $5.50 US/$6.50 CAN

Dorchester Publishing Co., Inc.
P.O. Box 6640
Wayne, PA 19087-8640

Please add $1.75 for shipping and handling for the first book and $.50 for each book thereafter. NY, NYC, and PA residents, please add appropriate sales tax. No cash, stamps, or C.O.D.s. All orders shipped within 6 weeks via postal service book rate. Canadian orders require $2.00 extra postage and must be paid in U.S. dollars through a U.S. banking facility.

Name_____
Address_____
City_____State_____Zip_____
I have enclosed $_____ in payment for the checked book(s).
Payment <u>must</u> accompany all orders. ❑ Please send a free catalog.
        CHECK OUT OUR WEBSITE! www.dorchesterpub.com

Wink & A Kiss

The Bewitched Viking
Sandra Hill

'Tis enough to drive a sane Viking mad, the things Tykir Thorksson is forced to do—capturing a red-headed virago, putting up with the flock of sheep that follow her everywhere, chasing off her bumbling brothers. But what can a man expect from the sorceress who put a kink in the King of Norway's most precious body part? If that isn't bad enough, he is beginning to realize he isn't at all immune to the enchantment of brash red hair and freckles. But he is not called Tykir the Great for nothing. Perhaps he can reverse the spell and hold her captive, not with his mighty sword, but with a Viking man's greatest magic: a wink and a smile.

___52311-6 $5.99 US/$6.99 CAN

THE Last Viking

SANDRA HILL

He is six feet, four inches of pure unadulterated male. He wears nothing but a leather tunic, speaks in an ancient tongue, and he is standing in Professor Meredith Foster's living room. The medieval historian tells herself he is part of a practical joke, but with his wide gold belt, callused hands, and the rabbit roasting in her fireplace, the brawny stranger seems so... authentic. Meredith is mesmerized by his muscular form, and her body surrenders to the fantasy that Geirolf Ericsson really is a Viking from a thousand years ago. As he helps her fulfill her grandfather's dream of re-creating a Viking ship, he awakens her to dreams of her own until she wonders if the hand of fate has thrust her into the arms of the last Viking.

___52255-1 $5.99 US/$6.99 CAN

Dorchester Publishing Co., Inc.
P.O. Box 6640
Wayne, PA 19087-8640

Please add $1.75 for shipping and handling for the first book and $.50 for each book thereafter. NY, NYC, and PA residents, please add appropriate sales tax. No cash, stamps, or C.O.D.s. All orders shipped within 6 weeks via postal service book rate. Canadian orders require $2.00 extra postage and must be paid in U.S. dollars through a U.S. banking facility.

Name_____
Address_____
City_____State_____Zip_____
I have enclosed $_____ in payment for the checked book(s).
Payment <u>must</u> accompany all orders. ❑ Please send a free catalog.
CHECK OUT OUR WEBSITE! www.dorchesterpub.com

THE LOVE POTION
SANDRA HILL

Get Ready . . . For the Time of Your Life!

A love potion in a jelly bean? Fame and fortune are surely only a swallow away when Dr. Sylvie Fontaine discovers a chemical formula guaranteed to attract the opposite sex. Though her own love life is purely hypothetical, the shy chemist's professional future is assured . . . as soon as she can find a human guinea pig. The only problem is the wrong man has swallowed Sylvie's love potion. Bad boy Lucien LeDeux is more than she can handle even before he's dosed with the Jelly Bean Fix. The wildly virile lawyer is the last person she'd choose to subject to the scientific method. When the dust settles, Sylvie and Luc have the answers to some burning questions—Can a man die of testosterone overload? Can a straight-laced female lose every single one of her inhibitions?—and they learn that old-fashioned romance is still the best catalyst for love.

___52349-3 $5.99 US/$6.99 CAN

Cinnamon and Roses
Heidi Betts

A hardworking seamstress, Rebecca has no business being attracted to a man like wealthy, arrogant Caleb Adams. Born fatherless in a brothel, Rebecca knows what males are made of. And Caleb is clearly as faithless as they come, scandalizing their Kansas cowtown with the fancy city women he casually uses and casts aside. Though he tempts innocent Rebecca beyond reason, she can't afford to love a man like Caleb, for the price might be another fatherless babe. What the devil is wrong with him, Caleb muses, that he's drawn to a calico-clad dressmaker when sirens in silk are his for the asking? Still, Rebecca unaccountably stirs him. Caleb vows no woman can be trusted with his heart. But he must sample sweet Rebecca.

Lair of the Wolf

Also includes the second installment of *Lair of the Wolf*, a serialized romance set in medieval Wales. Be sure to look for future chapters of this exciting story featured in Leisure books and written by the industry's top authors.

___4668-7 $4.99 US/$5.99 CAN

DESPERADO
SANDRA HILL

Major Helen Prescott has always played by the rules. That's why Rafe Santiago nicknamed her "Prissy" at the military academy years before. Rafe's teasing made her life miserable back then, and with his irresistible good looks, he is the man responsible for her one momentary lapse in self control. When a routine skydive goes awry, the two parachute straight into the 1850 California Gold Rush. Mistaken for a notorious bandit and his infamously sensuous mistress, they find themselves on the wrong side of the law. In a time and place where rules have no meaning, Helen finds Rafe's hard, bronzed body strangely comforting, and his piercing blue eyes leave her all too willing to share his bedroll. Suddenly, his teasing remarks make her feel all woman, and she is ready to throw caution to the wind if she can spend every night in the arms of her very own desperado.

_52182-2 $5.99 US/$6.99 CAN